16 Weeks to Weight Training Success: A Basic Approach

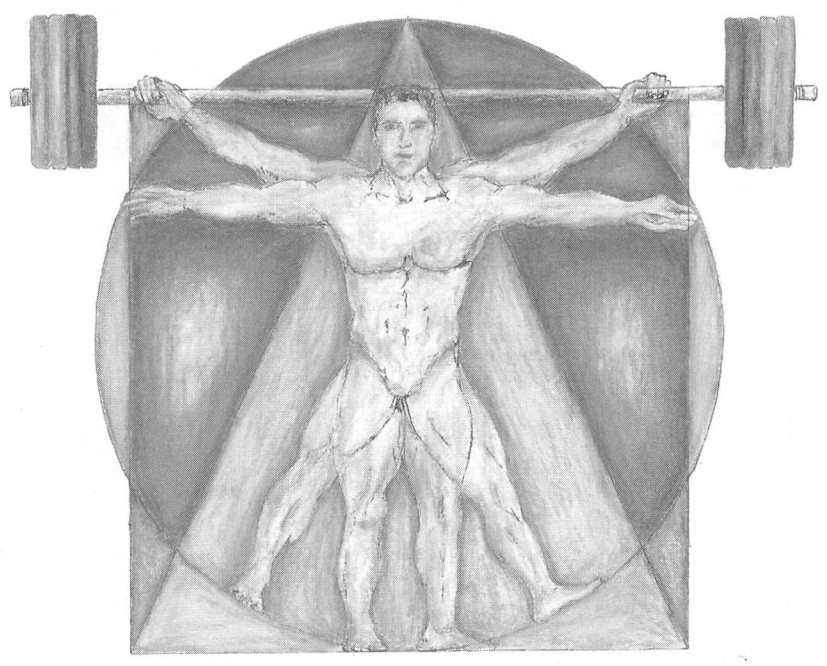

Doug Briggs

New Mexico State University

KENDALL/HUNT PUBLISHING COMPANY
4050 Westmark Drive   Dubuque, Iowa 52002

Title page art courtesy Monica Rabel.

DEDICATION I

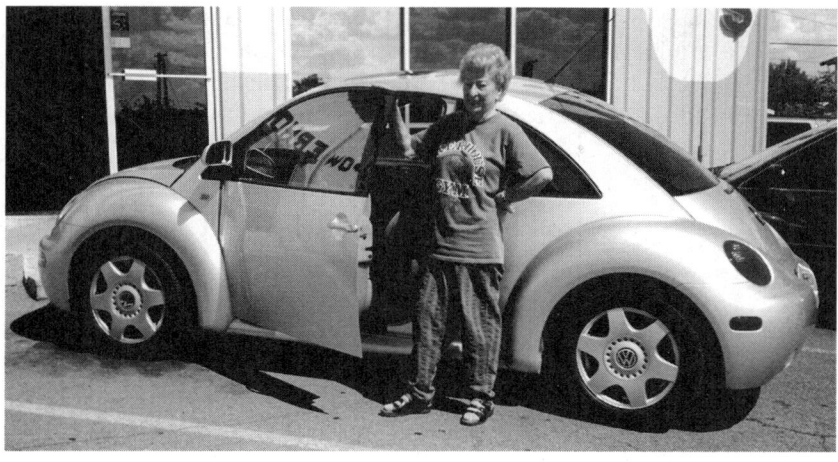

This book is dedicated to my mother and father, Josephine O. and Lloyd C. (Gunner) Briggs. My mother, who will be 93 years young when this book is published, still works out with weights five days a week. I remember their living the healthy lifestyle long before it was popular or the "in thing" to do. It was never a fad to them. Our diet consisted of natural foods that were not refined, enriched, processed, sprayed with pesticides or injected with hormones. We grew as many vegetables and fruits as possible in our garden. We canned or juiced everything we could find to provide the variety that we as humans so often need and desire. In fact, we still have the original juicer purchased in the early 1960s. It is a Stur-Dee Deluxe Juicer and I juice to this day. There was no such thing as "fast food" or "junk food," because every meal was balanced and prepared with care. We took vitamins. This exposure piqued my interest in vitamins and supplements, and to this day I am constantly researching and experimenting with different concoctions and combinations.

My mother would start every morning with exercises taught by Jack LaLanne, and finish everyday with a bicycle ride. My parents encouraged me to participate in any and all kinds of sports, which for me were baseball, basketball, football, martial arts, running, weights, and a couple of oddities, namely hang gliding and scuba diving. Sports participation was important, but never at the cost of academics. Life is a balancing act, they told me. The mind and body are connected, and if you abuse one, you abuse the other. Everything in moderation, and my favorite: "Your body is a temple; treat it with respect, dignity, hard work, and a good diet." The body is meant to work. I finally settled on individual sports because I didn't like leaving my fate to others, as is done in team sports. Olympic weightlifting became my love.

My parents' examples in nutrition and exercise have led to a long and happy life for them. I only hope that I can be as happy and productive for as many years as they have been. Thank you for life's lessons on living and the sacrifices you have made for me. I truly appreciate it, will never forget it, and will pass it on to my son.

—*Doug Briggs*

DEDICATION II

To my wife Margaret, for lending your knowledge of physical therapy and sports rehabilitation to my textbook, and being my best friend, as well as the best mother my son could ever have. To my son Alexander Maximus, for all the help and fun I have had with you while writing this book. You have been an inspiration to me, not only in life but also in weightlifting, and you are the most valuable gift I have ever received.

—*Doug Briggs*

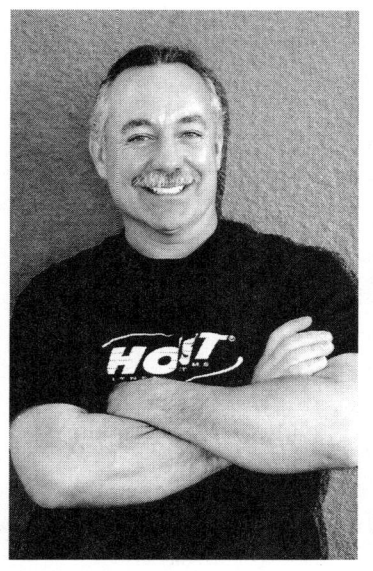

Doug Briggs, Ph.D., CSCS has been involved in weight training for 25 years. He is a competitive Olympic weightlifter who won the 2002 Pan American Masters Championships, setting a new Pan American Masters Snatch Record, and was named the Male Athlete of the Year for 2002 in the New Mexico State Games. He has held over 100 state records in Olympic weightlifting. Doug currently teaches in the Physical Education, Recreation, and Dance Department at New Mexico State University in Las Cruces, New Mexico. Subjects that he teaches include anatomy, motor development, principles of strength training & conditioning, and tests and measurements, as well as beginning, intermediate, advanced, women's, and Olympic weightlifting. Doug also writes for *Pure Power Magazine* and will finish his Ed.D in Sport Management/Finance at the U.S. Sports Academy in 2004.

Doug owned a Powerhouse Gym for 12 years and also owned a personal training studio that eventually became an Olympic-style weight training facility that has produced numerous collegiate national champions and national level athletes. Doug has acted as an Assistant Coach for the men's and women's teams of USA Weightlifting at the World University and College Championships and the Young Louis Cyr Competition in Canada in 2000. He is a USA Weightlifting International Coach and Treasurer of the New Mexico Local Weightlifting Committee (LWC). He has previously served as President for three terms, and as Secretary.

In addition to teaching and weightlifting, Doug owns the American Weightlifting Association, Inc. (AWA), and is involved in restoring Olympic-style weightlifting to the nation of Jamaica. The AWA is a grass roots organization devoted to developing Olympic-style weightlifters.

Doug is married and has one son. His wife, Margaret, is a physical therapist specializing in sports rehabilitation. Margaret is featured on the cover of this textbook and is also a competitive Olympic-style weightlifter who was named Female Athlete of the Year for 1999 in the New Mexico State Games. Their son Alexander Maximus is the youngest registered weightlifter in the world, and competed in the New Mexico State Games in 2000 at the age of 11 months.

Theirs is truly a fitness family. Doug does not believe in the hype that surrounds the fitness industry or the promises of rapid weight loss and massive muscle gains; in fact, he states that 90-95 percent of the supplements on the market are an absolute waste of money. Doug tells it like it is, with no hype, and does not promote any product. What he presents in this book is the culmination of 25 years of real-world experience from working in the trenches of the fitness industry.

CONTENTS

CHAPTER 3

Back Muscles and Exercises 29

CHAPTER 4

Shoulder Muscles and Exercises 41

FOREWORD

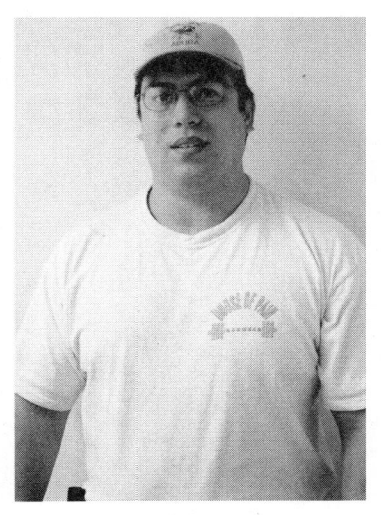

It is with great pleasure that I am given this opportunity to express my respect and appreciation for all Doug Briggs has given me. Doug has been something of a mentor to me since my career in the fitness industry began. He is also my coach, an honor I am not quick to bestow. I have been lifting weights since I was twelve and had to sneak behind my parents' back to do it, because "weightlifting stunts your growth!" I have always trained on my own and I first learned about weightlifting through trial and error, magazines, books, and any advice I could get from others in the gym. In the first years of my training, I trained like all the magazines and professional bodybuilders said was the correct way for "massive growth and strength." I very quickly came to a plateau and nothing seemed to work. Then I met Doug Briggs. He helped me change my program to start growing again and gain strength.

At about the same time, he exposed me to powerlifting. I began competing for Briggs' Barbell Club and won the state and regional championships in the teenage and junior division. I also finished second at the Natural Athlete's Strength Association (NASA) World Cup of Powerlifting. Doug was always there to offer advice and encouragement to help me train and compete. At Doug's suggestion, I became a certified personal trainer, and currently make my living by training others.

I moved to Los Angeles to do personal training. Even after moving, I called Doug with questions about training, diet, and business. It was his example after which I patterned my business philosophy. After competing and winning numerous odd titles, I developed new training systems, and trained clients using these systems. The results of these systems were fantastic. These systems of training were based on things I learned from Doug.

When I decided to compete in Olympic weightlifting, I again sought advice from Doug. I was living in Albuquerque, New Mexico, and would drive 225 miles one way to train with Doug. Under his guidance, I became the NM State record holder in the 105+ kilo class in the snatch, clean & jerk, and total in my first year. I have since finished in the top 10 of USA Weightlifting (USAW) American Open, and won the American Weightlifting Association National Championship in the 105+ kilo class in 1999. Doug's advice not only covered weightlifting, but nutrition as well. His sometimes demented thoughts on nutrition usually end up being very effective, with positive results utilizing overlooked products or products that have not been properly applied.

In judging the quality of a book, you must examine the author's track record, credentials, and the book itself. Doug is also a national-caliber athlete in Olympic weightlifting, and coach of many national-caliber weightlifters. He has been selected to coach at the national and international levels, and is a high-caliber personal trainer. He has been in the fitness industry longer than many of his students have been alive. Doug is an International Coach for USA Weightlifting and a Certified Strength and Conditioning Specialist (CSCS) with the National Strength and Conditioning Association. He has more than 100 State records in Olympic weightlifting. If this isn't enough, he teaches at New Mexico State University, and has owned a gym for more than 12 years.

I have read almost everything about fitness, and to find a no-nonsense, straightforward textbook on the subject of weight training is refreshing. It demonstrates many exercises, covers the essentials in starting a workout program, and even covers the history of resistance training. It is not the latest, overnight dream body program found in every other exercise magazine and book on the market, but rather a book about the basics of weight training. No pie in the sky here. I use only one standard to judge a trainer or coach—results. The basic tenets described in this book will lay the foundation that will yield results. Doug's programs have always yielded results. This book is no exception.

In my work as a trainer, I would be aided in educating my clients by a quality, factual book about exercise. Until now, I have not found one I will distribute to my clients. I am proud to offer my congratulations to Doug and my endorsement of this book.

Richard Kahle, USAW Club Coach
ISSA Certified Sports Conditioning Specialist
AWA National Champion 1999

Doug Briggs is a great coach, person, and friend. My name is Rhena Mills and it is definitely a great opportunity to actually show my appreciation for everything he has done for me. I have been involved in various sports throughout high school, such as volleyball, basketball, and track, all giving me a little background in lifting weights. I always thought of lifting weights as a way to improve in different sports, not as a sport itself. Doug was quick to show me differently. For my first two years here at New Mexico State University I "worked out" at his Powerhouse Gym. I constantly asked him many questions related to my workouts and my nutrition. To my surprise, no matter how many questions I asked, he never got annoyed. From then on I knew he was a very patient, well respected individual in his gym.

Around March of 2000, he somehow talked me into trying Olympic weightlifting. He was very patient and showed me the technique of the sport. About three months later, he entered me into my first competition. Not sure where I stood, he made sure that I knew he had all the confidence in the world for me. In this competition I not only placed first, but also set three new state records for the junior division in the 63 kg. weight class. From then on I knew I wanted to continue training with Doug. He then offered me a job at his gym so I would have more time to train. He was always willing to help.

It is now August of 2001 and I am still lifting with Doug. I am continually improving my performance using his programs and advice, and (most important) feeding off of the encouragement and confidence he is never reluctant to give. He has helped me to become the 2001 Collegiate National Champion in the 63 kg. weight class and set a total of 12 state records. With his positive attitude he has also helped me to become the National Champion in the American Weightlifting Association for the year 2000.

I am also proud to be an athlete competing beneath the great coaching of Doug Briggs. My name is Kandy Presser, and I compete in the Senior 53 kg. class. Olympic weightlifting is something I never heard of until I became a member at Powerhouse Gym. Doug convinced me to give the sport a try. I, being a mom, never thought I would be able to give the time and dedication that a sport requires, but the patience and time that Doug put into helping me allowed me to accomplish many goals that seemed out of reach. Not only does Doug take time out of his lifestyle for me, but he also enjoys coaching my eight-year old son, who also loves weightlifting.

I have acquired two state records for the 53 kg. class and am constantly training to improve my performance. I also had the opportunity to compete in the National Collegiate Competition, and thanks to the great coaching, programs, and dedication from Doug I was able to place first and become the Collegiate National Champion for the 53 kg. weight class. Doug has been an inspiration to my family and me, in both weightlifting and my personal life. He has shown me how to be more confident in everything I do. His time and energy is greatly appreciated, and I look forward to continuing lifting under his coaching strategy.

Doug is not only a coach for the sport but an awesome athlete as well. He carries over 100 state records in Olympic weightlifting and has competed in national and international competitions. Doug is also an international coach for USA Weightlifting and the Assistant Head Coach for the Jamaican team.

Reading fitness manuals, magazines, and other fitness books sometimes makes it more confusing than helpful. This book will cover the essentials in starting a workout program, the history of weight training, and even give step-by-step illustrations on the many different exercises that can be used. This book is meant to supply the reader with a background about the basics of weight training. Doug's programs will help yield fast and effective results.

We are proud to say "Congratulations" to a great coach, teacher, and awesome friend on his accomplishment of this book.

Rhena Mills, USAW Club Coach
President of NMSU AWA CLUB
President of New Mexico LWC   Kandy Presser, Member of Briggs' Barbell Club
National Collegiate Champion 2001   B.S. in Family and Child Science
AWA National Champion 2000   Full time student, mother, and wife
B.S. in Finance-2002

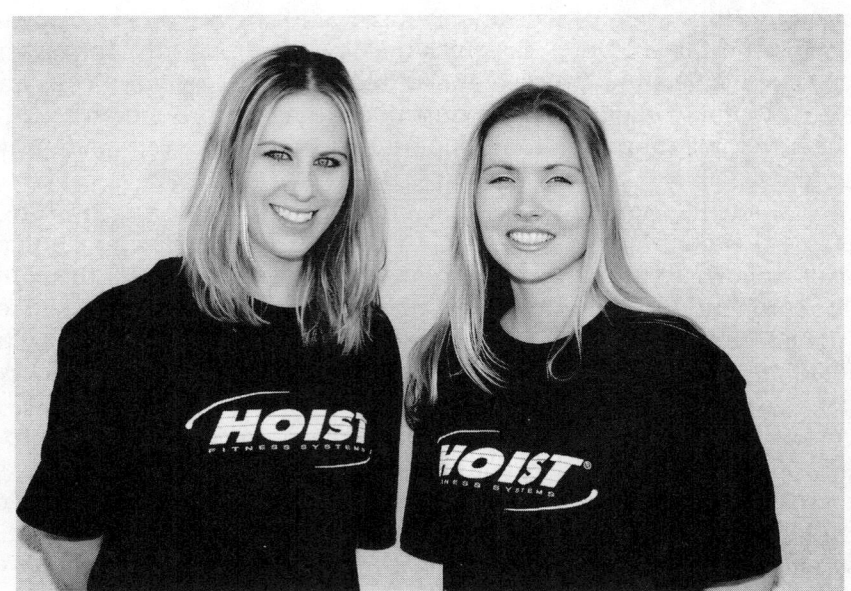

PREFACE

This textbook takes a unique approach to beginning weight training in that it is process-based, and guides the student through a 16-week semester of instruction. Most textbooks of weight training ignore the fact that most physical education classes are activity-based, and students take these classes to work out, not to listen to lengthy lectures. In many instances, students do not get to use the weights or machines until mid-semester, and by then they are either too bored to come to class or have already dropped the class. The opposite extreme is the instructor who doesn't use a textbook, but rather relies on handouts or the "just go work out" mentality. Typically, this kind of course will be unorganized and unable to convey the necessary information to the student. Either way, the student is cheated out of an experience that could inspire a lifetime of exercise and a pattern of good health. This textbook is designed to be covered one chapter per week or one chapter per class meeting through the first eight chapters, and then one chapter per two weeks. By the end of the eighth chapter, the student will have covered all of the information necessary to have a rudimentary idea of what is required to have a "good workout" and display proper gym etiquette.

Weight training has become enormously popular in the past 25 years, due to the broad appeal it has for everyone from professional athletes to those trying to remain youthful. This can be seen by the proliferation of health clubs, gyms, corporate fitness centers and a whole host of other workout venues. In many ways, gyms have become the "bars" of the new century, where people strive to look and feel good and at the same time incorporate the social aspect into their lives that is so often missing in this hectic world. Weight training has been shown to help reduce problems associated with aging, as well as improving athletic performance for all age groups and abilities. Weight training helps you reduce stress, be energetic, healthy, strong, and fit to meet the challenges that life has to offer, no matter how old you are.

While this textbook was written for use at the college level, it can be used by anyone with a desire to get in shape and learn more about these strange places we call "gyms" or "health clubs." Lift long and live long.

—Doug Briggs

ACKNOWLEDGMENTS

Without the help of my friends I would have never completed this textbook. As with most things in life, it is not the individual effort but the collaborative effort that makes all things possible. You will always be remembered for all the contributions, however subtle. If I have forgotten anyone, I apologize and want you to know it was not intentional.

Thank you to:

All of the models for the pictures on the covers and in the book. They have all been great friends of mine for a long time and great athletes as well. I especially want to thank Matt Rich and Carlos Wendler for their loyal and undying friendship. Training partners forever!

Bob and Tom Thaves of "Frank & Ernest." Bob was kind enough to allow me to use his comic strip during the six years it took me to write this textbook. www.thecomics.com.

Jeremy Halterman for the great cover designs. These are the best covers I have ever seen on a weight training book! Train on, dude!

Monica Rabel for her outstanding artwork on "The Weightlifter's Form." I have the framed original proudly displayed in my house.

Roy Patel for his friendship and sponsorship of my weightlifting team.

John Taylor, Head Strength Coach, and Tony McClure, Assistant Strength Coach at New Mexico State University (NMSU), for their friendship and use of their facilities over the years.

All the great people in the Physical Education, Recreation and Dance Department (PERD) at NMSU. I would especially like to thank Dr. Maud, and Betty Burgess for acting as reviewers for me.

My best friends and coffee-swilling partners Carolyn Aragon and Esther Valenzuela for their sense of humor, endless practical jokes, and e-mails. Without these two ladies, the PERD Department would not function.

Dr. Harvey White and Dr. Rick Powell, who have been great friends for the past 12 years in the PERD Department before retiring, moving to the Middle East and leaving me in El Paso to fend for myself. You have both been a great inspiration and resource for ideas and materials.

Joe Fedak and Sylvia Green of NMSU for allowing me to use the James B. DeLamater Activity Center for textbook pictures, and the friendships we have shared over the years.

John Hurst for the great photo finishing. I'm sure there were many times he would have liked to photo-finish me.

Martin Monzon of Fitness Superstores for his friendship and good advice on gym equipment, even though I still owe him a lunch from two years ago.

David Salisbury and Tom Orin of Hoist Fitness for the T-shirts the models wore in the pictures, and for the incredible deal on the Hoist 4400 gym.

Guy Andrews, M.A., Jeannie Patton, M.S., and Chris Marino, M.S., from Exercise ETC., Inc. for their great seminars in Houston, Texas on February 22 & 23, 2003. Your seminars gave me the finishing touches I needed for my textbook.

Dr. Wanda Eastman of NMSU for reviewing my nutrition chapter and teaching an oustanding sports nutrition class.

George and Laura Thomas for their moral support and great business advice. Hardbodies forever!

Chris Coffey of Fitness Masters for being a long-time friend and reviewer of this book.

Devon Lougee, my friend and philosopher, for all the great times we had discussing the "Apes around the Monolith." I hope you're still lifting weights and sailing the Caribbean!

Craig Sowers, Strength Coach for Velocity Sports Performance in Irvine, CA, for the fun we had with Olympic weightlifting and our sons, Bo Sowers and Alexander Maximus Briggs.

Hugh Hammant, for his great skills as our team psychologist and his wife Beverly for her wonderful, healthy Caesar salads that fueled our many conversations about weight training.

Lee Peters and Lou Martinez, for their great legal advice, moral support, and continuing friendship over the years.

—*Doug Briggs*

ACKNOWLEDGMENTS II

I would like to offer a special thanks to the students of my PE P 411, Tests and Measurements class from the 2003 Spring Semester at New Mexico State University. As a class project in learning how to write tests and examinations, they undertook the Self Tests that you will see at the end of every chapter. We had fun writing the tests and proofing them, and I hope you enjoy taking them as you learn more about weight training. Below is a list of my students and the chapters for which they were responsible:

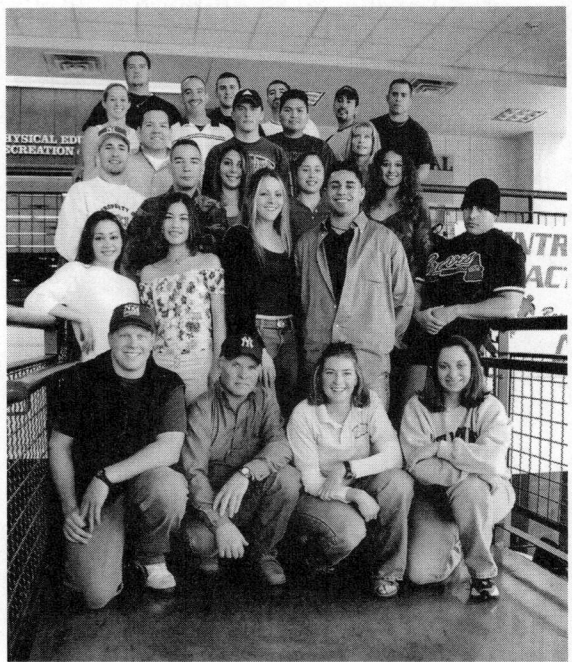

Chapter 1: Tyson Kloeppel, DeLoyd Landreth, Esther Woodward

Chapter 2: Stephan Arnold, Alicia Padilla

Chapter 3: Adrian Martinez, Adam Sinclair

Chapter 4: Claire Cozart

Chapter 5: Eric Adames, Shawna Angulo

Chapter 6: Kacie Boylan, Dan Tamminga

Chapter 7: Samantha May, Brennan Weir

Chapter 8: Jason Russell, Rick Thedford

Chapter 9: David Lujan, Rene Salazar, Crystal Wilson

Chapter 10: Danielle Adams, Kimberly Spitz

Chapter 11: Andrew Garretson, Ozzie Gonzales, Priscilla Jaramillo

Chapter 12: Priscilla Chaparro, Katie Penrod, Robin Quezada

Chapter 13: Stanson Begay, Susan Montoya

Chapter 14: Lori McNeely, Isaiah Nava

—Doug Briggs

INTRODUCTION

"The Apes around the Monolith" Syndrome

When I owned my gym, every time a new piece of equipment was added to the gym I would get a reaction I call the "apes around the monolith" syndrome. This is how it worked. When a new piece of equipment was installed in the gym, invariably no one would use it, even if it was a piece of equipment that the members had requested. Over the period of the first day, a few people would touch it, while other members watched, but no one would actually use it. Sometime during the second or third day, someone would actually use the new piece of equipment. After the first member used it and others saw them using it, they then decided to try the new piece of equipment. It reminded me of the movies of apes where they drag their knuckles around something new until one ape finally gets enough courage to actually reach out and touch the object and then run. Over time and with enough apes touching the object and running, they finally become accustomed to it and sit on it, pull on it, and generally just play with the object. At this point the object becomes part of their environment and is included in their everyday play.

With this thought in mind, I encourage you to try new things when it comes to weight training. Try different exercises, sets, and rep schemes. Try different pieces of equipment in the gym. Talk to different people and ask questions. Train with different people. Train on different days and at different times. Become familiar with your body and what works with it, since no two of us are alike. In essence, become familiar with your surroundings and have fun doing it. The results and friendships you make will last you a lifetime. Who knows? Someone in the gym may not only make your day, but you may very well make his or her day as well! Here's to that great workout we all desire!

TEXTBOOK MODELS

The models that appeared in this textbook appear below in alphabetical order.

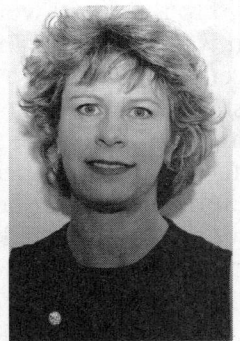

Margaret Briggs

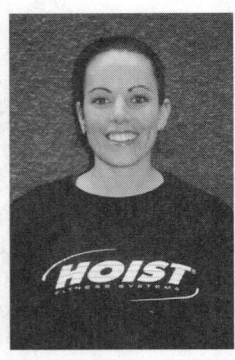

Liz Byrnes

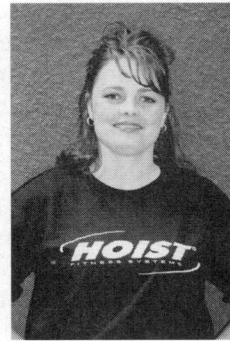

Alison Messick

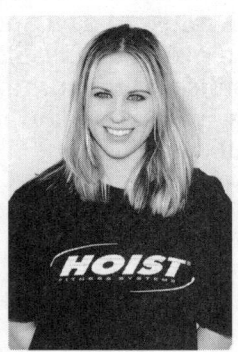

Rhena Mills

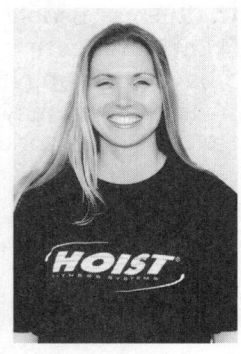

Kandy Presser

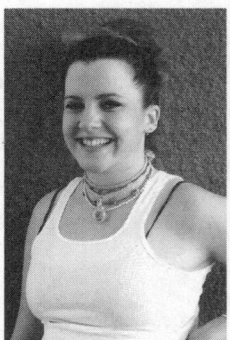

Monica Rabel

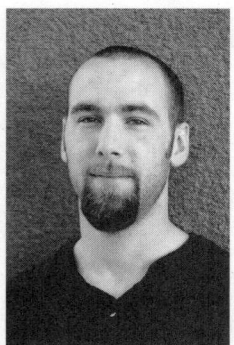

Matt Rich

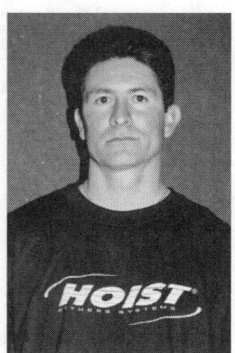

Joe Serna

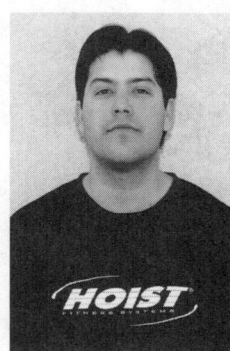

Carlos Wendler

Definition, Terminology, What to Wear, Equipment, Safety, Warming-up, Stretching, & Cooling Down

Frank and Ernest

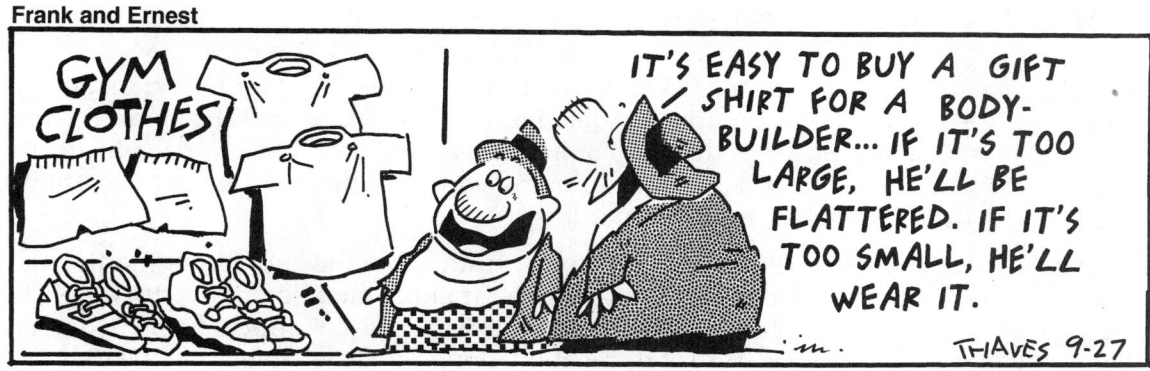

© 1999 Thaves / Reprinted with permission. Newspaper dist. by NEA, Inc.

Definition

Weight training is the use of progressive resistance for the purpose of increasing muscular strength, muscular size, or muscular endurance. This is accomplished by utilizing dumbbells, barbells, and weight machines that are either selectorized (machines that have a weight stack with a pin adjustment) or that are weight-plate loaded. Weight training may be used to accomplish the goals of strength, size, or endurance, either individually or in any combination, however, when one area increases, often times so do the others; that is, if you train for size, your strength and endurance may also increase.

Terminology

Working Out: What you will be doing as a non-competitive or recreational athlete. Most Americans are "weekend warriors" or recreational athletes.

Training: What a competitive athlete does. Training involves preparation for a sporting event where very specific programs are used, usually involving a concept known as periodization (chapter 8).

Types of Weight Training—Competitive

Olympic-style Weightlifting: The oldest competitive weightlifting sport. This sport features two lifts called the two-hands snatch and the two-hands clean & jerk. This sport is also known simply as "weightlifting." The contestants are the most powerful of the weight training sports participants. Mathematically, this would be expressed as Power = Force × Distance/Time, or $P = F \times D/T$, where Power is equal to the distance the weight is moved divided by the time it takes to complete the movement. See Chapter 8 for more on Olympic weightlifting.

Bodybuilding: A sport of illusion and muscle. The competitive part of bodybuilding is often referred to as a "male or female beauty pageant with muscles." In this sport, contestants compare musculature and, definition, and pose to music. Bodybuilders seek extreme musculature and train for hypertrophy. A panel of judges then subjectively rates the contestants. In the 1930s and 1940s the physique contests took place after the Olympic-style weightlifting meets, and the weightlifters posed for the best physique. Of the three weight-training sports, this sport requires the most discipline in terms of training and diet.

Powerlifting: A sport with its beginning around 1962. Three lifts are contested. The lifts are the squat, the bench press, and the dead lift. The contestants are the strongest of the three weight-training sports, with bench presses approaching 800 lbs. and squats breaking the 1000 lbs. barrier. The term "powerlifting" is a misnomer. The sport is actually based on maximum strength or absolute strength. Strength is equal to the maximal force that a muscle or muscle group can generate.

Other Types of Weight Training

Recreational: This term typifies most Americans who lift weights. They do it for recreation and social reasons, but derive the benefits of health from it. Sometimes referred to as "weekend warriors," the recreational athlete is the one who keeps the gyms of America in business. Recreational athletes also help keep the doctors and rehabilitation people in business, as many times they are not conditioned properly and tend to overdo exercises, resulting in injury.

Rehabilitation: The use of progressive resistance training in strengthening and reconditioning those who have been physically injured due to accident, improper training methods, or overtraining. The rehabilitation is normally done in conjunction with a physical therapist or athletic trainer who has advanced training in specific areas, such as sports rehabilitation, cardiac rehabilitation, neural rehabilitation, and the like.

Athletes: Those who use weight training both at the amateur and professional level as a tool for in-season and off-season conditioning for strength, endurance, and injury prevention.

Fitness Contestants: Persons who use weight training to seek such titles as Ms. Fitness USA. These contests stress coordination, strength, and athletic ability. Many routines are choreographed to music and feature evening gowns as well as swimsuits. The judging is similar to that of a bodybuilding contest.

What to Wear and Take to the Gym

When preparing to lift weights, it is important to be comfortable. Do not wear tight-fitting clothes that cause binding or discomfort. Cotton and many newer fabrics like spandex remove perspiration, which will keep you cool and dry. Not only is this clothing functional, but it is also attractive. It is a good idea to *never* work out in jeans or other bulky items that look like street clothes. Not only are they uncomfortable, but they could be dangerous as well. This means that you should wear and use the following:

Loose-Fitting Clothes: Tank tops and T-shirts in the summer, T-shirts and sweatshirts in the winter, and shorts or sweatpants as desired.

Athletic Shoes: Tennis, workout, cross trainers, weightlifting shoes, and such are good in the gym. The shoes should provide good support, with a wide and stable base. The soles should be firm and not spongy. *Never* wear anything that has exposed toes like sandals or Birkenstocks! A weight-plate, even a light one, falling from the end of a bar can chop a toe off or cause significant damage if it falls on your foot.

Gloves: A good idea if you don't like the idea of calluses. While this is a personal preference item and not required, they do sometimes give a better grip, especially on bars or equipment that might be smooth.

Weightlifting Belts: Another personal preference item that is not required. Weightlifting belts are generally overused and can lead to a weakening of the back and abdominal muscles. It should be recommended that they only be used when approaching or exceeding the 90 percent of maximum lift capability in the squat and deadlift, or in the Olympic lifts.

Weightlifting Wrist Straps: Once again, a personal preference item. The straps are good for gripping the bars and dumbbells when they are smooth, or for use in handling more weight when the handgrip strength is beginning to weaken from continuous sets or too much weight.

Wrist Wraps: Primarily used to support the wrist. If you don't have weak or injured wrists, don't use them.

Knee Wraps: Used for knee stability. There are many kinds of knee wraps, from simple slip-on ACE bandage types to very thick powerlifting types. These types of wraps are generally used by the competitive powerlifter, but are not necessary for the recreational lifter. Continued usage over an extended period of time can lead to knee problems.

Towels: A necessity. No one likes to work out or train in another person's sweat. Not only is it a matter of hygiene, but it is just plain rude not to use one. Always wipe up your sweat when you get off of any piece of equipment.

Water Bottles: Great for water or other beverages while working out. Keep the bottles tightly capped when not in use, and check with the gym to insure that it is all right to have them on the exercise floor. Many gyms will not allow beverages other than water, because some beverages leave sticky spots and permanently dye the carpeting in a gym because of the coloring used in the beverage.

Sports Bras: A very good idea for women, as they will help to support the breast while doing physical activities such as weight training and aerobics, making the activities more enjoyable and comfortable.

Equipment

There are various items of equipment, which are standard to any gym. These include, but are not limited to, bars of varying lengths and weight, weight-plates, dumbbells, handles, straps, and other pieces of miscellaneous equipment.

Weightlifting Bars: Two varieties. Standard bars usually weigh approximately 15 lbs., are 6 feet in length, and have a 1" diameter shaft. These bars are most often for home use, but can be found in gyms where there are sets of fixed barbells and EZ curl bars.

Olympic-style Bars: Any of the following, and usually with a 2" diameter shaft. Shaft lengths may vary.

> *7-foot bar:* Commonly referred to as an "Olympic Bar." This bar generally weighs 45 lbs. without the collars. The name comes from the use in Olympic- style weightlifting beginning around 1896.
>
> The *6-foot bar* generally weighs about 35 lbs.
>
> The *5-foot bar* generally weighs about 25 lbs.

EZ Curl Bars: The bars that are short and have the "zigzag" pattern to the handle. There are other similar bars, and most of them are used for curling or triceps work.

Plates: Two varieties: One has a 1" diameter hole in the center and is generally used in homes or on fixed barbells or EZ Curl bars; the other has approximately a 2" diameter hole in the center, which is the commercial standard. Plates range in weight from 2½ lbs. to 100 lbs. for commercial gym use. These plates are called "Olympic plates"; however, this term is incorrect. True "Olympic plates" are made of different materials that encase a metal inner core. These plates allow for the dropping of the weights without damaging the floor or surrounding area, and are quite expensive if you have to buy them.

Dumbbells: Various weights, with some as low as 1 lb. and many as high as 200 lbs. Some dumbbells do not include the weight of the handle in the weight stamped or stenciled on the dumbbells.

Handles: Manufactured to allow for different width of grips, hand positions, and variety in order to hit a muscle in different ways. The handles usually go on various pieces of selectorized equipment like the lat machines, cable crossovers, and rowing machines.

Ankle Straps: Used primarily for selectorized machines and cable crossover machines to attach the ankles to the cable for doing adduction, abduction, flexion, and extension exercises.

Collars: For holding the weight-plates on the bars. There are many varieties of collars; however, the most popular are known as "spring lock" collars.

Safety

1. Always use collars on the bars to keep the weights from sliding off the bars and injuring you or someone else. Weight-plates falling off of bars are dangerous.
2. Always use a spotter when lifting weights that are heavier than you normally use, or when "maxing out." It is a good idea to use a spotter anytime you go over 80% of your one rep max.
3. Never wear sandals or go barefooted in the gym. The toes you save may be your own.
4. Do not unload weightlifting bars one side at a time, the plates may fall off the other side and injure someone nearby. Unload the bar in an even fashion.

Why People Do Things Wrong in the Gym

If you go to any gym in the world, you will invariably see people doing all kinds of strange things in a misguided attempt to develop the perfect body or increase their strength and power. According to Guy Andrews, M.A. of Exercise ETC., Inc. there are three main reasons: (1) "This is the way I have always done it."; (2) "This is how I was taught."; and (3) "I saw somebody in the gym doing it this way and they were in really good shape and had a good body, so I decided to do it myself." Don't be a part of the "monkey see, monkey do" crowd. Educate yourself.

Eating Before Working Out

Always eat something about 1 to 1½ hours before working out. If you have no fuel for your body to burn, you will run out of energy early in your workout. Imagine this: You start out on a trip in your car with an empty tank of gas. Not too far down the road, you run out of gas. This is what happens to the body when you have nothing to fuel it during a workout. Not eating can lead to a blood-sugar imbalance and cause light-headedness, and in extreme cases, fainting. When eating before a workout, do not eat a heavy meal or anything that can cause gas or bloating. Many foods, while enjoyable for a meal, make a terrible pre-workout meal. Something easy to digest is ideal.

Water

There can't be enough said about water. Water makes up approximately 70 percent of your body weight. Therefore, it is extremely important to replenish it continuously. The water in your body controls your body temperature, aids in the production of energy, lubricates joints, transports nutrients, and removes toxins. Water helps detoxify the body; when you don't drink enough water, your body will actually retain water. If you wait until you are thirsty, you have waited too long. By the time your body tells you that you are thirsty, you are already deficient in water. Drink plenty of water before, during, and after working out. Generally, at least ½ to 1 gallon a day spread throughout the day. Coffee, tea, soda, etc., don't count as a water replacement and can actually have a diuretic effect causing the body to lose water. The VERY FIRST thing you should do upon waking in the morning is drink 8 to 16 ounces of water to replenish what you lost due to bodily functions during the night. Typically, the time you spend sleeping will be the longest period of the day that your body will not intake any fluids, and can be the time you are most dehydrated.

Your urine is a good indicator of hydration. If your urine is clear or only slightly yellow you are probably hydrated. It should appear like this 4 to 6 times a day. If your urine is dark yellow and odoriferous, then you are probably dehydrated and need to concentrate on rehydrating. Some B & C vitamins can cause the urine to be very bright.

Warming Up

One of the most important aspects of lifting weights or exercising in general is warming up. The warm-up will reduce your chances of injury by increasing your heart rate and blood flow. This increase in heart rate and blood flow will cause an increase in muscle and body temperatures, and will aid your body in lubricating the joints. A thorough warm-up should last approximately 5 to 10 minutes and may be done utilizing a bike, treadmill, stepper, or any other piece of cardiovascular equipment. You may prefer to run in place, jump rope, or just walk briskly between classes and before working out. There are any number of ways to warm up, and it is generally a good idea to incorporate variety in warming up. By doing this, you prevent boredom or stagnation. Be sure to always warm up *BEFORE* stretching. Stretching with cold muscles is a good way to injure yourself. If you only have time for one or the other, warming up is the choice.

To Stretch or Not to Stretch, That Is the Question!

As an athlete I have never stretched and I have never been injured. Something about stretching and then lifting weights just never made any sense to me. Why would I want my muscles to be relaxed when I am about to lift weights? Wouldn't I want them to be tighter? In an article by Dr. Bob O'Connor, the whole idea of stretching is considered.[1] Some of the findings indicate that stretching may actually cause injury and reduce muscular power. Consider this:

1. Muscles function poorly after stretching due to a reduction in the stiffness required for maximal force production.
2. Muscular power is reduced anywhere from 2–8%.
3. Among athletes who stretch, muscle and connective tissue injuries are higher.
4. Damage can be produced at the cellular level by stretching.
5. Stretching can mask muscular pain.
6. Stretching will do nothing to decrease the incidence of delayed onset of muscle soreness (DOMS) either before or after the pain of weight training has set in.

The bottom line is this: Do not stretch before weight training, but instead increase the amount of time you would normally spend warming up. If you want to stretch, do it after your workout, when the connective tissue is warmer and you should still be able to increase your flexibility.

Breathing When Lifting Weights

Breathing is very important when lifting weights. If you hold your breath while lifting weights you will become dizzy, and quite possibly pass out. The best way to breathe is to inhale during the least strenuous part of each repetition, and exhale on the most strenuous part of each repetition. For example, if you were bench-pressing, you would inhale as the bar lowers to your chest (least strenuous) and exhale as you press the bar back to the starting position (most strenuous). Cycle your breathing so that you inhale on the downward phase of the lift and you exhale on the upward phase of the lift. NEVER HOLD YOUR BREATH!

Valsalva Phenomenon

Holding your breath can initiate what is known as the Valsalva phenomenon, named after the seventeenth-century anatomist. As you lift the weight, the pressure in the intrathoracic cavity is increased, which causes a rise in the blood pressure and thus prevents the return of venous blood to the heart. When the blood doesn't return to the heart, there is a sudden drop in blood pressure and the person may feel dizzy or faint.

Cooling Down

Once you have completed your workout, it is time to cool down. This will help return your body to its pre-exercise state. Cool-downs should last approximately 5 to 10 minutes at a low-intensity level. You could again use the cardiovascular equipment, or just slowly lessen the intensity on whatever exercise you are doing.

Eating After Working Out

Be sure to always eat a small meal or have a protein drink immediately after working out. This nutrition will replenish what you have taken from your body during the training session and start the recovery process. It is a good idea to eat something containing carbohydrates and protein. The carbohydrates will help to replenish the body's carbohydrate stores, and the protein will help with muscle tissue growth and repair. A protein drink containing whey with milk and egg protein would be ideal.

Etiquette for the Weight Room

After 13 years of owning a gym, these are my recommendations to making weight training an enjoyable experience for all concerned.

1. Do not drop weights or bang weight-plates or dumbbells together.
2. Put dumbbells and weight-plates back in their proper place.
3. Do not leave weight-plates on the bars.
4. Wipe up any sweat that you may leave on benches, machines, or equipment.
5. Spot for other lifters if they need the help; don't wait to be asked.
6. Do not sit on equipment for long periods of time; let others work in.
7. Stay home if you are sick; no one wants your illness and you will recover faster.
8. Do not make loud and obnoxious noises when lifting, i.e., grunting, screaming, farting, etc.
9. Do not use profanity, tell dirty jokes, or make rude comments about gym members, male or female.
10. The gym is not a bar or nightclub, do not go on the prowl for your weekend date here.
11. Do not chew gum in the gym, and definitely do not stick it on equipment.
12. Use chalk sparingly and clean up any that is left after use.
13. Take a shower, brush your teeth, and wear clean gym clothes for every workout.
14. Ladies, the gym is not a fashion show, so go easy on the make-up.
15. Always notice those around you and be careful around them.
16. Do not tie up the gym phone, and for goodness sake, do not talk on a cell phone.
17. Pay your membership on time.

Myths

1. "No Pain, No Gain." This is probably one of the dumbest myths around. Muscle soreness is normal; "pain" is not.
2. Muscle-boundness. There is no such thing. The lack of flexibility usually results from improper training technique.
3. Women will get "big" like the men. Women do not produce enough testosterone to get "big."
4. "I only need to do aerobics, yoga, spinning, Pilates, etc." Aerobics and all the other forms of exercise are highly overrated when done by themselves. You need to do a combination of activities to be in peak physical condition.
5. More is better. Train smart, not long.
6. "I can eat any and everything I want if I work out." You can't, but nice try.
7. Muscle turns to fat. Muscle cannot turn to fat and fat cannot turn into muscle.
8. I don't have the time to work out." Simple enough: "Make the time."
9. Slim down, then tone up. Lifting weights while slimming down will help you accomplish this faster.
10. "I get enough protein daily." You probably don't. The Recommended Daily Allowance (RDA) is designed for sedentary Americans.
11. Doing cardio is better for losing weight. It isn't. The more muscle you build, the more calories you burn.
12. Performance-enhancing steroids are legal. Steroids are not legal unless you have a valid prescription from a physician. Simple possession of steroids without a prescription is a Class 4 felony. Steroid use is just plain dumb.
13. "I want to lose weight only on my thighs." There is no such thing as "spot reducing."

Muscle Dysmorphia

This is a newly identified psychiatric disorder that is characterized by a practitioner's preoccupation with being lean and muscular. This disorder was discovered and identified by Dr. Harrison G. Pope, Jr., a psychiatrist at McClean Hospital in Belmont, Massachusetts, and his graduate student Roberto Olivardia of Brown University School of Medicine in Providence, Rhode Island.[2] The researchers believe that this disorder comes from the same genetic predisposition that can cause other forms of obsessive behavior. The disorder can be a dangerous obsession where the participants work out five to six hours a day. They risk losing their jobs and loved ones, and abuse steroids, but they still don't feel big enough compared to how large they think they should be. Rarely is this life-threatening, and it is possibly treatable with drugs like Prozac.

How to Buy a Gym Membership

How to buy a gym membership is included in this chapter because many students will choose to work out at a health club that is off-campus. When working out at a facility off-campus, it is best to know what to expect in terms of price and product.

1. Work out at the gym during the time you normally work out, and observe whether or not the gym is crowded. Is it stuffy? Is there enough equipment to work out on with all the other people working out? Is it pleasant and fun? Is it noisy, smelly, or messy?
2. Can the gym provide you with a printed price list? Many gyms will base your membership price on how you look, how you dress, how you act, and so on. This is especially true of initiation fees. If the gym cannot give you a printed price list, chances are the prices are variable based on the above-mentioned items.

3. Does the gym charge an initiation fee? If they do, ask them to waive it. If they are unwilling to waive it, find another gym. At many gyms the salespeople work for whatever initiation fees they can collect. At other gyms a good-looking woman might pay no initiation fee and a man may pay a considerable amount for the initiation fee. Sometimes, it will be impossible to get out of paying an initiation fee, especially at clubs that feature tennis courts, racquetball, basketball, running tracks, massage therapy, hair cuts, and so on.

4. Does the club have a contract? Contracts should be an option, not a requirement. The average person joining a gym quits working out within two to three months of joining, but the contract continues for a year or more, and some renew automatically for life or until you provide the gym with written notice canceling the contract. Is there a cancellation period in which you can change your mind? Many states give you five working days to change your mind with no penalty. Check with the attorney general of your state if you have a problem, or contact the Better Business Bureau (BBB) and file a complaint. Ask them to allow you to take a contract home and read it. If they won't, find another gym. You may have no choice but to sign a contract.

5. READ THE FINE PRINT. Many contracts renew automatically for life unless the member cancels them. Usually, the contract is for one year, at which time you must cancel it or it automatically renews. Most of the time the gyms require 30 days written notice to cancel a contract at the conclusion of one year. Add it up. This ends up being 13 months . . . NOT 12! If you fail to make your payments on time or you quit paying, this will appear on your credit report! Of course, you will get the annoying calls from bill collectors also.

6. Does the gym require an EFT? Electronic Funds Transfers (EFTs) allow the gym to get into your bank account directly and deduct funds from it. Some unscrupulous gym owners and employees will tap into your account more than once a month until caught, or take out an extra payment right before they close the doors on the gym forever. Do not allow an EFT to be taken out of your account, or set up an account strictly for the gym to deduct from keeping a minimal amount in the account.

7. Watch out for gimmicks. There is no such thing as a "Win a Free Week Contest" or "Free Membership." They use the free come-ons to build mailing lists and referrals. If you go in for your "free membership," be prepared for the "hard sell." You'll be lucky to get out without a membership you didn't want.

8. Does the gym rely on volume? Gyms using the "volume principle" will offer extremely low membership prices to get you to join, and they will pay a lot of attention to you UNTIL you join. After you join, they hope you go away, because if everyone shows up to work out, there will be no equipment to work out on.

9. Is the gym clean? The gym should be clean and the equipment well maintained. There shouldn't be any holes in the equipment upholstery or carpeting, or broken mirrors on the walls. If there is, find another gym.

10. Is the staff friendly, but not pushy? Are the staff members salespeople? Be ready for the "hard sell" if the staff members are salespeople. They make their living on commission. If they have you in an office before you even see the workout areas, run for your life and find a different gym!

11. Are their personal trainers and aerobics staffs certified? Many gyms will tell you they are when in fact they are not. Ask for the certifying agency and call the agency to find out if they are certified. Many times you will find out that the staff is not certified. Do not use any personal trainers or take classes from any instructor that is not certified.

12. Does the staff know CPR/First Aid? Your life may depend on it.

13. Visit all the gyms in your area before making a decision. Ask for a free workout. Check with the BBB and/or the State Attorney General to see if any complaints or lawsuits have been filed against the gym. Report any gym that uses deceptive marketing tactics, "double dips" into your bank account, or tries to scam you.

14. Once you make the decision on which gym to join, enjoy it and use it to the fullest!

Medical Clearance

Before starting any exercise program, check with your physician to insure that you are physically able to begin a workout routine. Always discuss with your physician any concerns or problems you have. This is no time to hold back any information that could negatively impact you when you start your exercise program. If you have any restrictions, be sure to inform the class instructor or club owner, and have the restrictions in writing.

The First Workout

Don't be intimidated. Everyone in the gym started out in exactly the same way. Take it easy, get acquainted with the gym and the people, and enjoy yourself. Ask questions of others. Chances are they will be glad to help. Do not do too much too soon. One or two sets when using machines or free weights will give you the feeling of working out, but will not make you so sore that you can't move. This will prevent you from hating the gym and the experience. Use proper technique when lifting weights and you will see results faster than when you use improper technique. You will also have less risk of injury.

Doug's Words of Wisdom on Training with Weights

As you begin your journey into the world of weight training, I would like to bestow on you the wisdom that only a lifetime of experience can bring: *"The exercises you don't like to do will invariably be the ones that you NEED to do!"* If you don't believe me, think about all the guys you know who wear baggy pants to the gym to cover up their scrawny legs. Do you ever see them doing squats? If you do, it is more like a "curtsy" than a squat, which is appropriate, since most guys who squat like this are sissies anyway. How about the guys by the pool or on the beach with the huge upper bodies and the little weebly-wobbly legs that don't look like they can support the massive weight of the upper body? Instead of having a pleasing, balanced, and symmetrical body, they have shapes like light bulbs or keyholes! Balance your workouts so that you have exercises that work all parts of the body, and you will not only have a body that is pleasant to the eye, but a body that will be functional in the everyday demands of life and living, not to mention how good you will look in your clothes! This is the truth, as Doug knows it!

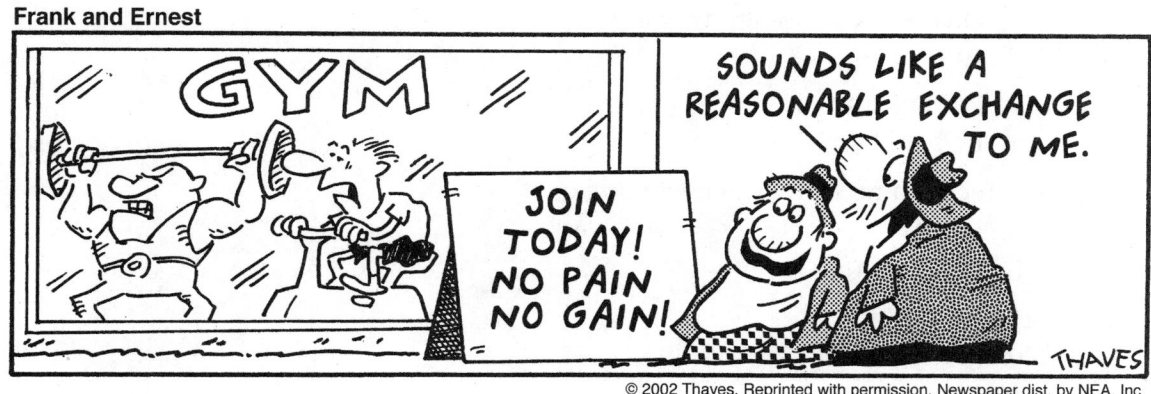

Frank and Ernest

© 2002 Thaves. Reprinted with permission. Newspaper dist. by NEA, Inc.

1. O'Connor, R. (January 2003). Stretching the Truth, It is No Bargain! *Coach & Athletic Director*, 46–47.
2. Bilger, B. (Jan-Feb 1998). Barbell Blues. *The Sciences* [On-line], *vol. 38 n1p10*. Available: http://www.findarticles.com/cf_dls/m2379/n1_v38/20136389/p1/article.jhtml

CHAPTER 1 SELF TEST

Please feel free to write on this page

True or False

1. _____ Olympic-style weightlifting is the oldest competitive weightlifting sport.

2. _____ Athletics use weight training at both the amateur and professional levels.

3. _____ Olympic style bars are used for EZ curls.

4. _____ Collars should be used when doing heavy weight training.

5. _____ Wait until you are thirsty before drinking water.

6. _____ You should always eat 1½ hours prior to the workout.

7. _____ You should NOT go to gyms with printed price lists.

8. _____ The average sedentary person consumes enough protein throughout the day in what they normally eat.

9. _____ Weight training is the use of progressive resistance for the purpose of increasing muscular strength, muscular size, or muscular endurance.

10. _____ A thorough warm-up should last approximately 5–10 minutes and may be done utilizing a bike, treadmill, stepper, or any other piece of cardiovascular equipment.

11. _____ Muscles function poorly after stretching due to a reduction in the stiffness required for maximal force production.

Multiple Choice

12. _____ Which of these is NOT a competitive type of weight training?
    a. Olympic-style weight training
    b. Weight training
    c. Powerlifting
    d. Bodybuilding

13. _____ Which is a necessity when working out?
    a. towel
    b. knee straps
    c. wrist straps
    d. gloves

14. _____ Upon awakening in the morning, it is recommended to consume _____ ounces of water.
    a. 8–10 oz
    b. 8–16 oz
    c. 17–20 oz
    d. both a and b

15. _____ What are the types of equipment which are standard to any gym?
   a. bars of varying lengths and weights
   b. weight-plates and dumbells
   c. handles and straps
   d. all of the above

16. _____ Standardized 1″ weightlifting bars weigh approximately _____ pounds.
   a. 10
   b. 15
   c. 25
   d. 30

17. _____ When is stretching most appropriate and beneficial for weight training?
   a. prior to warm-up
   b. during warm-up
   c. after working out
   d. all of the above

Fill in the Blank

18. When purchasing a gym membership, always _____ print.

19. Cool-downs last approximately _____ minutes at a low-intensity level.

20. The best way to breathe when lifting weights is to _____ on the most strenuous part of each repetition.

Please feel free to write on this page

The Male
MUSCULAR AND SKELETAL SYSTEM

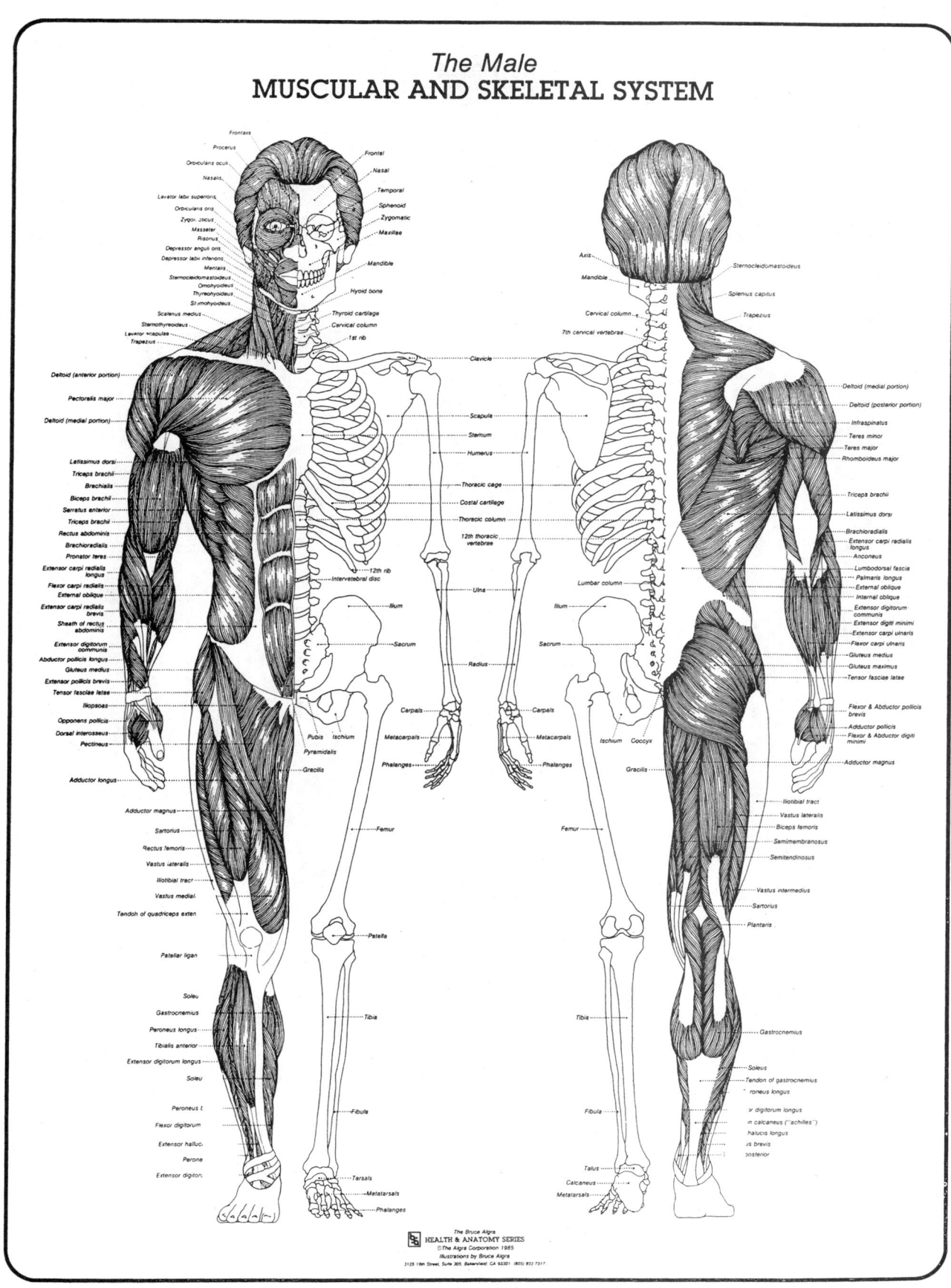

The Female
MUSCULAR AND SKELETAL SYSTEM

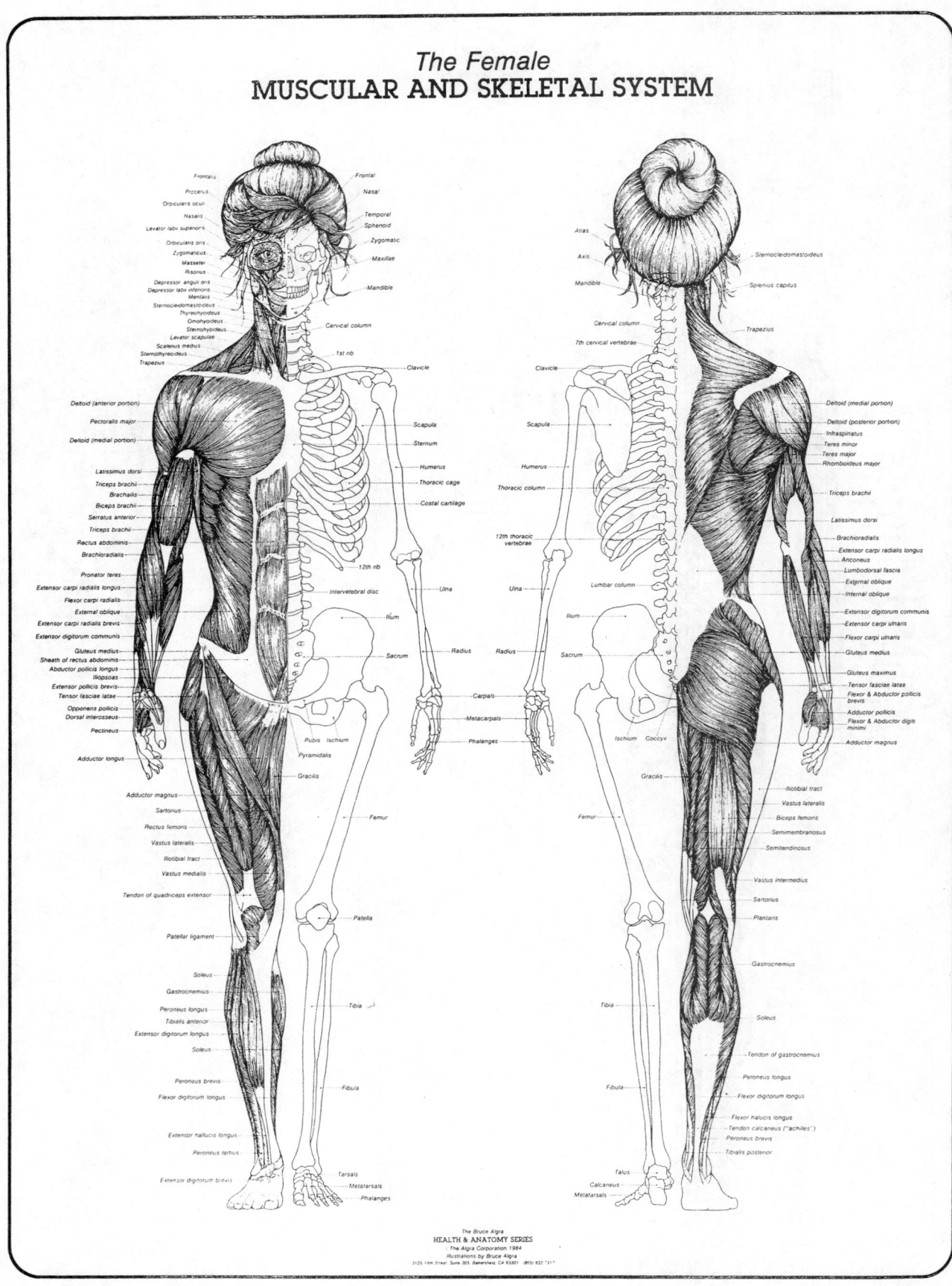

The Bruce Algra
HEALTH & ANATOMY SERIES
The Algra Corporation 1984
Illustrations by Bruce Algra
3125 19th Street, Suite 305, Bakersfield CA 93301 (805) 832 "31"

Chest Muscles and Exercises

Frank and Ernest

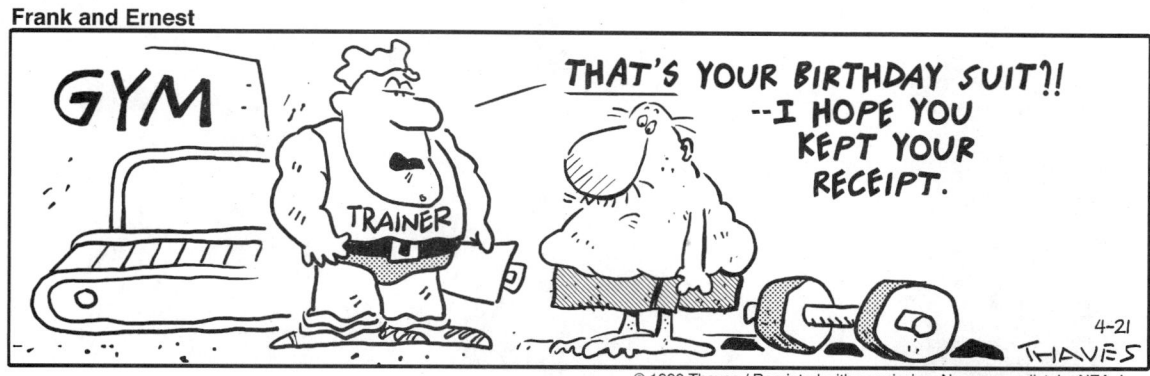

© 1999 Thaves / Reprinted with permission. Newspaper dist. by NEA, Inc.

Muscles of the Chest

The muscles of the chest are the pectoralis major and the pectoralis minor. The primary purposes of these muscles are shoulder flexion, shoulder internal rotation, and shoulder horizontal adduction.

Adduction refers to moving a limb toward the centerline of the body, while abduction refers to moving a limb away from the centerline of the body. Isn't it amazing? Surveys have shown that 56 percent of men are unhappy with their chests, but only 43 percent of women are unhappy with their chests.

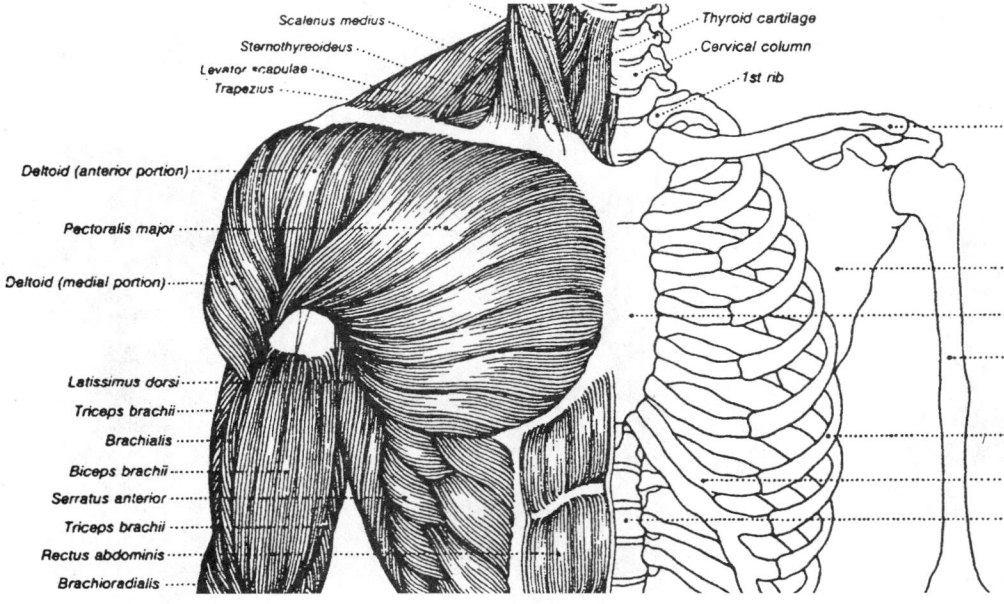

© Algra Corporation www.algra.com Used with permission.

Other Muscles Involved in Chest Exercises

Other muscles involved in chest exercises are the anterior deltoid, serratus anterior, and the triceps brachii.

Hand Positions Used in Weight Training

There are five hand positions commonly used in weight training. They are the pronated grip, supinated grip, alternating grip, neutral grip, and false grip.

Pronated Grip: With the forearms parallel to the floor, the palms will be facing the floor.

Supinated Grip: With the forearms parallel to the floor, the palms will be facing the ceiling.

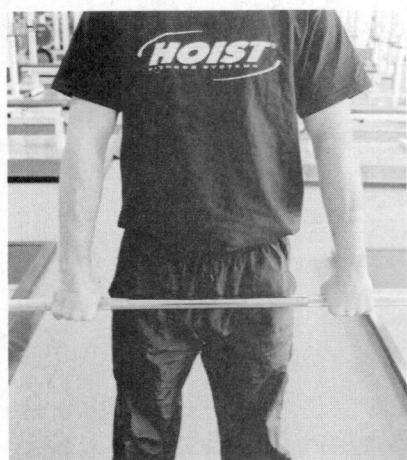

Pronated Grip

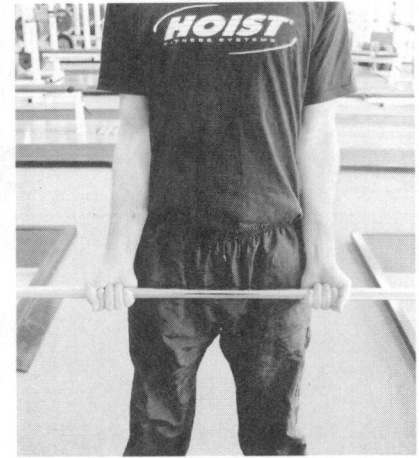

Supinated Grip

Alternating Grip: With the forearms parallel to the floor, one palm will be facing up; the other will be facing down. If the arms are held to the side, one palm will face forward, one palm will face backward.

Neutral Grip: Both palms are facing each other. If the arms are held to the side, both palms will face the legs.

False Grip: The thumbs are not locked around the bar or dumbbell. This is not a safe grip for anyone to use, and especially not for beginners.

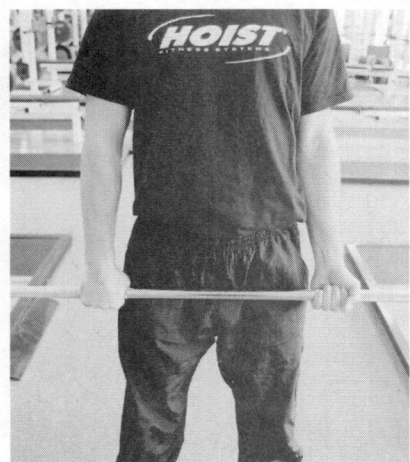

Alternating Grip

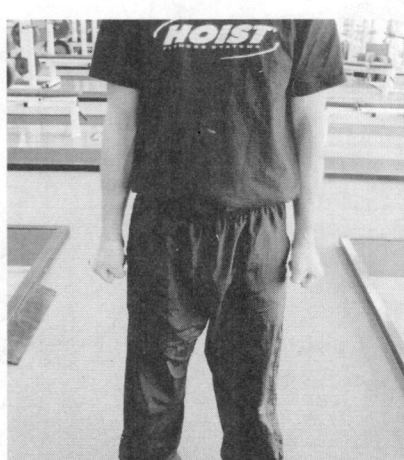

Neutral Grip

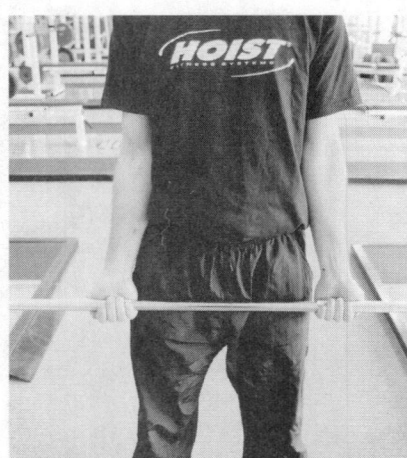

False Grip

Hand Spacing for Various Grips

Normal Spacing: This grip will place the hands on the bar approximately shoulder-width apart. The normal grip will stress the overall muscle.

Narrow Spacing: This grip will place the hands on the bar approximately 4 to 12" apart. The narrow grip will stress more of the inner part or origin of the pectoralis major, anterior deltoid, and the triceps.

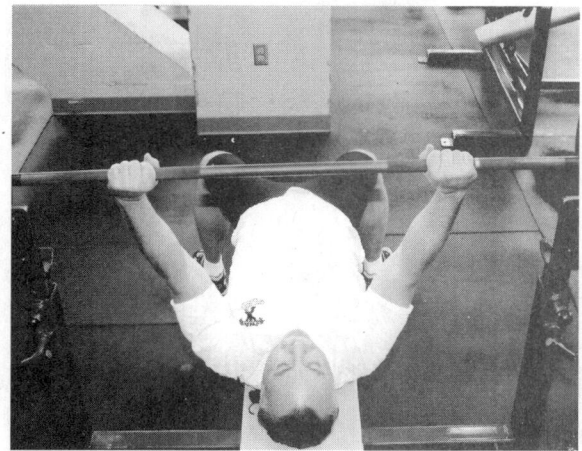

Normal Spacing

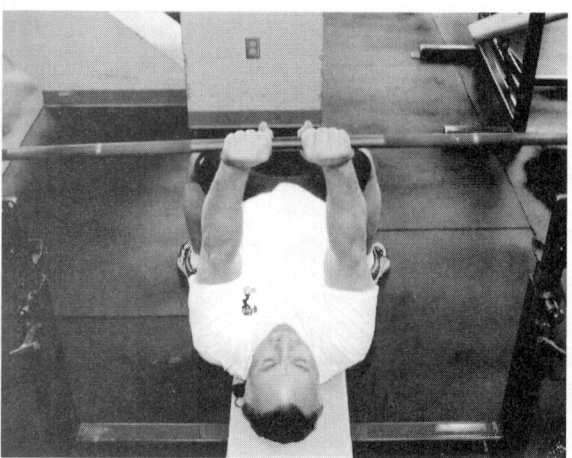

Narrow Spacing

Wide Spacing: This grip will place the hands on the bar approximately 24 to 36" apart. The wide grip will stress more of the outer part of the pectoralis major.

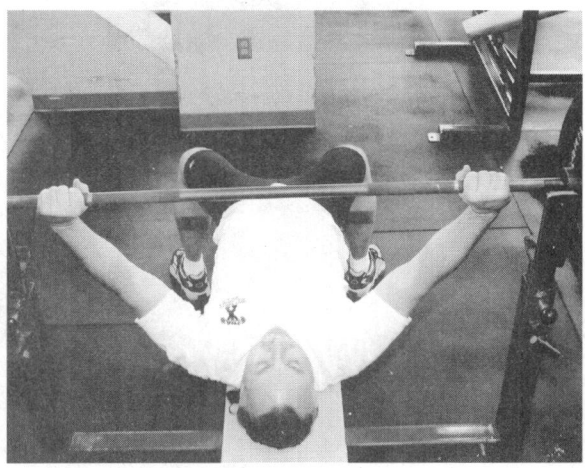

Wide Spacing

Elbow Placement

By bringing your elbows to your side, you will place more stress on the anterior deltoid and triceps.*

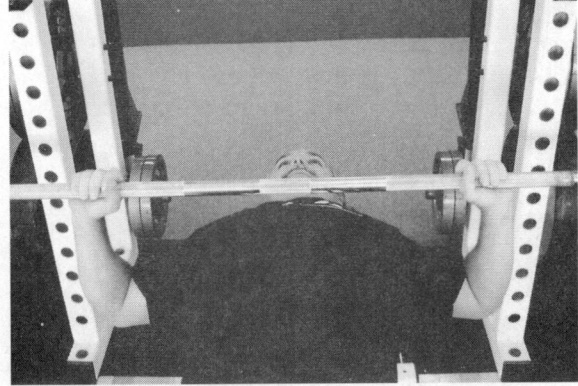

Out

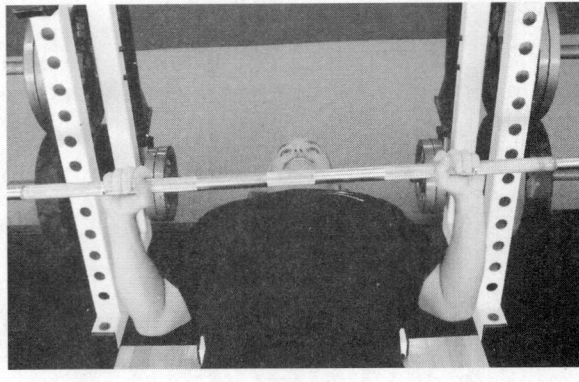

In

Spotting for Chest Exercises

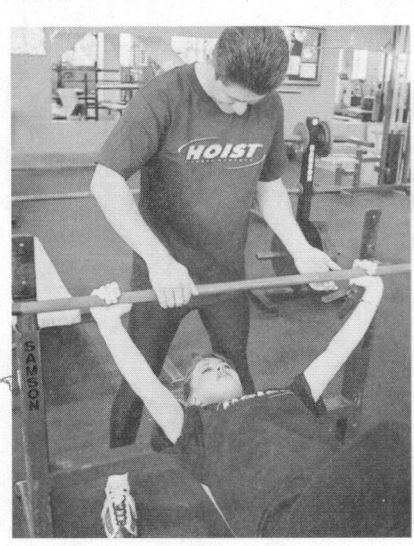

Correct

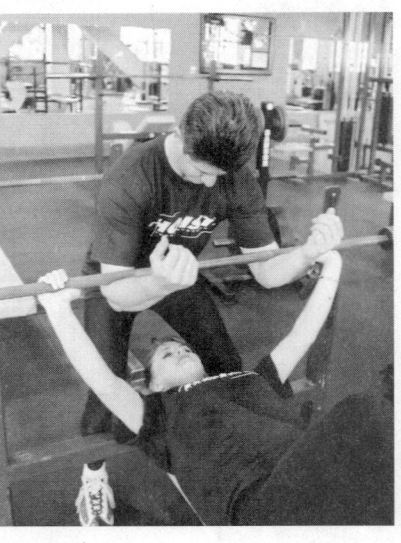

Incorrect

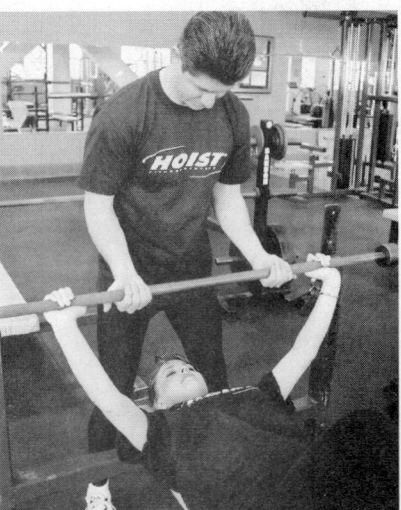

Incorrect

When spotting a person using dumbbells, it is usually best to spot them by gripping their wrists. By doing this, the possibility of having the dumbbell hit them in the face is reduced as the elbow will not be able to bend in an out-of-control manner.

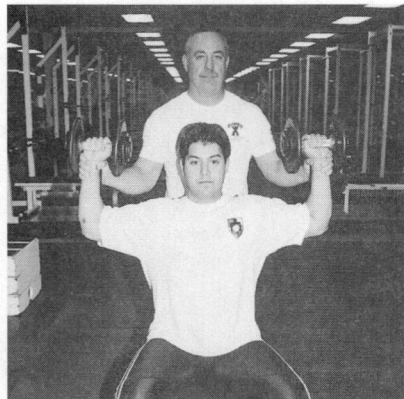

Spotting—Wrists Correct

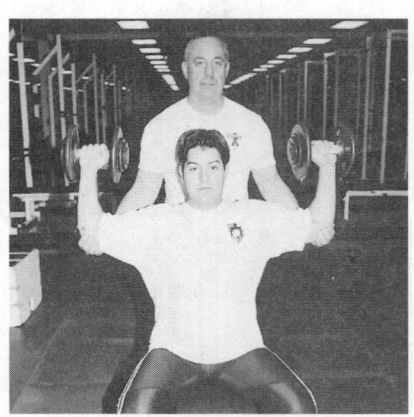

Spotting—Elbows Incorrect

Free Weight Exercises for the Chest

Barbell Pressing Exercises: Barbell pressing exercises will work the pectorals, triceps, anterior deltoid, and serratus. The incline bench press will place more stress on the upper pectorals, while the decline bench press will place more stress on the lower pectorals.

Bench Press:

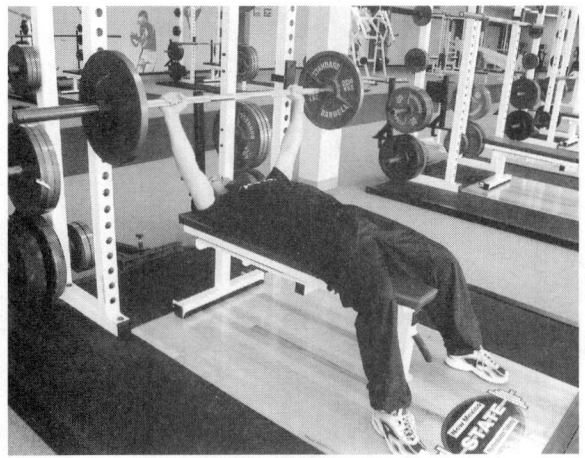 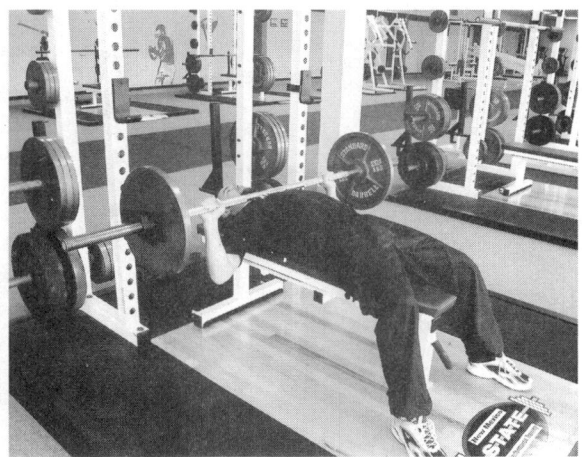

Incline Bench Press: Adjust the bench to 10 to 45 degrees from vertical.

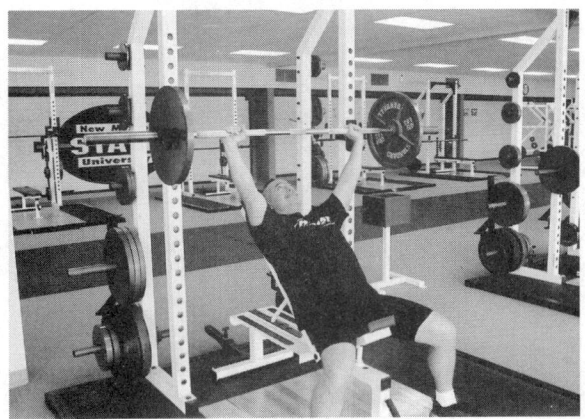 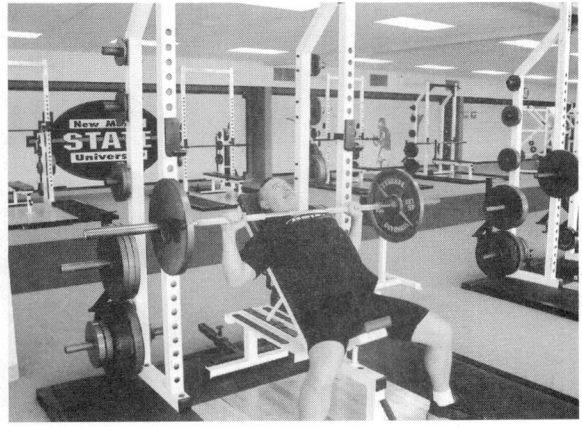

Decline Bench Press: When adjusting the bench, try to get the bench about 10 degrees below horizontal. This will emphasize the lower chest without placing the undue stress on the shoulders that is found when the head of the bench is dropped down significantly below parallel. This is an excellent exercise for people with shoulder problems, impingement, bursitis, and tendinitis. This is not a good exercise for those with hypertension or heart problems, or for pregnant women or older adults.

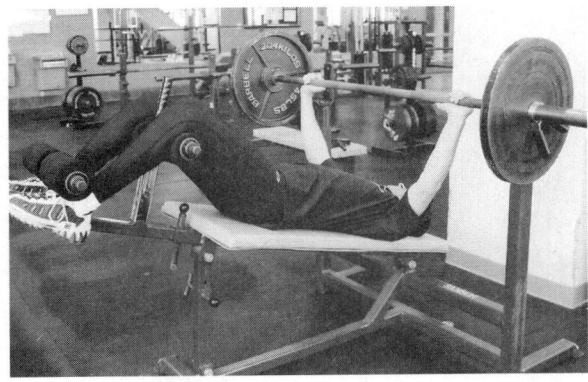 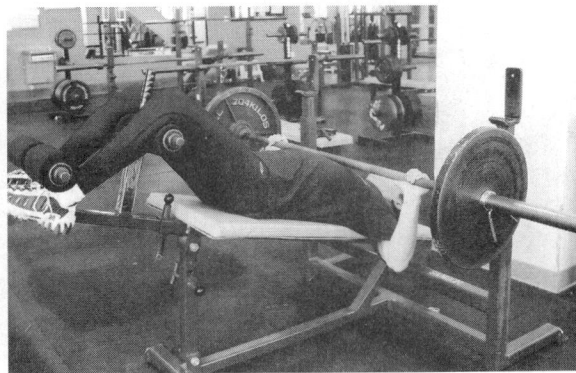

All of the above exercises can also be done on a Smith Machine with a moveable bench.

Dumbbell Pressing Exercises

Dumbbell presses involve the pectoralis, the triceps, and the anterior deltoid.* Dumbbells allow for a greater range of motion and thus more stretch than would a barbell; however, the maximum weight you use will be greater with a barbell. The angle of the bench will affect the muscles as described above in the barbell section.

Dumbbell Bench Press

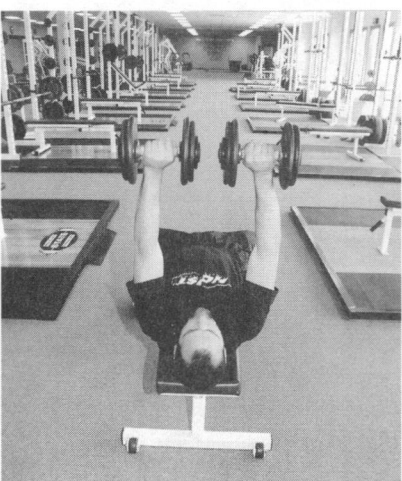 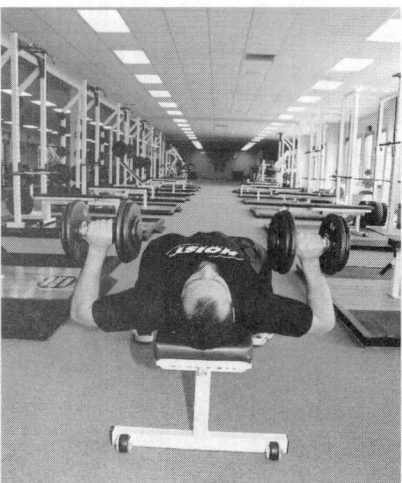

Dumbbell Incline Bench Press: Same rules apply as in barbell incline bench press.

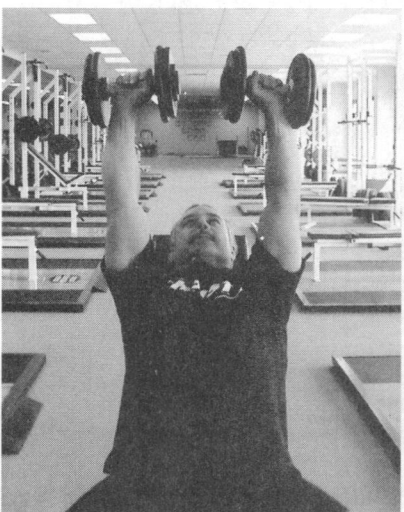 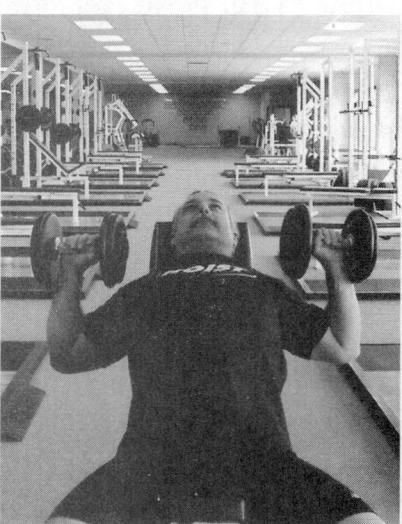

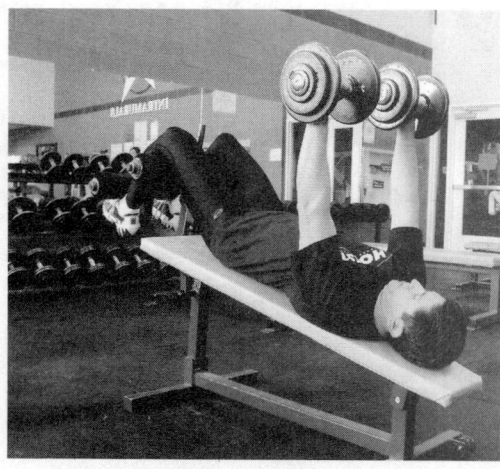 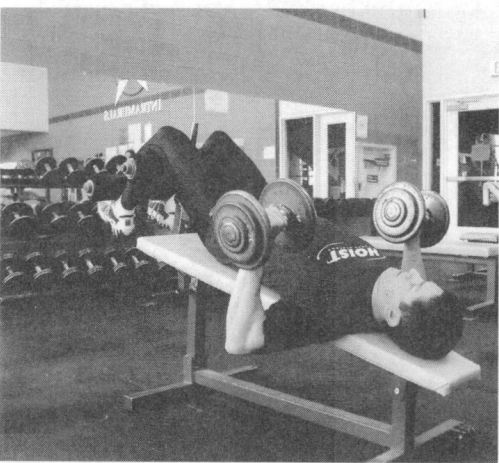

Dumbbell Decline Bench Press: Same rules apply as in barbell decline bench press.

Dumbbell Flyes

Dumbbell flyes isolate the pectoralis major. Typically, when the weight is light, the arms will be more outstretched (greater angle between the upper and lower arm), but as the weight used increases, the arms will move closer together through the range of motion (lesser angle between the upper and lower arm). * Dumbbell flyes should not be done with heavy weight.

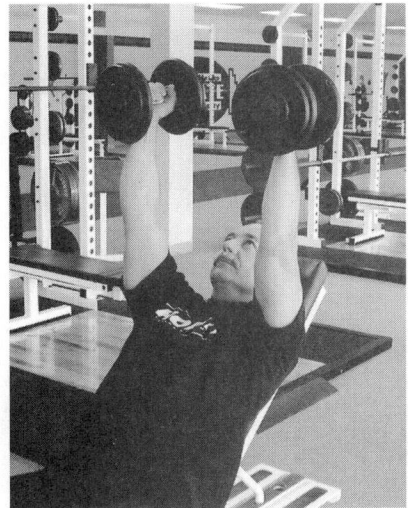 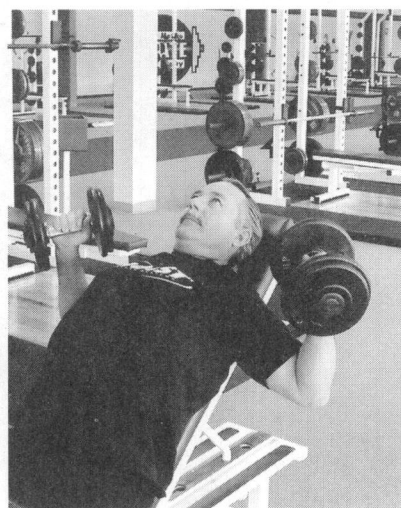

Dumbbell Incline Flyes

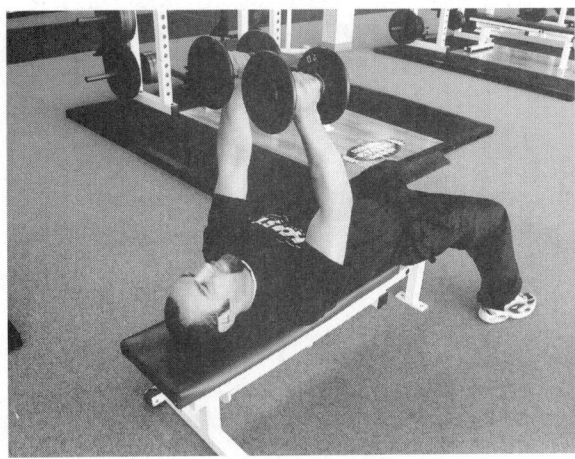 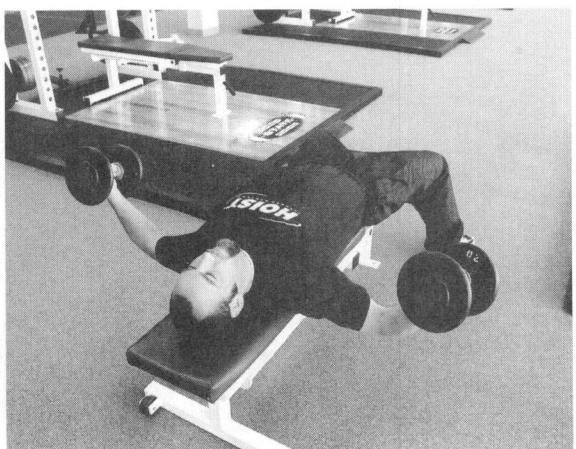

Dumbbell Flat Flyes

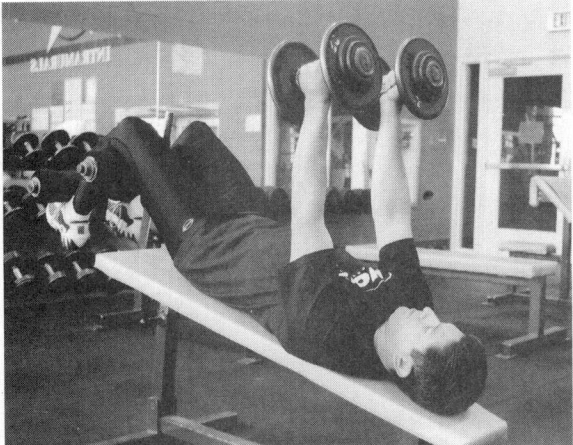 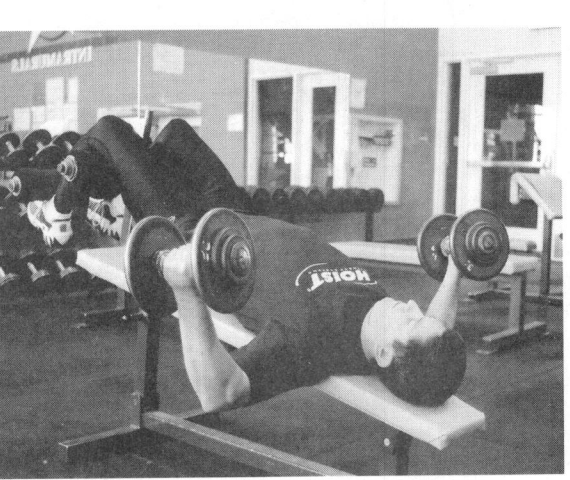

Dumbbell Decline Flyes

Selectorized Machine Exercises for the Chest

Decline Chest Press: A great exercise for the women that have had a mastectomy and removal of pectoralis minor.

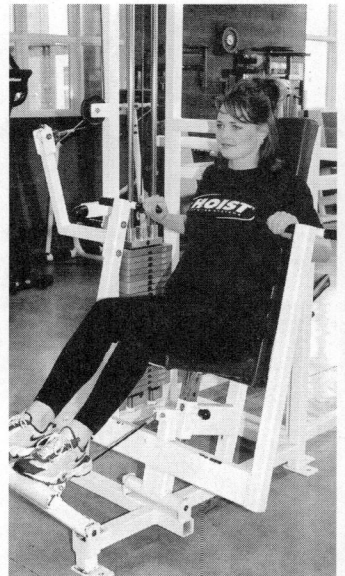 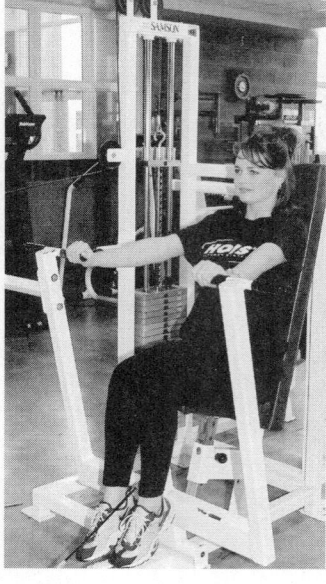 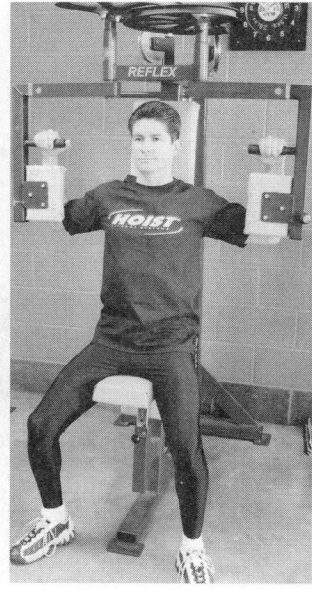 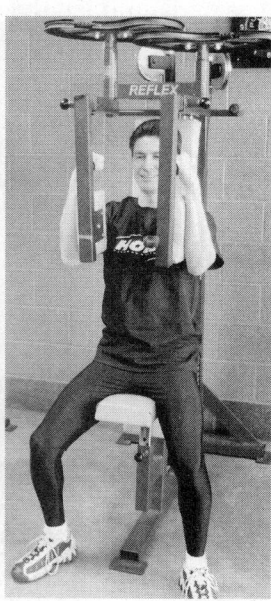

Chest Press – Start   Finish   Pec Deck – Start   Finish

Pullovers

Pullovers using either the barbell or dumbbell are excellent exercises and will work the pectoralis major and minor, triceps, lats, teres major, serratus anterior, rhomboids, and (to a lesser degree) rectus abdominous.*

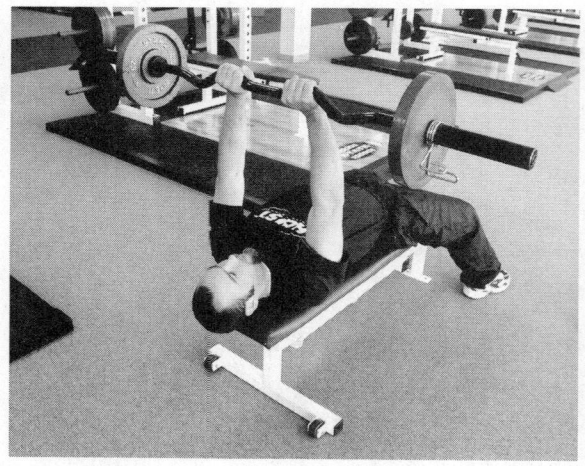 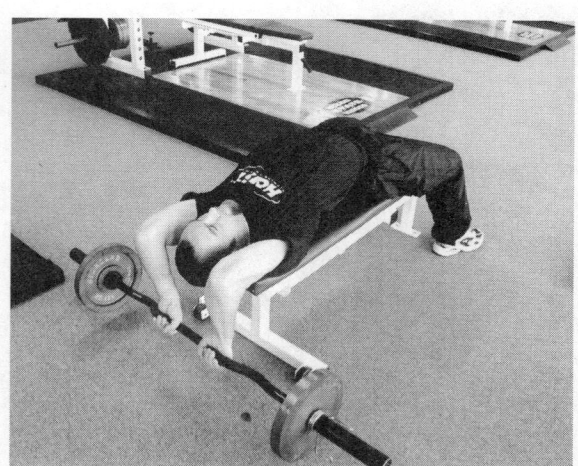

EZ Curl Bar Pullovers

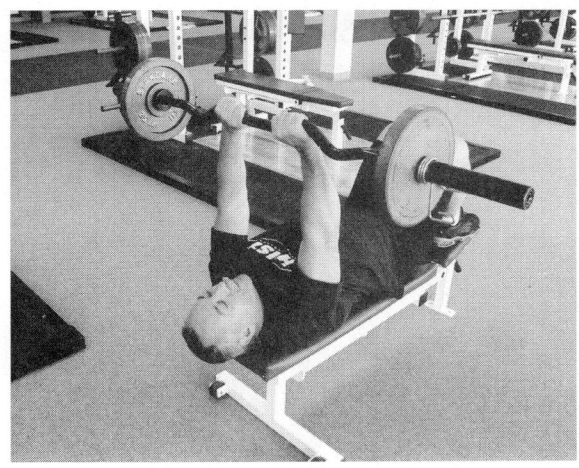
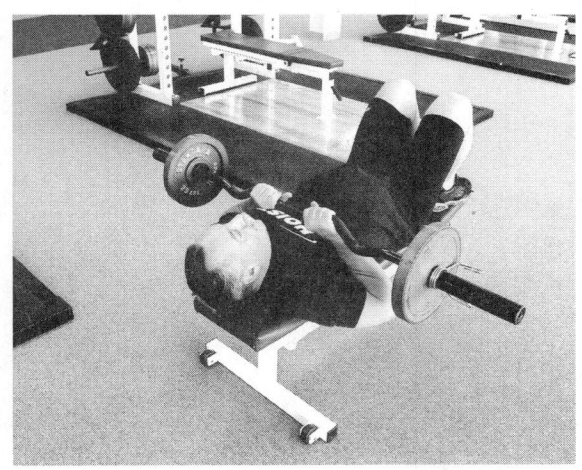

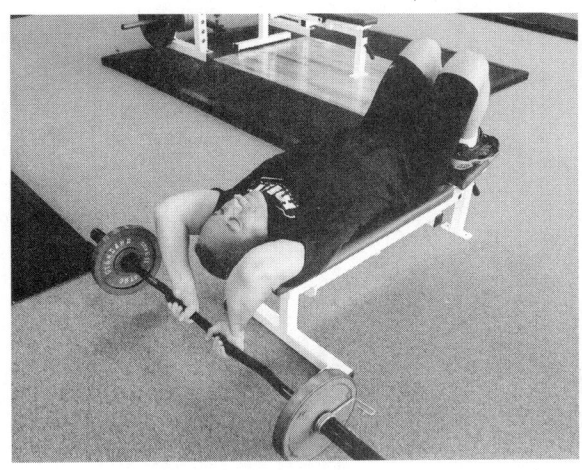
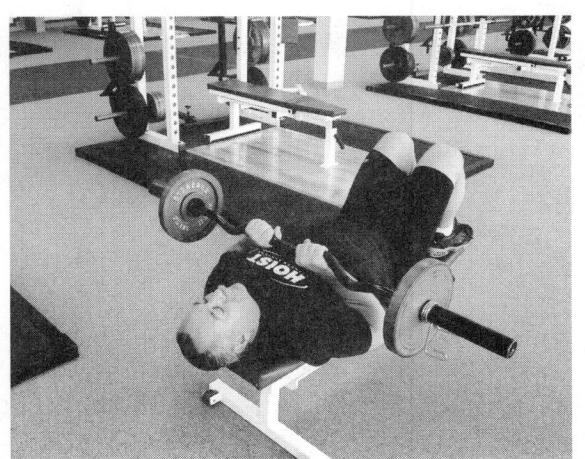

EZ Curl Bar Pullovers with Press

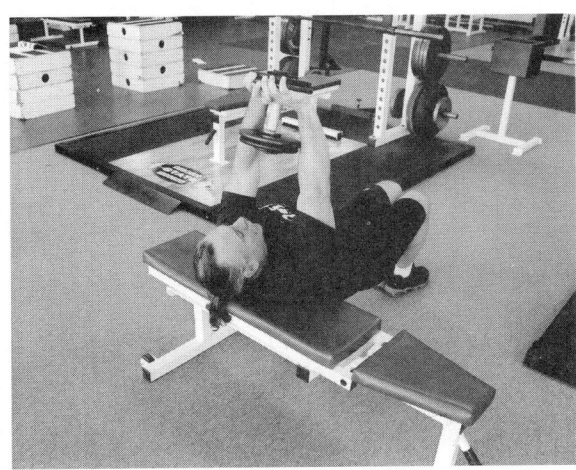
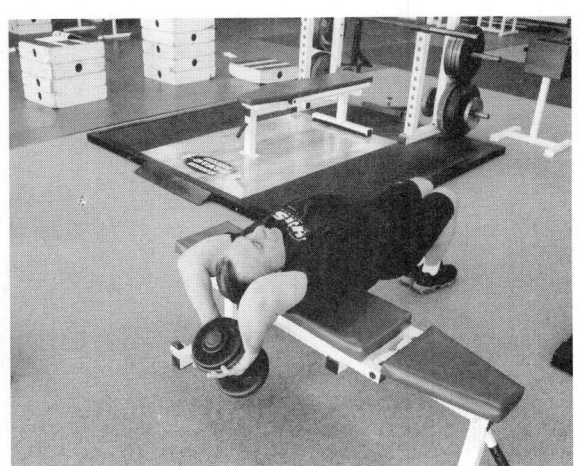

Dumbbell Pullovers

Dips

Dips Work the Chest and Triceps: In leaning forward, more work is placed on the pectoralis, while leaning back to an almost an upright position will shift the emphasis more to the triceps.*

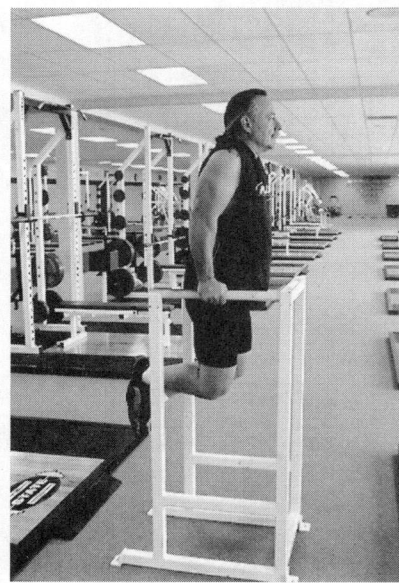 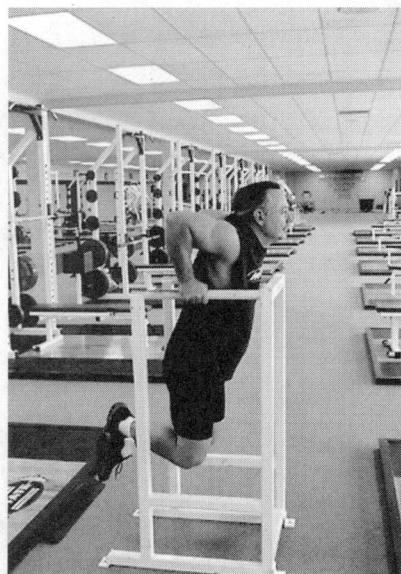

Legs Back

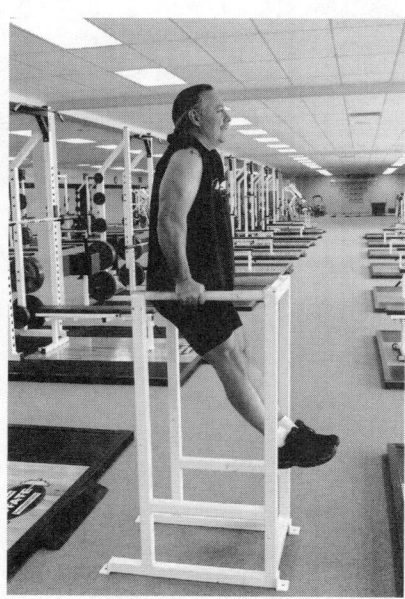 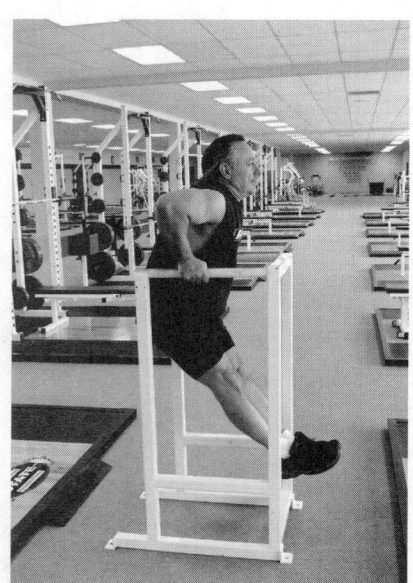

Legs Forward

(*Asterisk indicates information from "Strength Training Anatomy" by Frederic Delavier, Human Kinetics. This information is used as reference material.)

Cable Crossover Flyes

Cable crossover flyes will work the pectoralis major and minor. By changing the amount of forward bend in the waist, the emphasis can be changed to upper, overall, or lower pectoralis. Crossing the arms at the end of the movement will place the stress on the upper pectoralis.

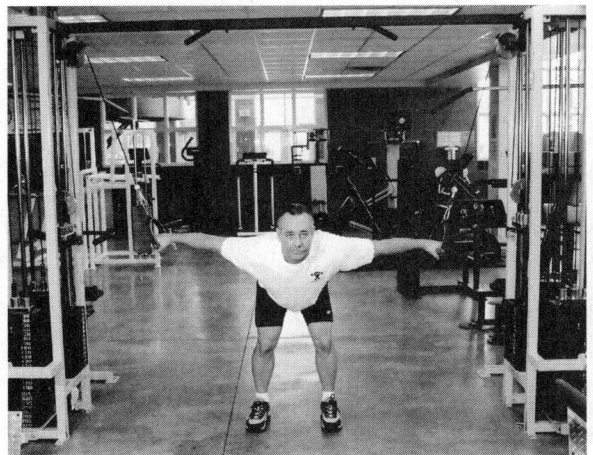 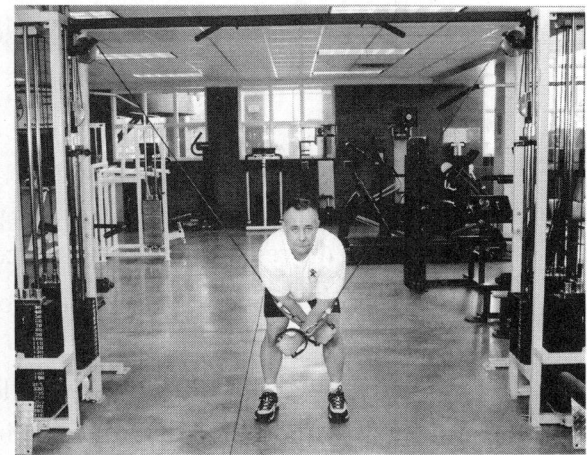

Squeeze

When doing chest exercises, "squeeze" the muscle at the completion of the movement. By "squeezing," the muscle is tightened to the point that you can feel the muscle pulling together at the end of the movement and thus working on upper pectorals. The squeeze is felt when you maximally contract the pectoralis muscle.

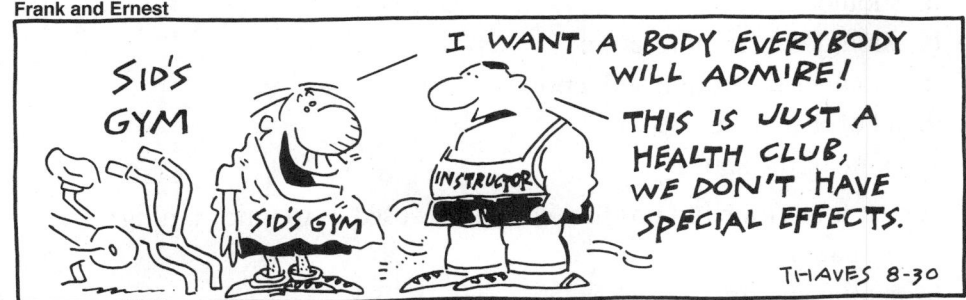

CHAPTER 2 SELF TEST

Please feel free to write on this page

True or False

1. _____ When doing chest exercises, "squeeze" the muscle at the completion of the movement.

2. _____ Adduction refers to moving the limb away from the centerline of the body, while abduction moves a limb toward the centerline of the body.

3. _____ When spotting a person using dumbbells, it is usually best to spot them by gripping their elbows.

4. _____ Using a normal spacing of a hand grip on a bar will stress the overall muscle.

5. _____ You can use more weight with dumbbells than with a barbell.

Multiple Choice

6. _____ Which of the following exercises work the chest muscles?
   a. cable crossover flyes
   b. pullovers
   c. dips
   d. dumbbell flyes
   e. all of the above

7. _____ The primary purpose of the chest muscles are:
   a. shoulder flexion
   b. shoulder internal rotation
   c. shoulder horizontal adduction
   d. all of the above
   e. none of the above

8. _____ Which is NOT a hand position commonly used in weight training?
   a. pronated grip
   b. supinated grip
   c. alternating grip
   d. frontal grip

9. _____ What are the names of hand spacing used for lifting?
   a. narrow
   b. wide
   c. normal
   d. all of the above

10. _____ By bringing your elbows to your side, you tend to put more stress on the anterior deltoids and the _____ .

a. biceps

b. triceps

c. pectoralis major

d. pectoralis minor

11. _____ When doing chest dips, leaning forward will work the _____ , while leaning back works more the _____ .

a. triceps, biceps

b. deltoid, trapezius

c. pectoralis, triceps

d. latissimus dorsi, serratus

12. _____ Which muscle group will the incline bench press place more stress on?

a. anterior deltoids

b. serratus

c. upper pectoralis

d. biceps brachii

13. _____ What do dumbbell flyes isolate?

a. pectoralis major

b. pectoralis minor

c. biceps brachii

d. triceps brachii

14. _____ When doing crossover cables, what will change the emphasis on the upper, overall, and lower pectoralis?

a. heavier weight

b. lower weight

c. bending forward

d. bending backward

15. _____ Which exercise is not effective if done with heavy weight?

a. pullovers

b. dips

c. dumbbell flyes

d. cable crossover flyes

Please feel free to write on this page

Answers: 1. True 2. False 3. False 4. True 5. False 6. e 7. d 8. d 9. d 10. b 11. c 12. c 13. a 14. c 15. c

CHAPTER 3

Back Muscles and Exercises

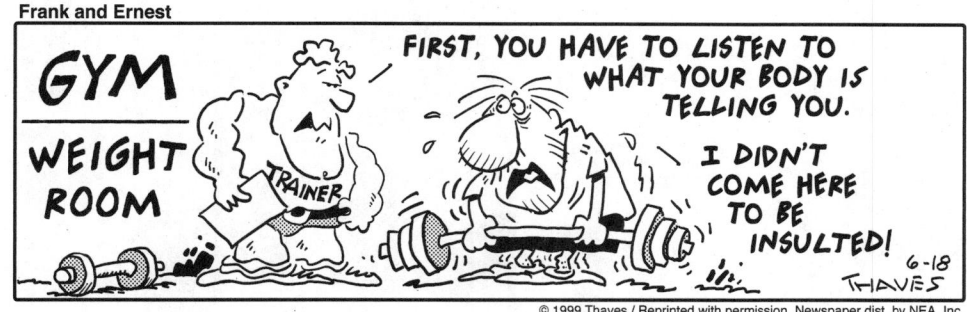

Frank and Ernest

GYM
___
WEIGHT
ROOM

FIRST, YOU HAVE TO LISTEN TO WHAT YOUR BODY IS TELLING YOU.

I DIDN'T COME HERE TO BE INSULTED!

6-18
THAVES

Back Muscles

Upper Back Muscles: The muscles of the upper back are the rhomboids, the trapezius, and the latissimus dorsi. The rhomboids are used to squeeze your shoulder blades together in conjunction with the trapezius. The trapezius is responsible for elevation, depression, and rotation of the scapula. The latissimus dorsi (lats) are the largest muscles in the back, and are responsible for extension, adduction, and internal rotation of the arm, as well as shoulder depression. The latissimus dorsi acting bilaterally hyperextends the spine. The erector spinae is a deep muscle of the back that extends from the sacrum to the base of the skull, and is responsible for extension of the spine.

Lower Back Muscles: The lower back muscle group that we are concerned with is the erector spinae. The erector spinae is responsible for back extension and stabilization of the torso. Stabilization of the torso is done in conjunction with the abdominals.

Scapular muscles are the latissimus dorsi, trapezius, teres major, and rhomboids.

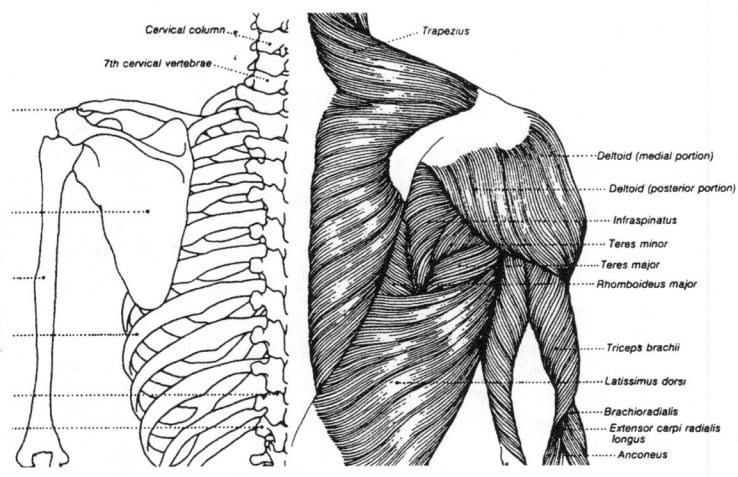

Cervical column

7th cervical vertebrae

Trapezius

Deltoid (medial portion)

Deltoid (posterior portion)

Infraspinatus

Teres minor

Teres major

Rhomboideus major

Triceps brachii

Latissimus dorsi

Brachioradialis

Extensor carpi radialis longus

Anconeus

Free Weight Exercises for the Back

Barbell Exercises

Stiff-Legged Deadlifts: Work the erectors of the back, gluteus maximus, hamstrings (biceps femoris, semimembranosus, and semitendonosus). This exercise stretches the hamstrings. Many people will perform this exercise standing on a bench or step, to further allow for stretching or to increase the range of motion.

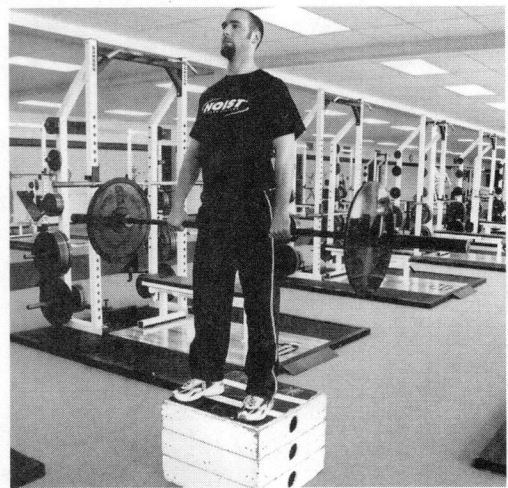
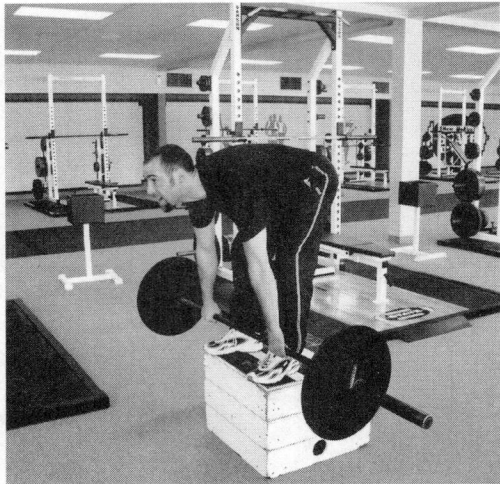

Bent Over Rowing: Works the muscles of the lats, teres major, posterior deltoids, arm flexors, biceps, brachialis, brachioradialis, rhomboids, and trapezius.* This exercise can also be done using a supinated grip and with wide or narrow hand spacing.

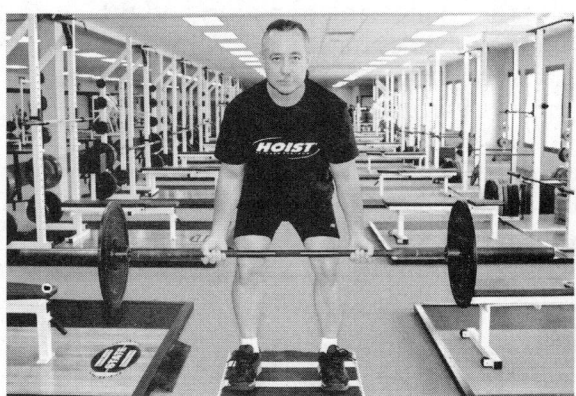
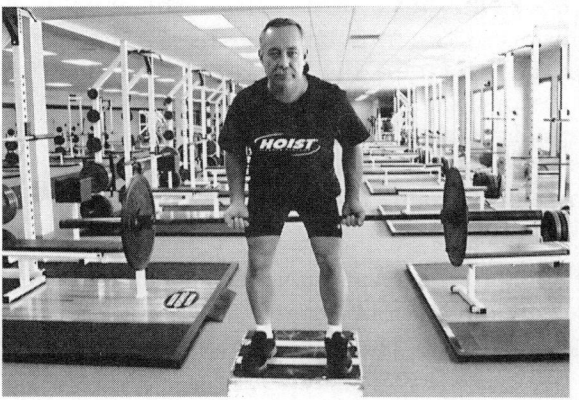

Supinated Grip

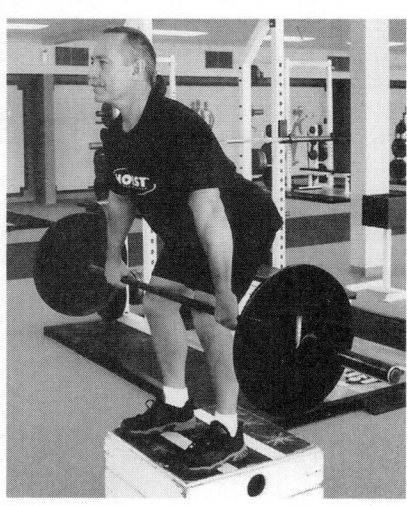
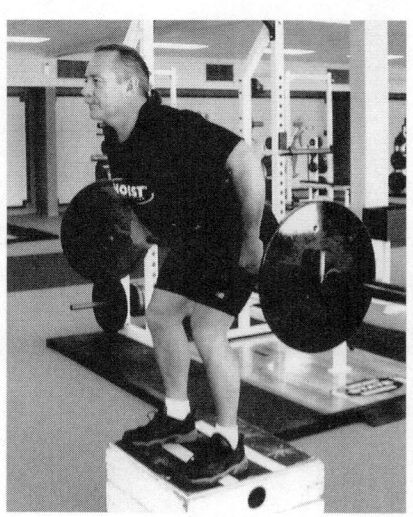

Pronated Grip

Barbell Pullovers: Pullovers using the barbell are excellent exercises and will work the pectoralis major and minor, triceps, lats, teres major, serratus anterior, and rhomboids.*

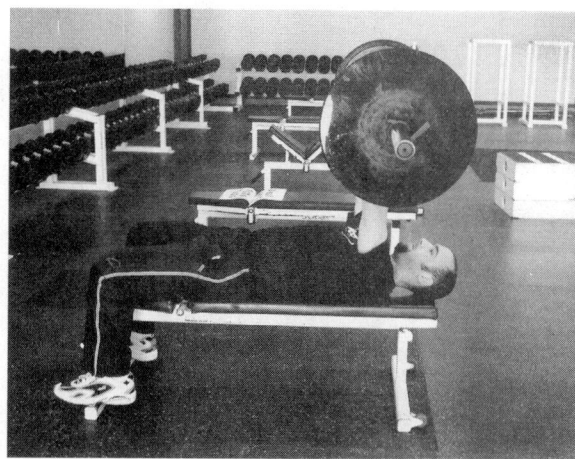 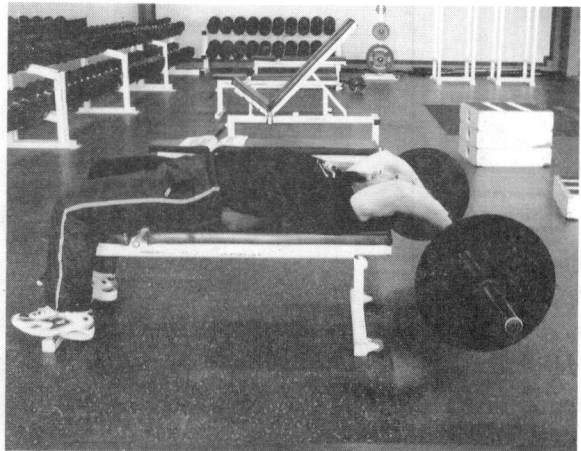

Deadlifts: Work about every muscle in the body. When beginning this exercise, drive with the legs. The upper body should remain upright and the hips and shoulders should come up at the same rate. You will be stronger using an alternating grip, as compared to a pronated grip, in this exercise.

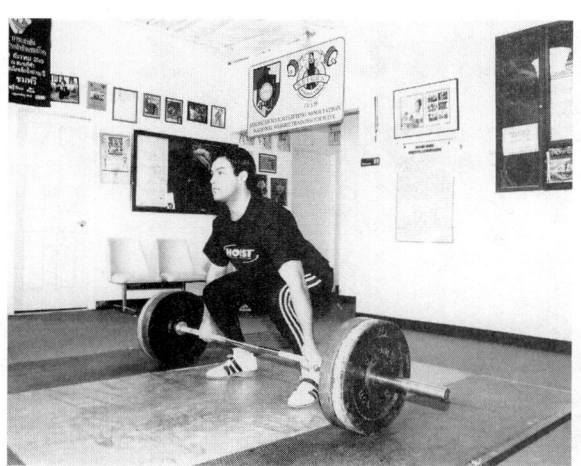 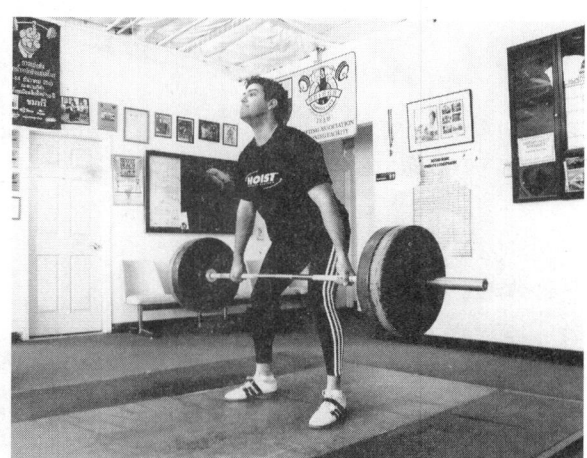

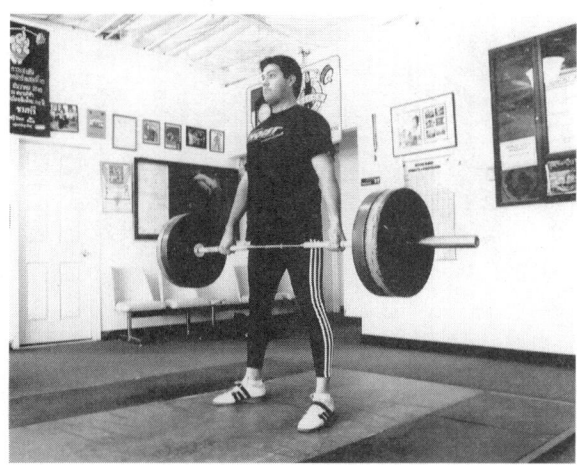

Dumbbell Exercises

One-arm Dumbbell Rows: Primarily work the lats, teres major, posterior deltoids, trapezius, and rhomboids.

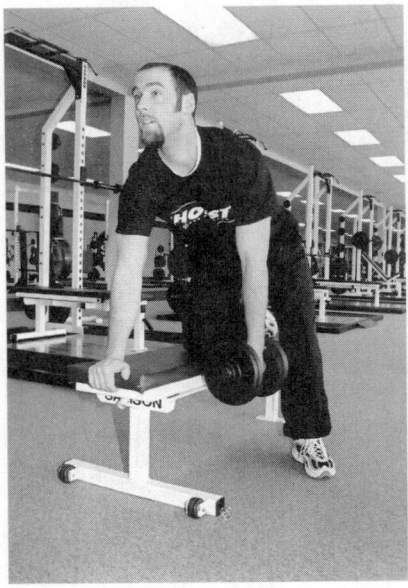 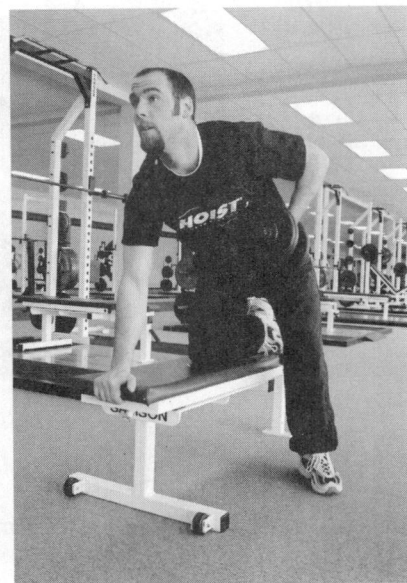

Dumbbell Pullovers: Pullovers using dumbbells are excellent exercises and will work the pectoralis major and minor, triceps, lats, teres major, serratus anterior, and rhomboids.*

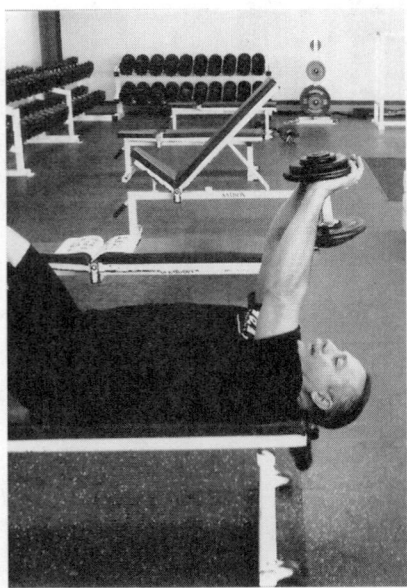 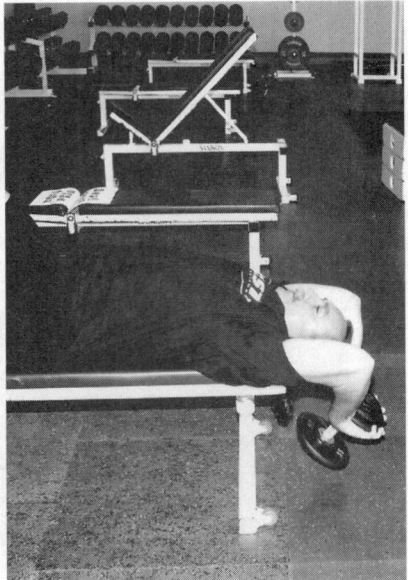

Machine Exercises

Does It Matter if I Do Lat Pull-downs to the Front or to the Rear?

According to research done by researchers at the University of Miami, it does. The research involved 10 males and the use of electromyography (EMG). Muscle activity was measured in the latissimus dorsi, pectoralis major, teres major, posterior deltoid, and the long head of the tricep while the subjects did either a front lat pull-down or a rear lat pull-down. Results of the study show that an anterior lat pull-down produced more muscle activity in the latissimus dorsi than did a posterior lat pull-down. This was true for both the concentric and eccentric phases.[1]

And if this isn't enough reason to do lat pull-downs to the front, then how about the stress that doing them to the rear can place on the rotator cuffs? What happens is when the exercise is done to the rear of the head, shoulder abduction and external rotation occurs, which could lead to injury.

Front Lat Pull-downs: Work the latissimus dorsi, teres major, brachialis, and biceps brachii. Also worked to a lesser degree are the trapezius, rhomboids, and pectorals.* This exercise can also be done using a wide or narrow hand spacing.

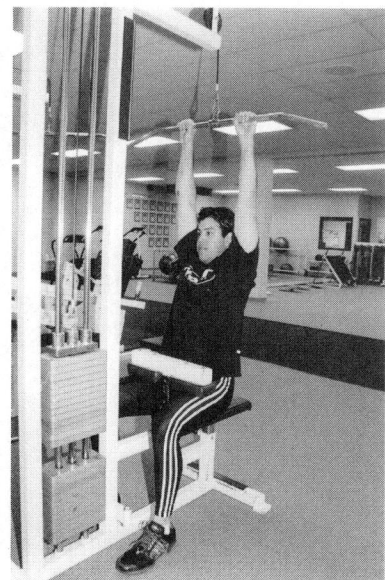
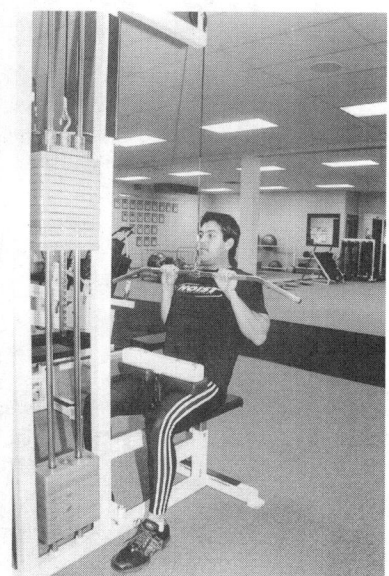

Pronated Close Grip

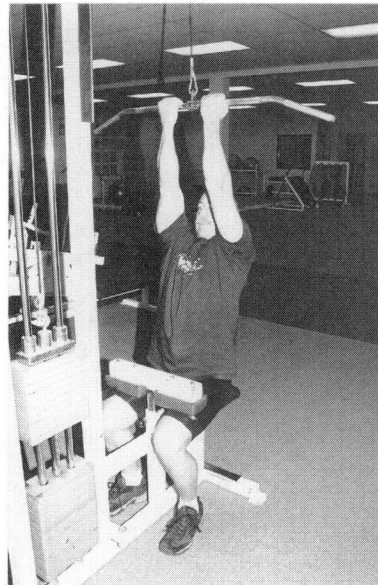
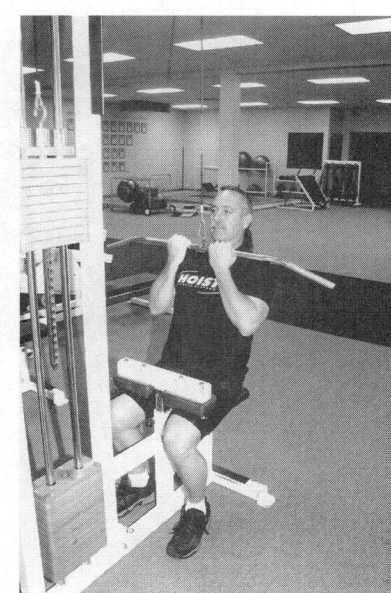

Supinated Close Grip

Wide-grip Front Lat Pull-downs: Work the latissimus dorsi, teres major, rhomboids, trapezius (scapular muscles), posterior deltoids, biceps, brachialis, and brachioradialis. This exercise can be done with a narrow supinated grip to place more emphasis on the bicep.

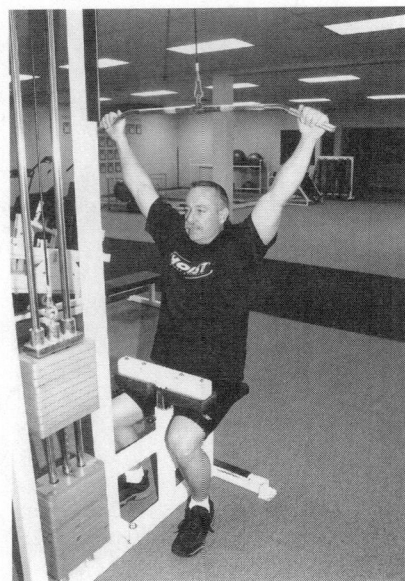 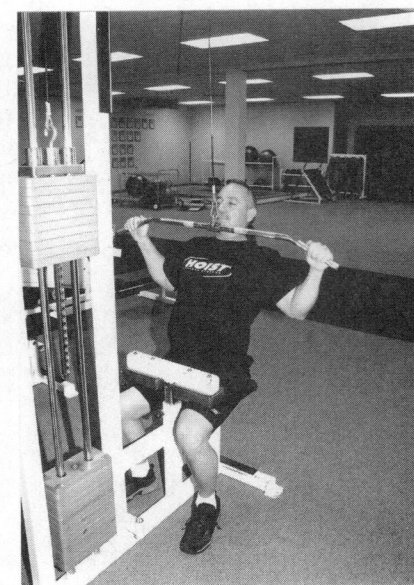

Rear Lat Pull-downs: Work the latissimus dorsi, forearm flexors, biceps, brachialis, brachioradialis, rhomboids, and trapezius.*

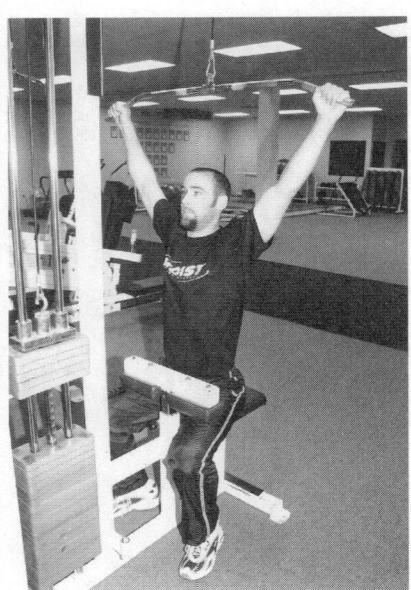 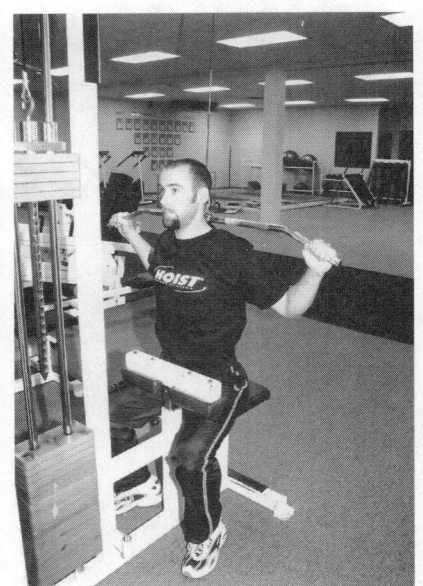

Other Items to Consider When Doing Lat Pull-downs

When gripping the bar with a pronated grip to do a lat pull-down, the wider the grip you use the more posterior deltoid you will use. A narrower grip will utilize more of the latissimus dorsi.

Also, if you use a supinated grip with your arms held close to your sides, you will use more of the bicep brachii muscle and the weight will seem lighter due to the strength of the biceps muscle.[2]

Low Rows (also called Seated Rows): Work the latissimus dorsi, teres major, trapezius, rhomboids (scapular muscles), posterior deltoids, biceps, brachialis, brachioradialis, and erectors.*

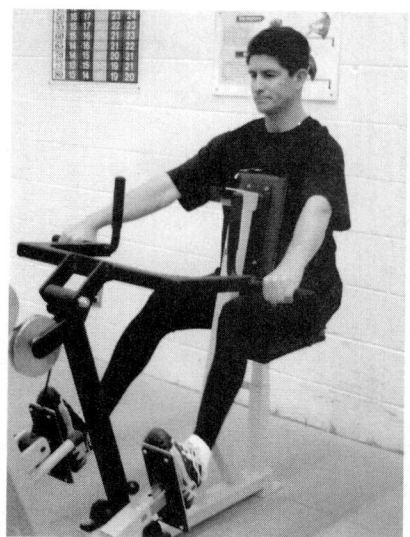 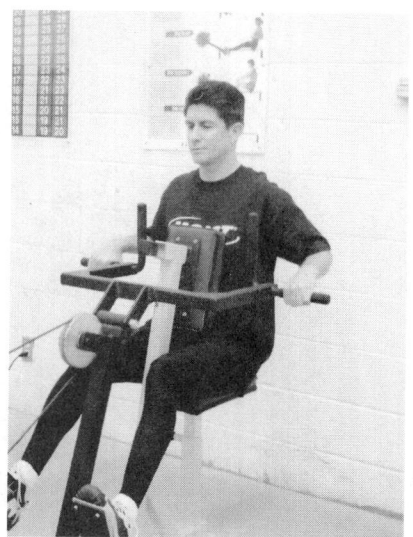

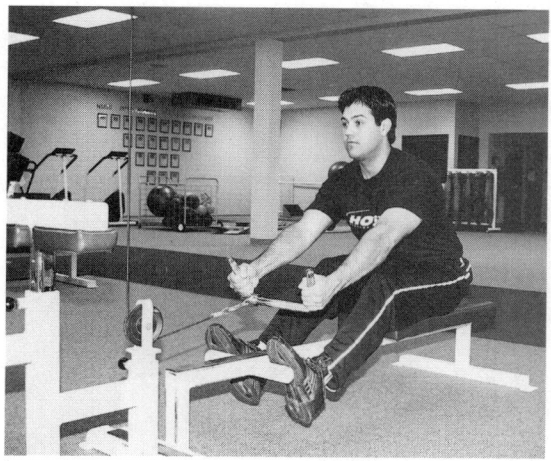 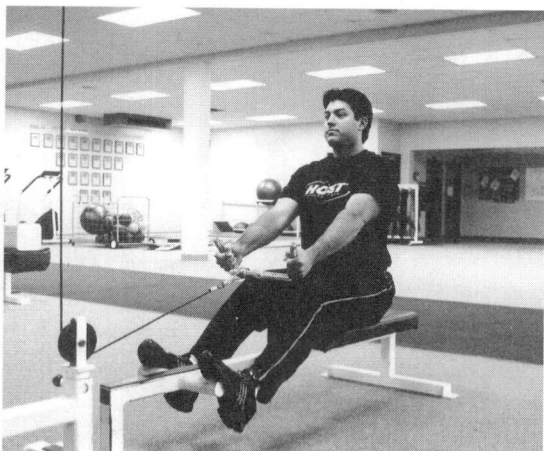

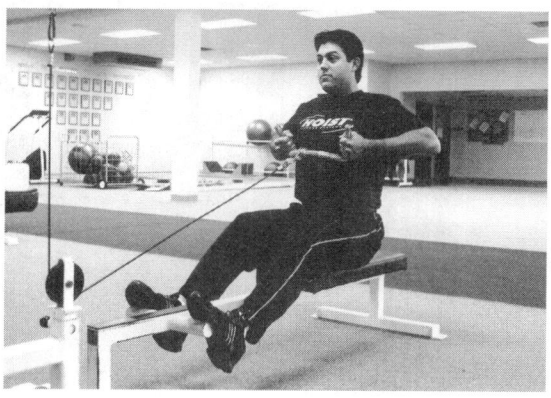

Exercises Utilizing Benches and Other Equipment

Incline Rowing and T-Bar Rowing: Works the latissimus dorsi, teres major, posterior deltoids, arm flexors, trapezius, and rhomboid muscles. The incline bench used in the exercise prevents the back from rounding and possible injury. By using a supinated grip, some of the work will shift to the biceps and upper part of the trapezius.*

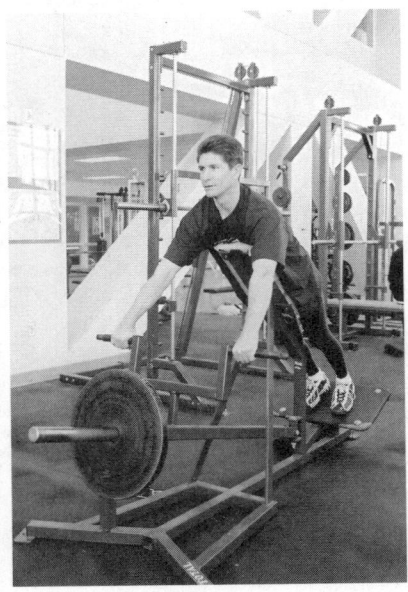
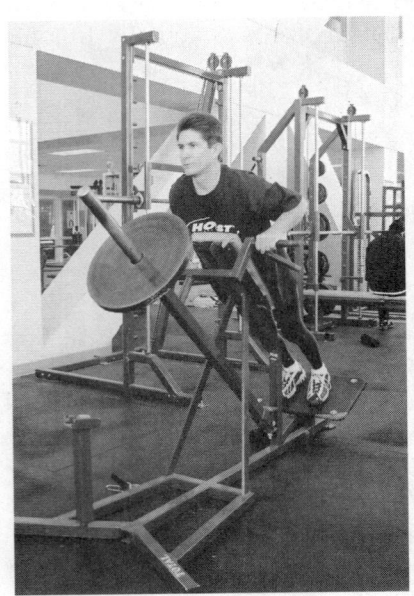

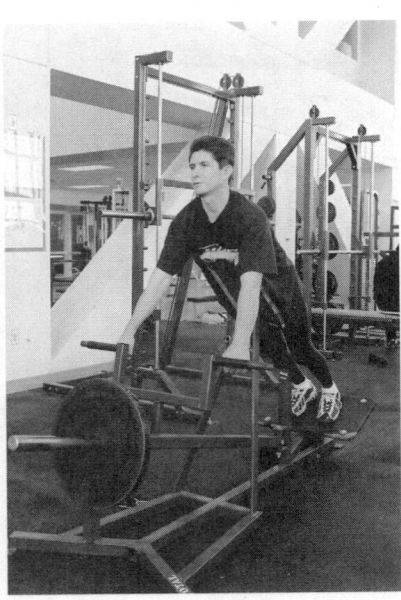
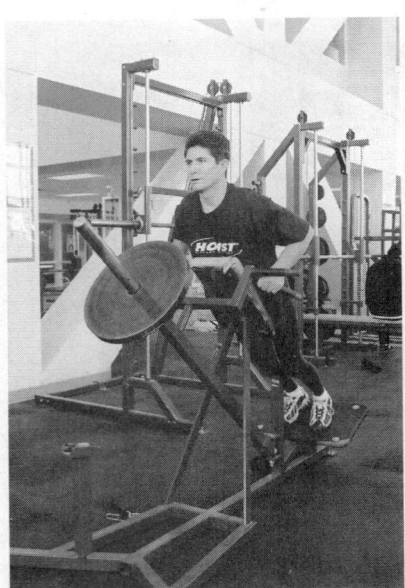

Chin-Ups: Work the latissimus dorsi, rhomboids, trapezius, teres major, biceps brachii, brachialis, brachioradialis, and pectoralis major.*

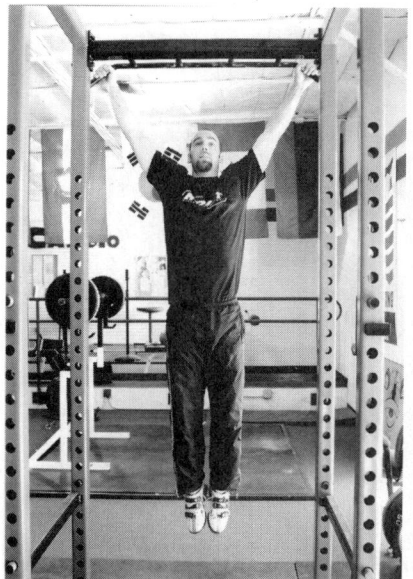 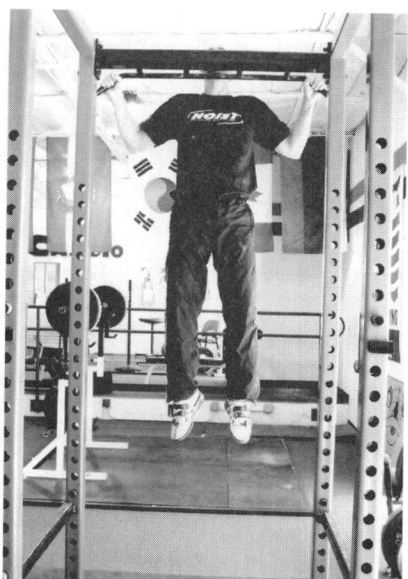

Pull-Ups (Reverse Chin-Ups): Work the latissimus dorsi, teres major, biceps, brachialis, trapezius, rhomboids, and pectorals.*

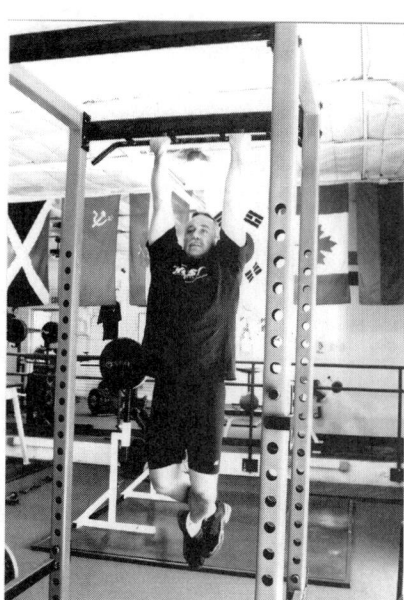 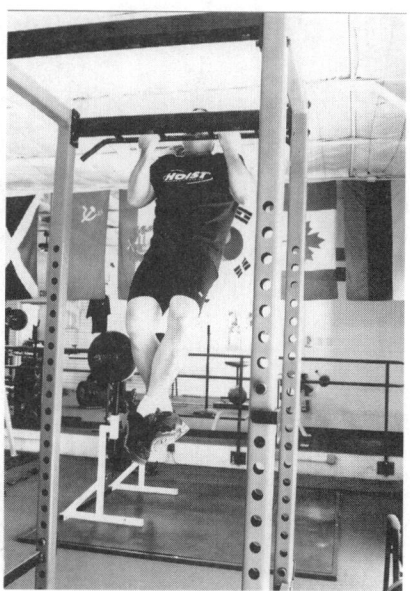

Other Items to Consider When Doing Barbell Rowing Exercises

A *narrow grip* will work more of the latissimus dorsi and teres major muscles, while a wide grip will focus more on the posterior deltoid. With narrow hand spacing the grip can be either pronated or supinated. Typically, wide hand spacing will utilize a pronated grip.

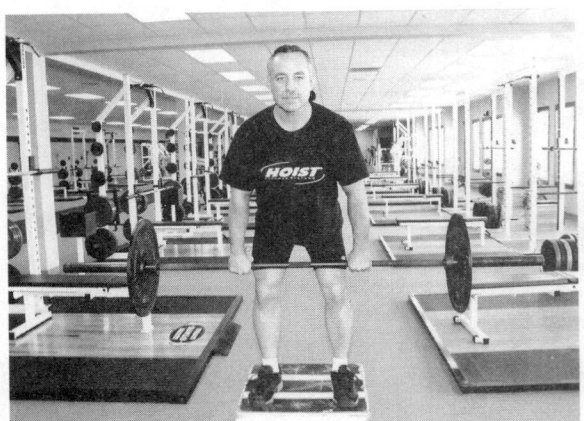

Narrow Pronated

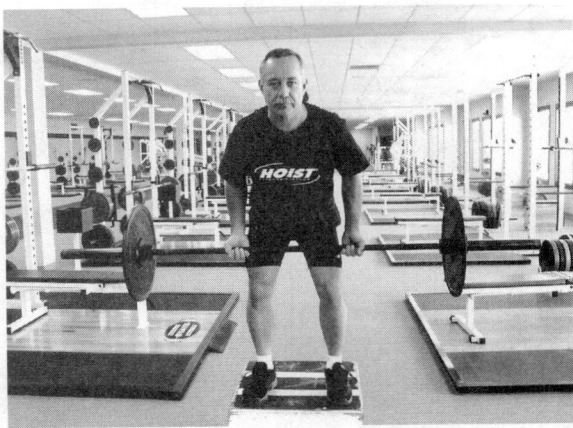

Narrow Supinated

A row using a *pronated grip* will focus more on the brachialis, a row using a neutral grip will focus more on the brachioradialis, and a row using a supinated grip will work more of the bicep brachii.[2]

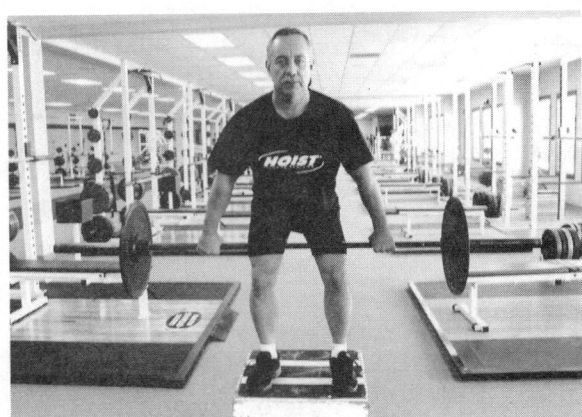

Wide Pronated

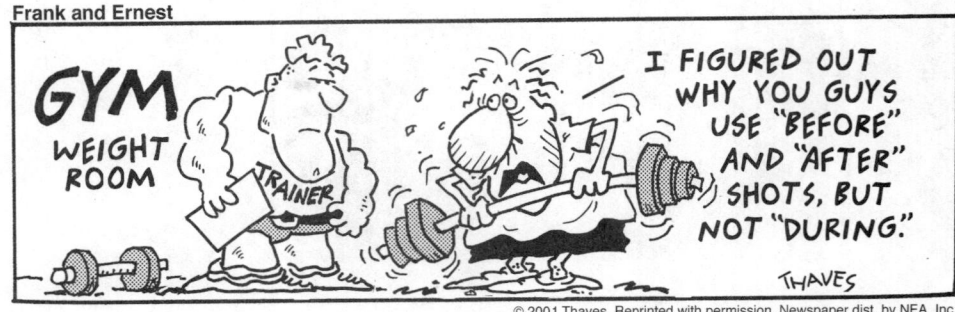

Frank and Ernest

GYM WEIGHT ROOM

TRAINER

I FIGURED OUT WHY YOU GUYS USE "BEFORE" AND "AFTER" SHOTS, BUT NOT "DURING."

THAVES

© 2001 Thaves. Reprinted with permission. Newspaper dist. by NEA, Inc.

1. Signorile, JF, Zink, AJ, Szwed, SP. (2002). A comparative electromygraphical investigation of muscle utilization patterns using hand positions during the lat pull-down. *Journal of Strength & Conditioning Research* 16 (4): 539–546.
2. Andrews, G. (September 2002). Angles, Positions and Variations. A thorough study of strength training. *Personal Fitness Professional*. 30–38.

(*Asterisk indicates information from, "Strength Training Anatomy" by Frederic Delavier, Human Kinetics. This information is used as reference material.)

Please feel free to write on this page

True or False

1. _____ The trapezius muscle is responsible for elevation, depression, and rotation of the scapula.

2. _____ Stiff-legged deadlifts workout the erectors of the back, gluteus maximus, and hamstring.

3. _____ Doing Lat Pulls to the rear have been shown to be more effective than doing Lat Pulls to the front.

4. _____ While doing Lat Pulls a wider grip will utilize more of the latissimus dorsi muscle.

5. _____ The erector spinae is responsible for back extension and stabilization of the torso.

Multiple Choice

6. _____ Of the muscles in the back, which is the largest?
   a. Rhomboids
   b. Teres major
   c. Latissimus dorsi (lats)
   d. Trapezius
   e. Levator scapulae

7. _____ Which of the following muscles are included in the scapular muscles?
   a. Rhomboids
   b. Teres major
   c. Latissimus dorsi (lats)
   d. Trapezius
   e. All of the above

8. _____ What is the purpose of people performing Stiff-legged Deadlifts standing on a bench or step?
   a. Allows further stretching
   b. To increase range of motion
   c. To make them look taller
   d. To increase their stance
   e. Both A & B

9. _____ Using a pronated grip while performing rows will focus primarily on what muscle?
   a. The brachialis
   b. The biceps brachii
   c. The brachioradialis
   d. The deltoid
   e. The triceps brachii

10. _____ Why is an incline bench used while performing Incline rowing?
   a. Because it causes the person to generate more force
   b. Because it prevents the back from rounding and causing a possible injury
   c. Because it helps to keep your legs in the proper position
   d. Because it prevents you from using other muscles other than the primary ones being worked
   e. Because it makes the muscles work that much more

Please feel free to write on this page

Answers: 1. True   2. True   3. False   4. False   5. True   6. c   7. e   8. e   9. a   10. b

CHAPTER 4

Shoulder Muscles and Exercises

Frank and Ernest

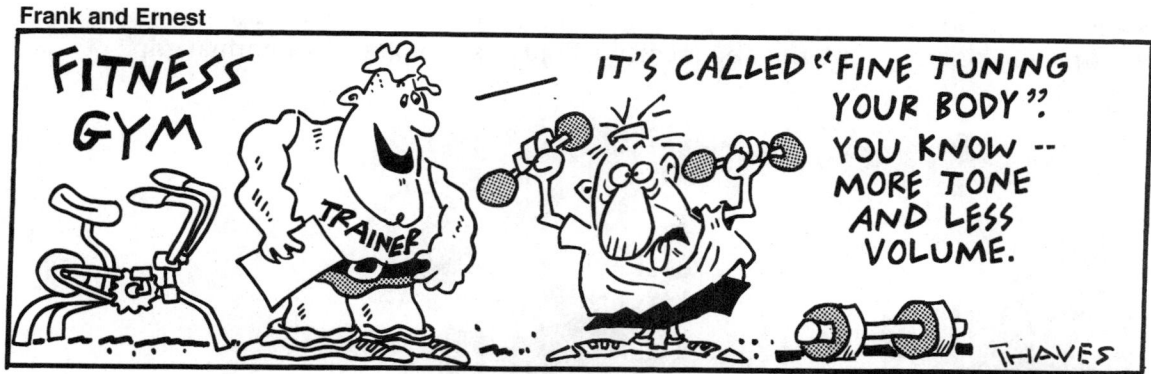

© 2001 Thaves. Reprinted with permission. Newspaper dist. by NEA, Inc.

Shoulder Muscles

The shoulder muscles are the deltoids (delts), rotator cuffs, trapezius (traps), and pectoralis major (pecs). The deltoids are composed of three muscles know as the anterior deltoid, medial deltoid, and the posterior deltoid. The rotator cuffs have four muscles known as the supraspinatus, infraspinatus, teres minor, and subscapularis. The trapezius muscle is composed of three sections; the upper, middle, and lower. The pectoralis major elevates, horizontally adducts, extends, and medially rotates the arm.

The deltoids are responsible for rotating and lifting the arms. The anterior deltoid lifts to the front, the medial deltoid lifts to the side, and the posterior deltoid lifts to the rear. The rotator cuff medially and laterally rotates the arm. The trapezius is responsible for shoulder elevation and depression as well as scapula adduction.

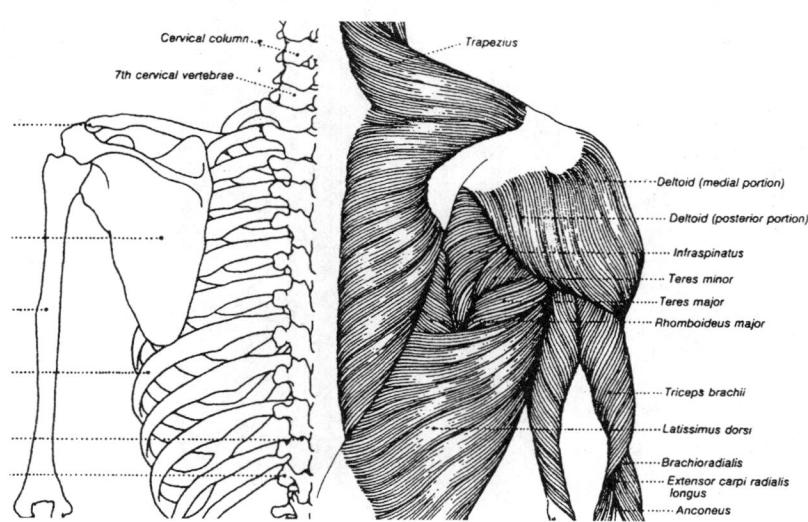

Free Weight Exercises for the Shoulder

The riskiest positions, and those most often associated with injury when doing shoulder exercises, are those that involve abduction above the line of the shoulder, or a combination of abduction with either external or internal rotation of the arm and forearm. Try to keep the shoulder healthy, and do exercises for the rotator cuffs.

Barbell Exercises

Military or Front Presses: Work the upper trapezius, anterior and medial deltoids, upper pectorals, triceps and serratus anterior. A narrower grip will work more anterior deltoid and upper pectorals. A wider grip will work more anterior and medial deltoids, as compared to a normal grip.*

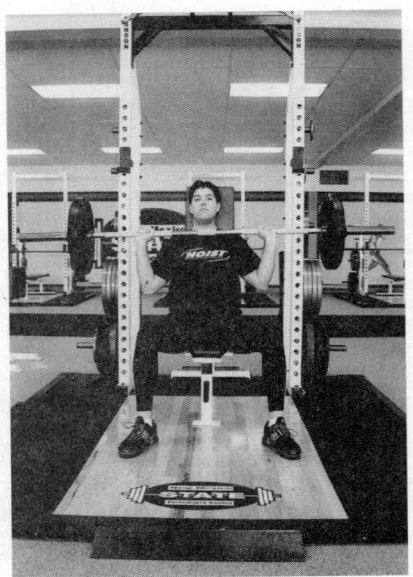 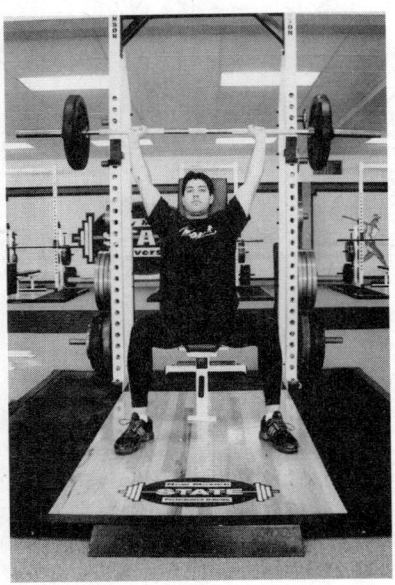

Seated

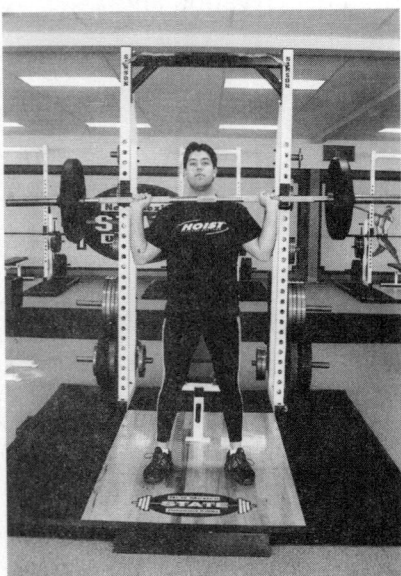 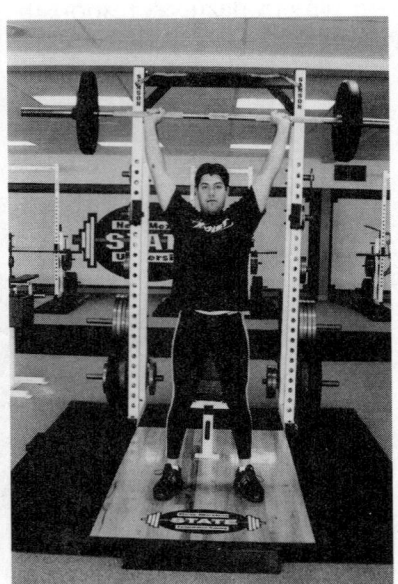

Standing

Behind the Neck Presses: Work the upper trapezius, medial deltoids, triceps and serratus anterior. This exercise also utilizes the rhomboids, infraspinatus, teres minor, and supraspinatus.* This exercise can put considerable strain on the rotator cuffs. If it doesn't feel comfortable, do the Military or Front Presses instead.*

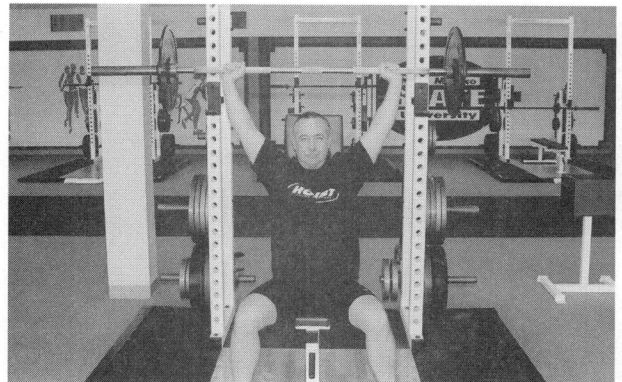 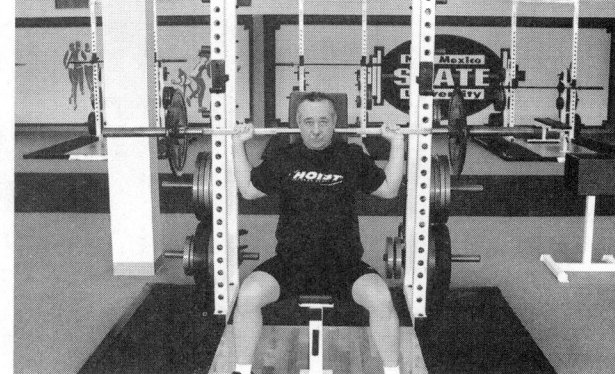

Seated

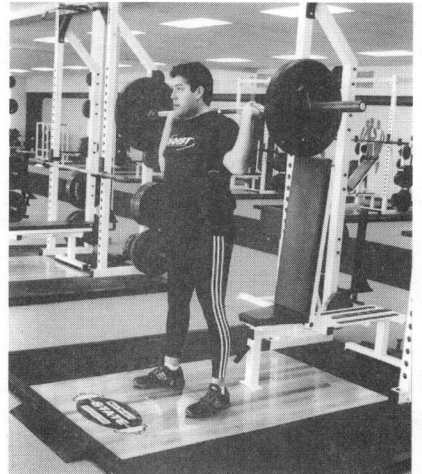 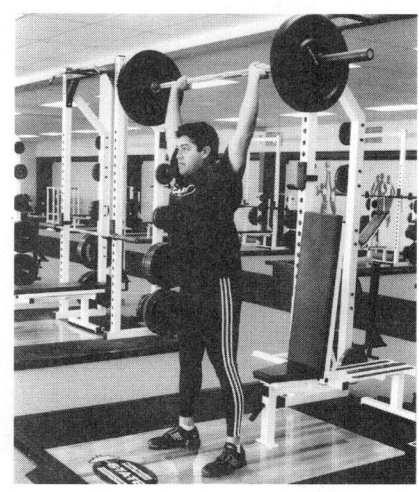

Standing

Other Items to Consider When Doing Presses

When using a wide grip in presses, the medial deltoid will be worked more. With a narrower grip, the anterior deltoid will receive more work.[1]

Barbell Upright Rows: Work the trapezius, deltoids, and biceps, with some action going to the forearm and abdominal muscles. Use a grip with approximately 12" between each hand to lessen the effects on the rotator cuffs, or for anyone who has tendonitis or any kind of impingement.[1]

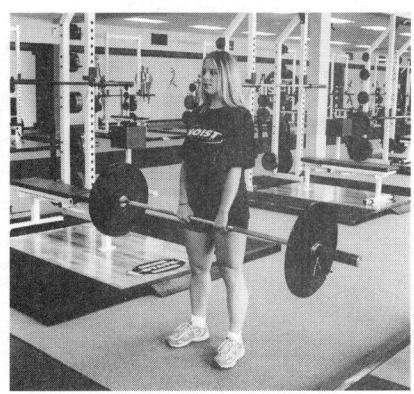 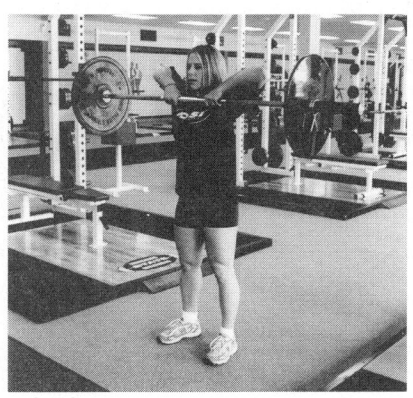

Barbell Shrugs: Work primarily the upper trapezius and deltoids.

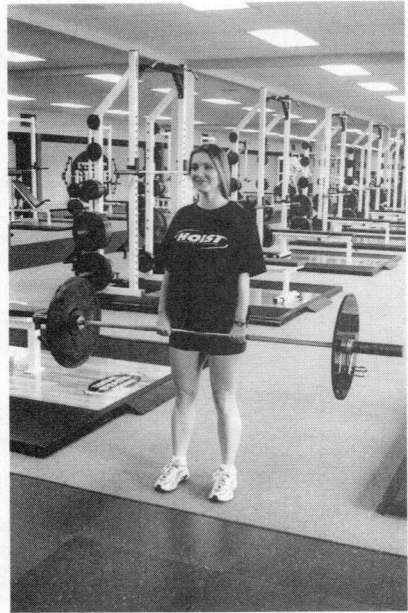 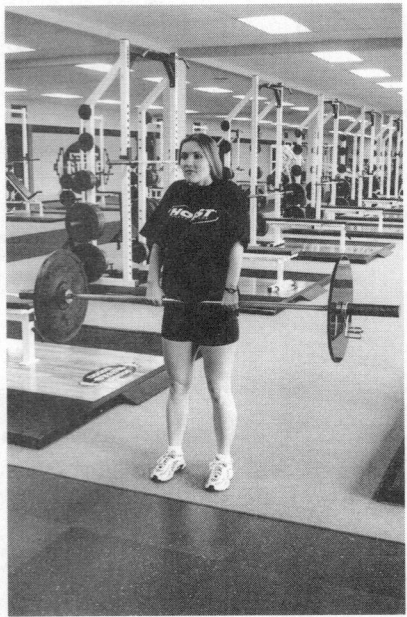

Barbell Front Lateral Raises: Work the anterior deltoids, upper pectorals, infraspinatus, and trapezius.*

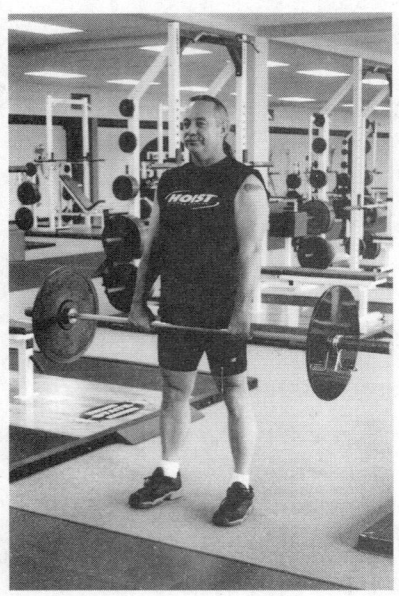 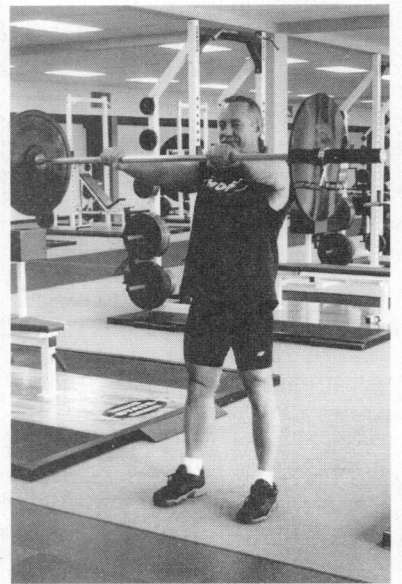

Dumbbell Exercises

Front Lateral Raises: Work the anterior deltoids, upper pectorals, and some medial deltoid. This exercise is a good alternate to doing the upright row, and does not place as much strain on the shoulders.

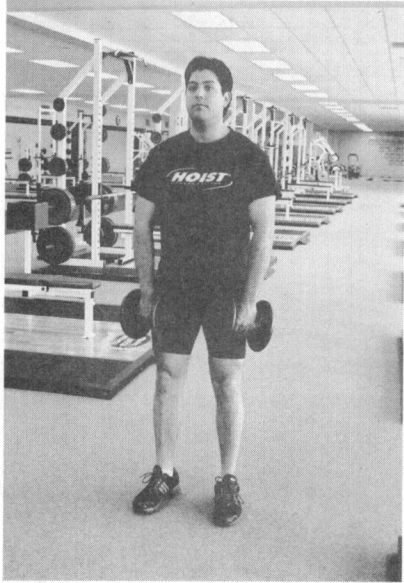
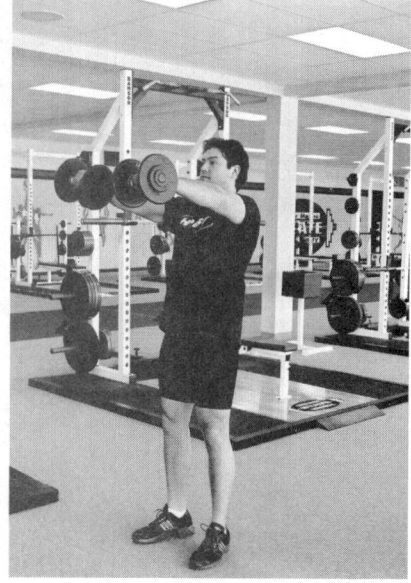

Front Lateral Raise

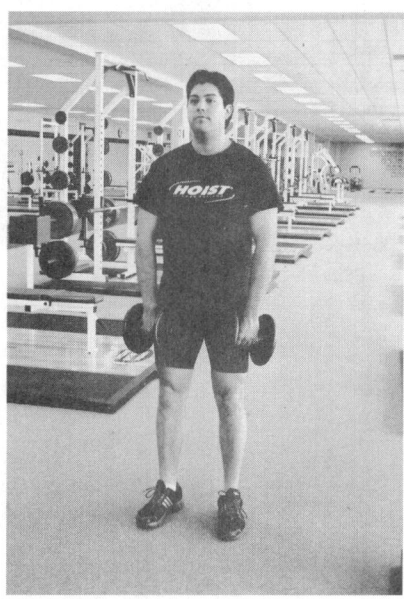
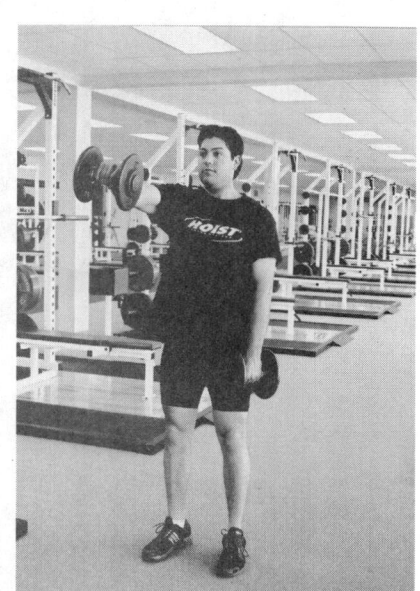

Alternating

Side Lateral Raises: Work the medial deltoids. By raising the dumbbells above shoulder level, you will make the trapezius work as well. Can be done seated or standing.

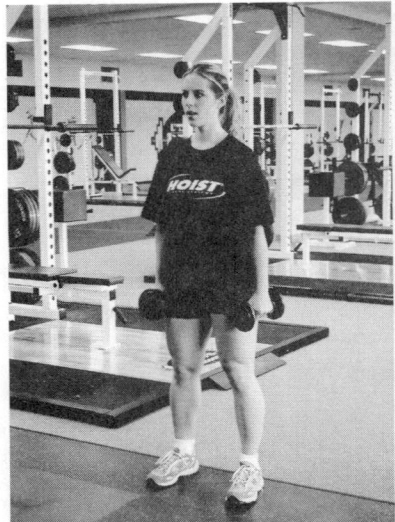 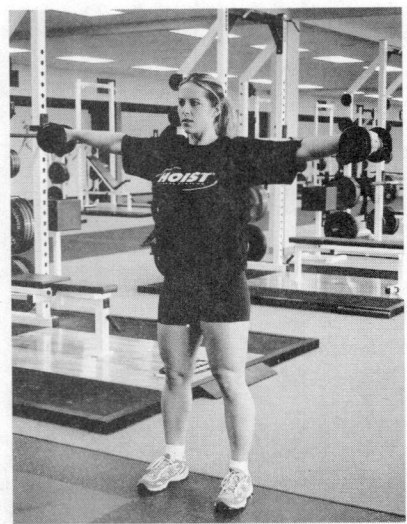

Bent Over Lateral Raises (Rear Lateral Raises): work the posterior deltoids, trapezius, rhomboids, teres minor, and infraspinatus.

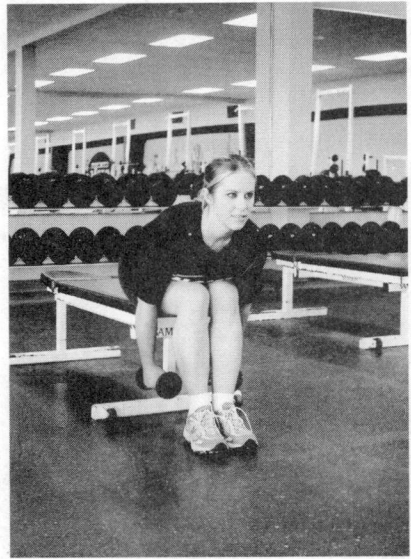 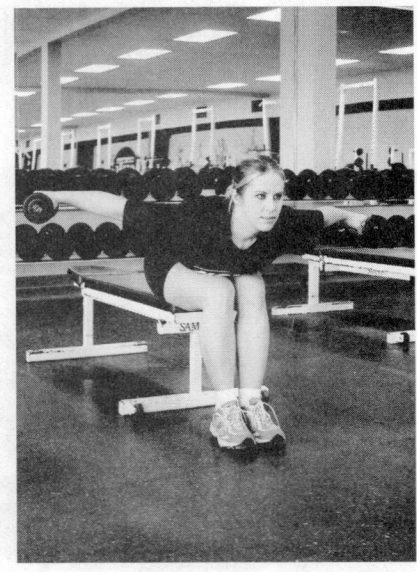

Seated

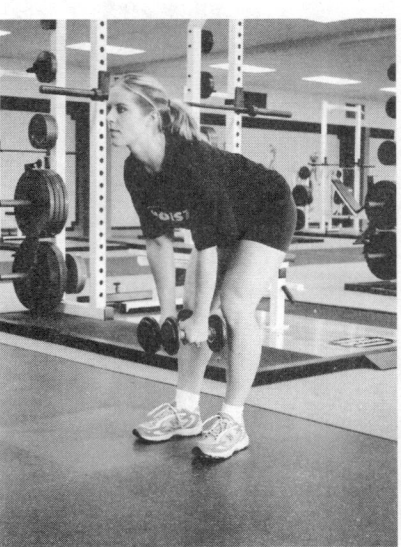 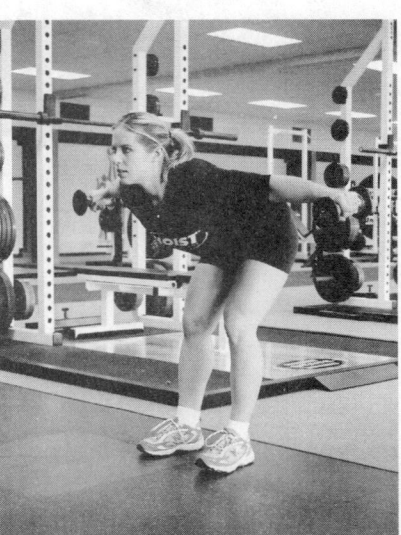

Standing

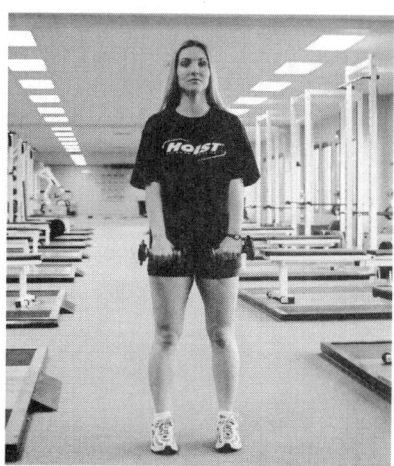 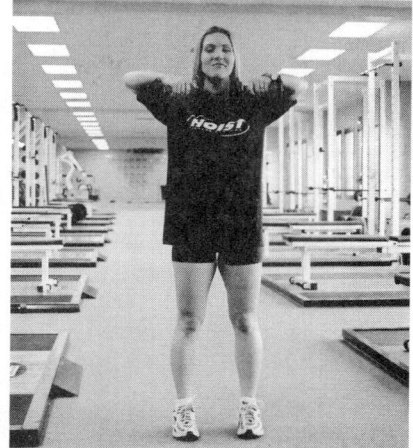

Dumbbell Upright Rows: Work the deltoids, trapezius, biceps, forearm, and abdominal muscles.

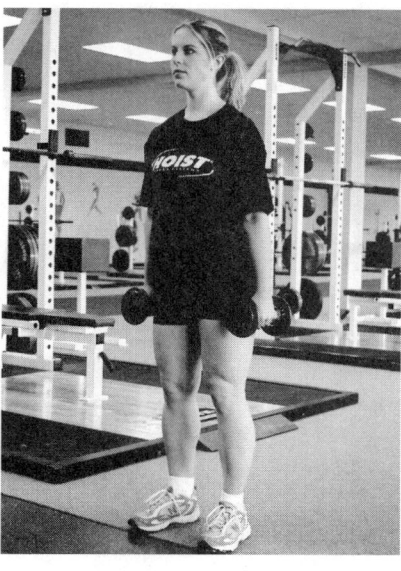 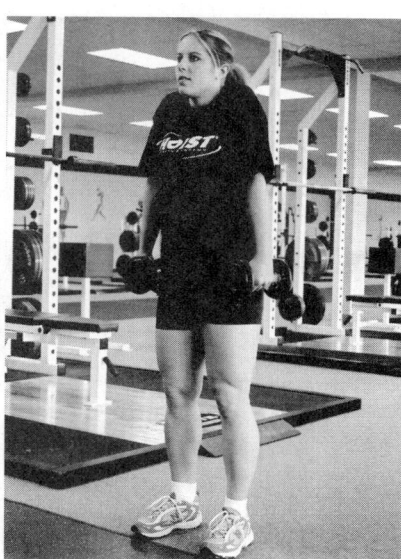

Dumbbell Shrugs: Work the trapezius and deltoids.

Dumbbell Shoulder Presses: Work the medial deltoid, the upper trapezius, serratus anterior, and triceps. This exercise will also work the anterior and posterior portions of the deltoids. Position the top of the bench 10 to 20 degrees back from vertical for maximum results.

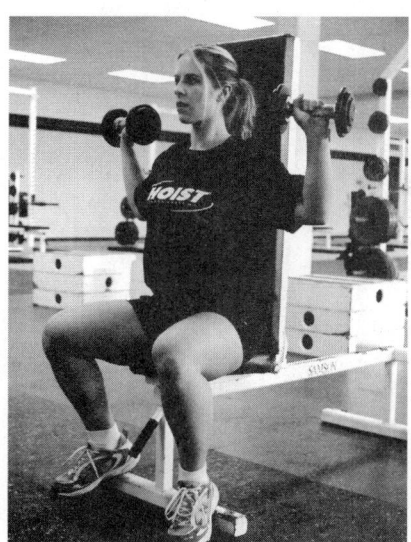 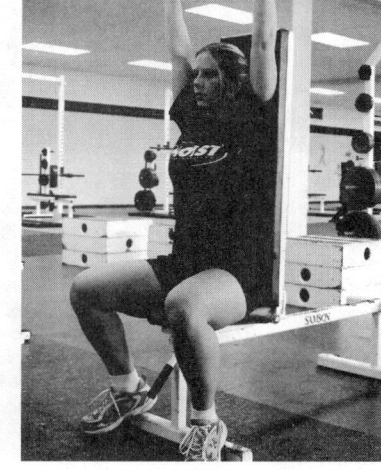 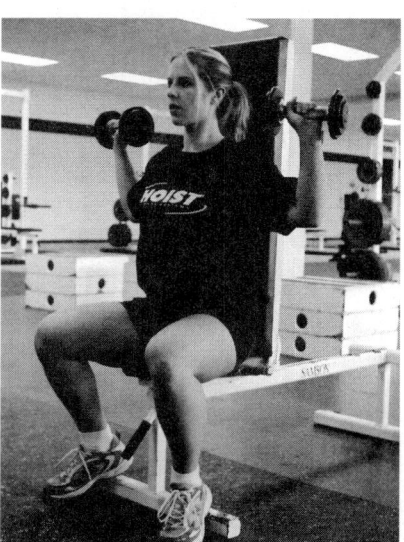

Seated

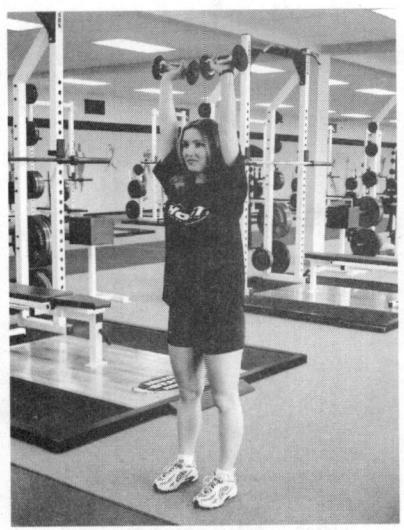 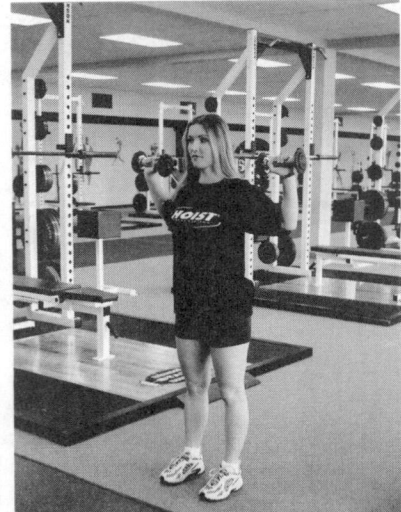 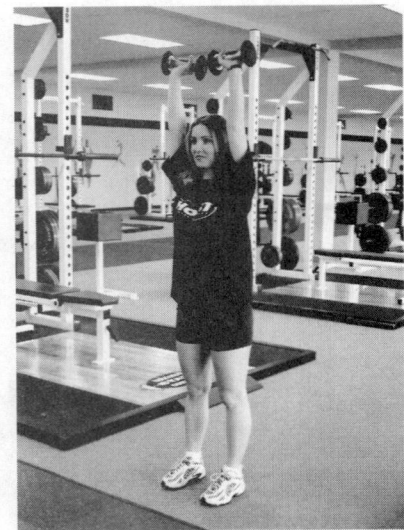

Standing Dumbbell Shoulder Press

Dumbbell Rotator Cuff Exercises

The most commonly injured muscle of the rotator cuff is the supraspinatus.

Dumbbell External Rotation

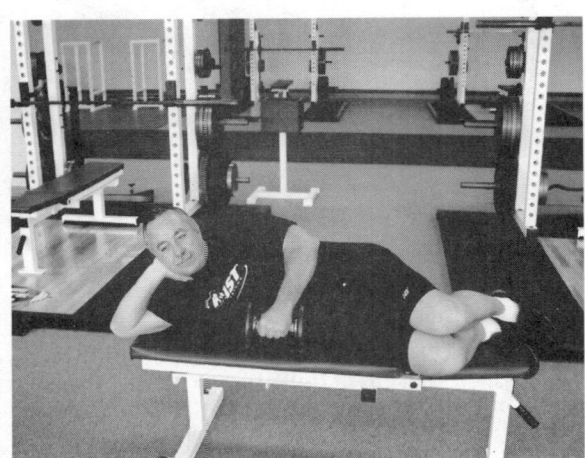 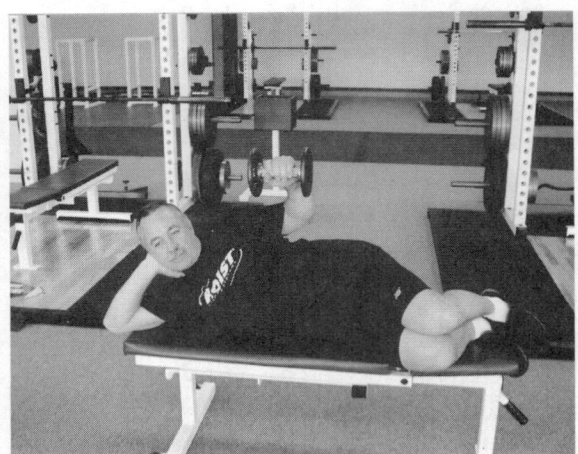

Dumbbell Internal Rotation

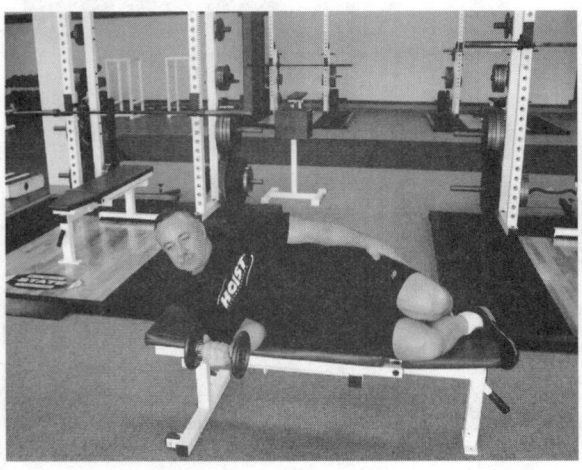 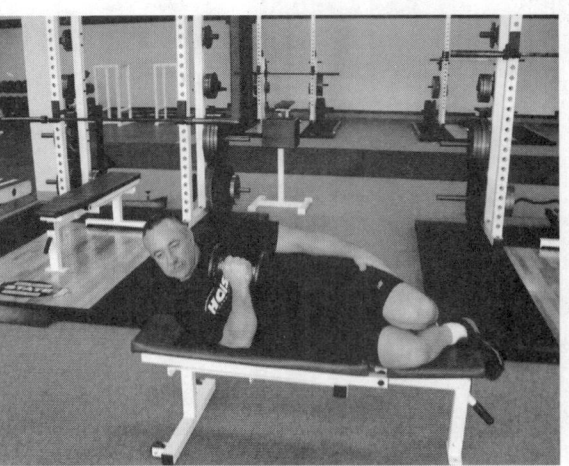

Standing Dumbbell External Rotation

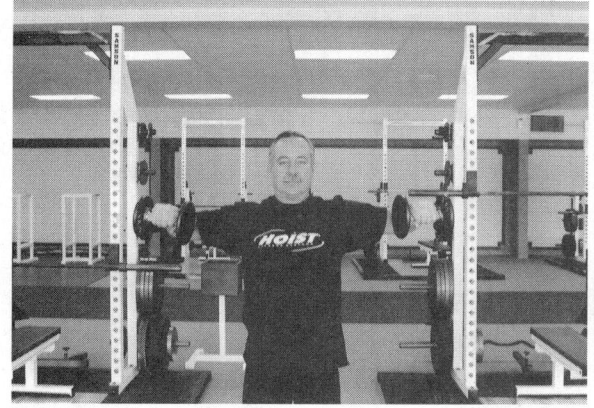 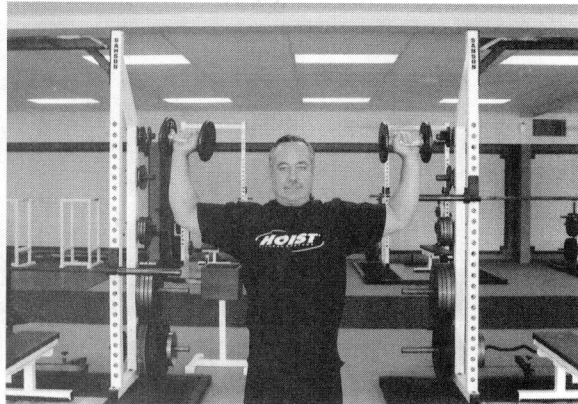

Machine Exercises

Lateral Raises: Isolate the medial deltoids and the upper trapezius if the arms are raised above the shoulders.*

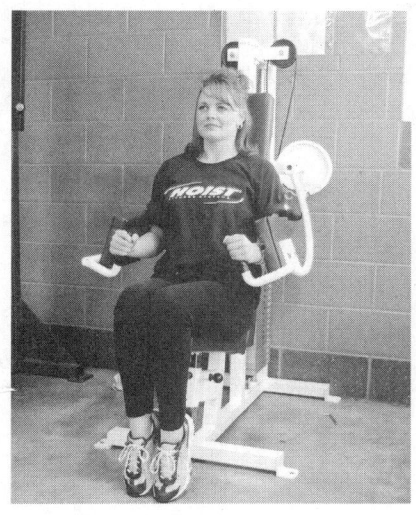 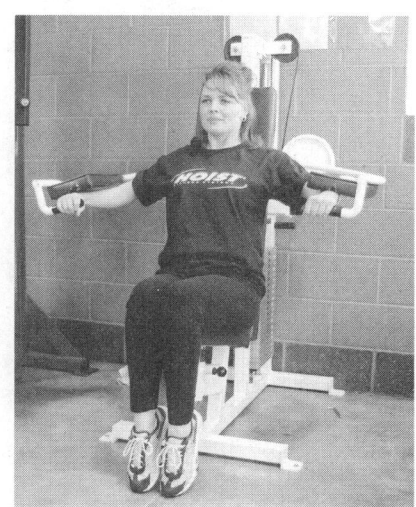

Shoulder Presses: Will work the deltoids, upper trapezius, triceps, and serratus anterior.

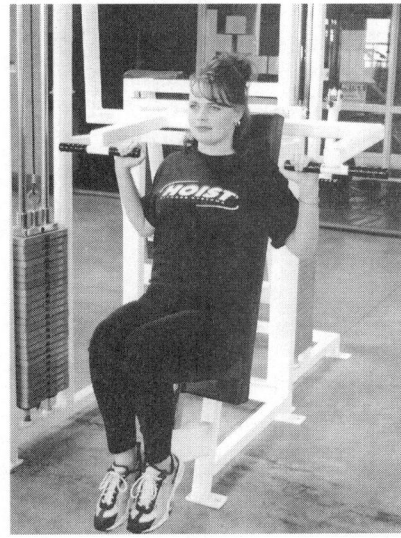 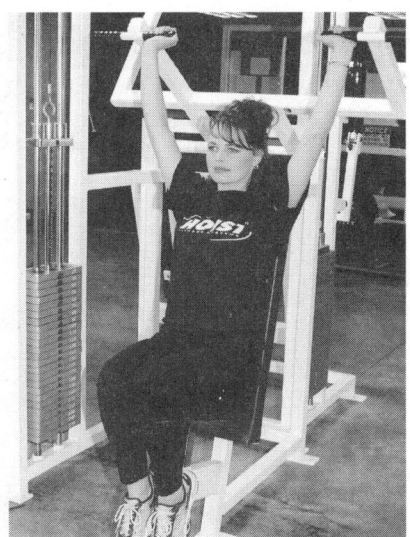

Shrugs: Work the trapezius and deltoids.

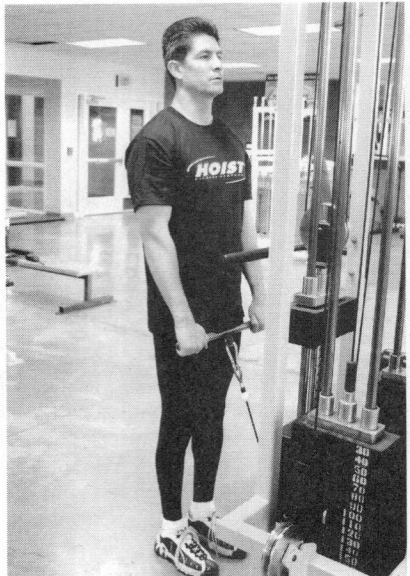 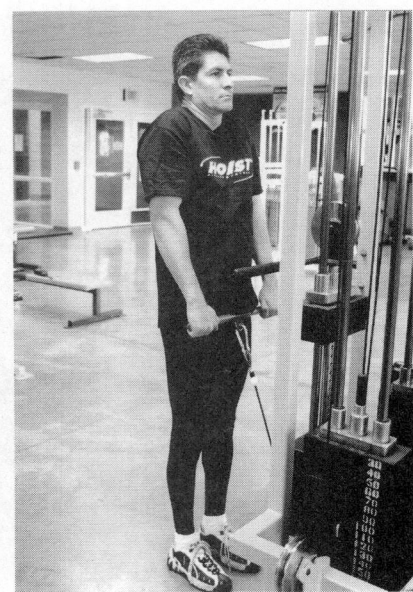

Cable Front Lateral Raises: Work the anterior deltoids, upper pectorals, and some medial deltoid.

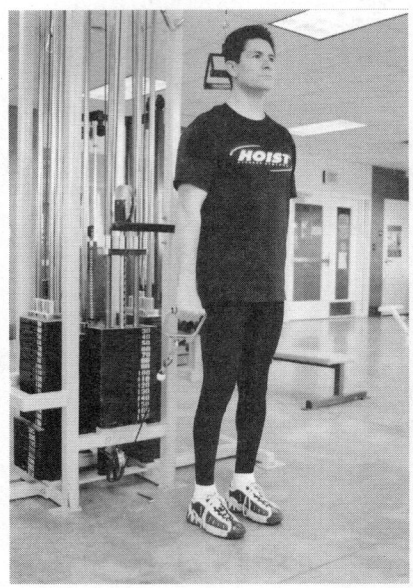 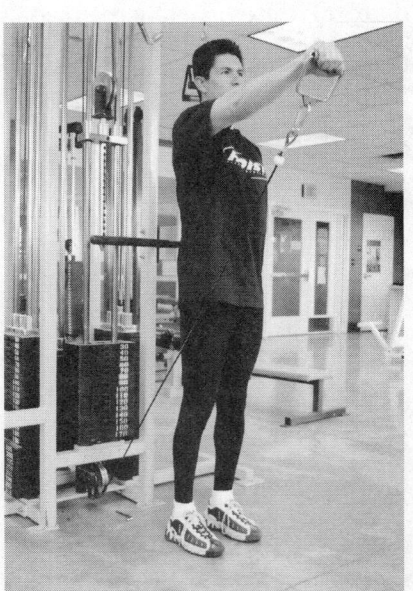

Cables are great for working the deltoids. Everything from front lateral raises, side lateral raises, and rear lateral raises can be done and everything in between, depending on the angle that you use to work the muscle. The most common piece of equipment for working the deltoids with cables is the cable crossover machine.

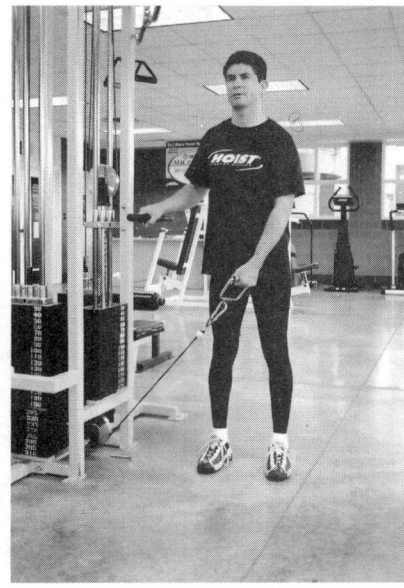 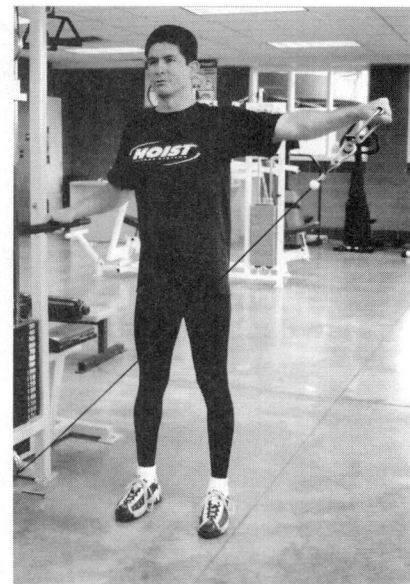

Cable Side Lateral Raises:
Work the medial deltoid.

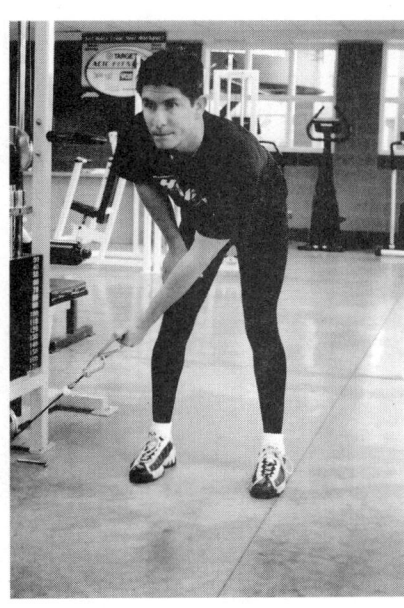 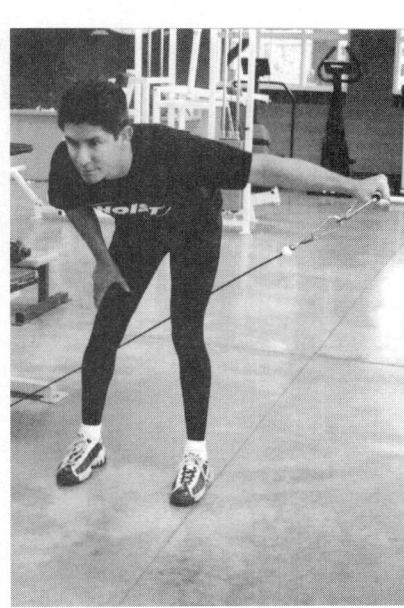

Cable Rear Lateral Raises:
Work the posterior deltoids, trapezius, rhomboids, teres minor, and infraspinatus.

Frank and Ernest

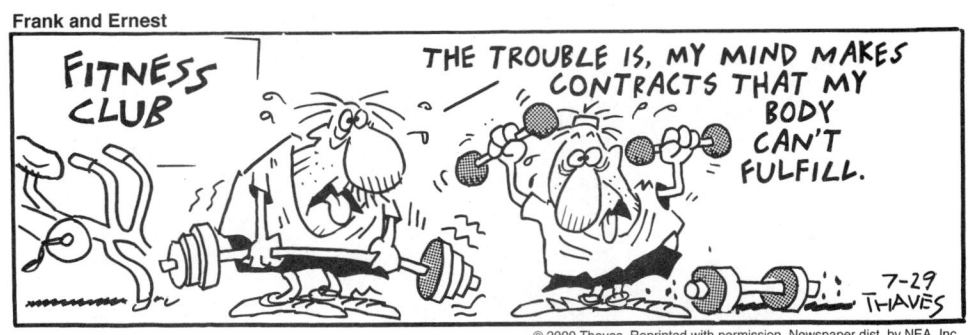

© 2000 Thaves. Reprinted with permission. Newspaper dist. by NEA, Inc.

(* Asterisk indicates information from, "Strength Training Anatomy" by Frederic Delavier, Human Kinetics. This information is used as reference material.)

1. Andrews, G. (September 2002). Angles, Positions and Variations. A thorough study of strength training. *Personal Fitness Professional.* 30–38.

CHAPTER 4 SELF TEST

Please feel free to write on this page

True or False

1. _____ A narrower grip will work more anterior and medial deltoids as compared to a normal grip.

2. _____ Behind the Neck Presses can put considerable strain on the rotator cuffs.

3. _____ Barbell Shrugs work primarily the deltoids and biceps.

4. _____ In doing Dumbbell Exercises, by raising the dumbbells above shoulder level, you will not make the trapezius work as well.

5. _____ Dumbbell shrugs work the trapezius and deltoids.

Multiple Choice

6. _____ Dumbbell Shoulder Presses work the media deltoid, the upper trapezius, serratus anterior, and triceps. This exercise will also work the
   a. Middle portion of deltoids
   b. Anterior portion of deltoids
   c. Anterior and posterior portions of the deltoids
   d. Middle, interior, anterior, and posterior portion of the deltoids

7. _____ Shoulder Presses will work the
   a. Deltoids
   b. Upper Trapezius
   c. triceps and serratus anterior
   d. All of the above

8. _____ In order to work the trapezius and deltoids, what exercise is needed?
   a. Shrugs
   b. Shoulder Presses
   c. Lateral Raises
   d. Dumbbell Side Laterals

9. _____ What machine is great for working the deltoids?
   a. Lateral Raises
   b. Rear Lateral Raises
   c. Cable Crossover Machine
   d. All of the above

10. _____ The most common piece of equipment for working the deltoids with cables is the
   a. Dumbbells
   b. Cable Crossover Machine
   c. Barbells
   d. Rear Cable Mechanism

Matching

Match with the lettered column below

11. _____ Trapezius Muscle

12. _____ Rotator Cuffs

13. _____ Shoulder Muscles

14. _____ Pectoralis Major

15. _____ Deltoids

A. elevates, horizontally adducts, extends, and medially rotates the arm

B. have 4 muscles known as the supraspinatus, teres minor, subscapularis, and infraspinatus

C. composed of 3 sections: the upper, middle, and lower

D. composed of 3 muscles known as the anterior deltoid, medial deltoid, and the posterior deltoid

E. the deltoids, rotator cuffs, trapezius, and the pectoralis major

NOTES

Please feel free to write on this page

CHAPTER 5

Arm/Forearm Muscles and Exercises

Frank and Ernest

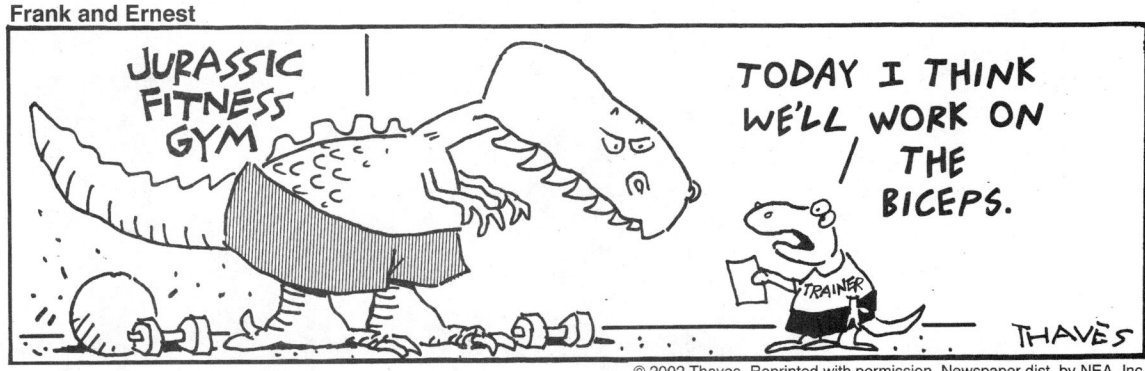

© 2002 Thaves. Reprinted with permission. Newspaper dist. by NEA, Inc.

Arm and Forearm Muscles

The muscles of the upper limbs can be divided into the arm and forearm muscles. The major arm muscles are the biceps (bi's) and triceps (tri's). The arm muscles are the biceps brachii (long and short heads). The tricep muscles are the triceps brachii, lateral head; triceps brachii, long head; and the triceps brachii, medial head. The major muscles of the forearm are the extensors—extensor carpi radialis longus, extensor carpi radialis brevis, extensor digitorum, extensor digiti minimis, extensor carpi ulnaris: and the flexors—flexor carpi radialis, palmaris longus, flexor digitorum superficialis, and flexor digitorum profundus, and flexor carpi ulnaris.

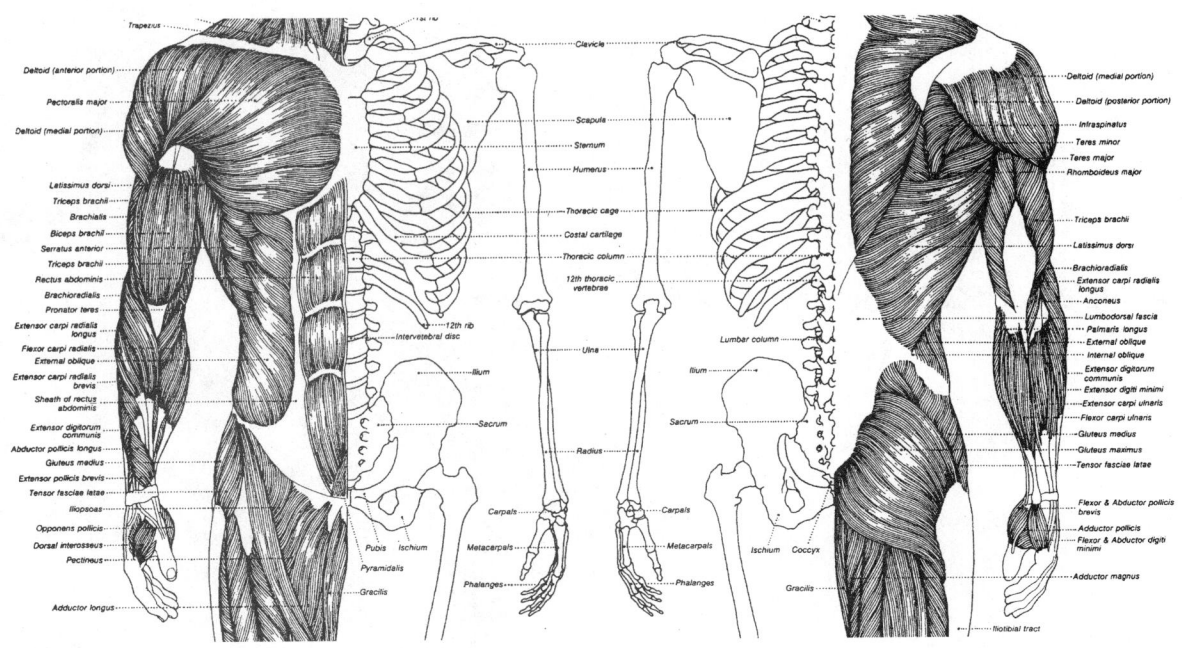

© Algra Corporation www.algra.com Used with permission.

The action of the biceps is to flex and supinate the forearm. The action of the triceps is to extend the forearm. In the forearm, the flexors are responsible for wrist flexion and the extensors are responsible for wrist extension. Both assist in deviation, supination, and pronation of the wrist.

Free Weight Exercises for the Biceps

Barbell Exercises

Barbell Curls: Work the biceps, brachialis, brachioradialis, pronator teres, and the flexors of the wrist and fingers.*

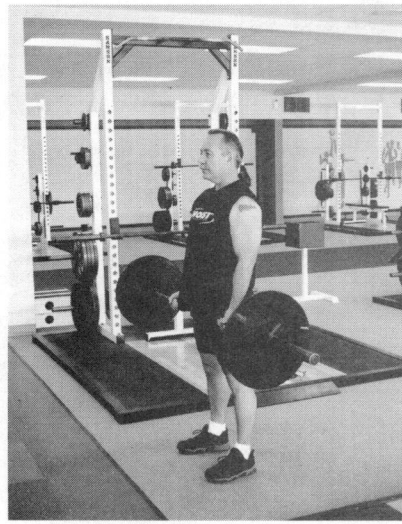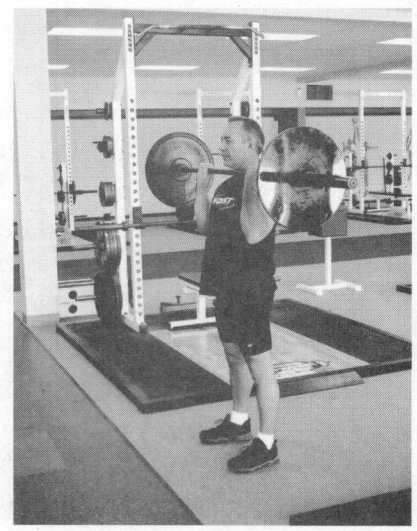

Narrow Grip Barbell Curls: Work the long head of the biceps.*

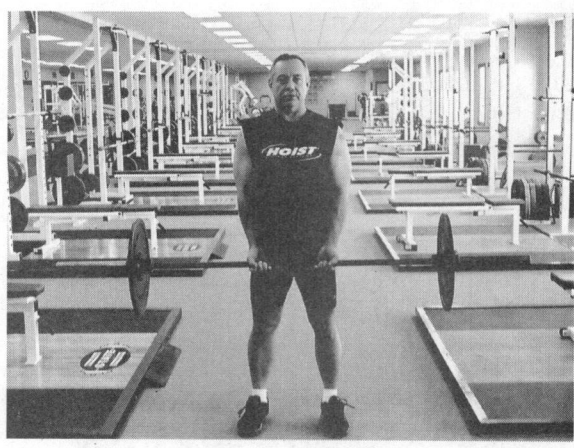

Wide Grip Barbell Curls: Work the short head of the biceps. *

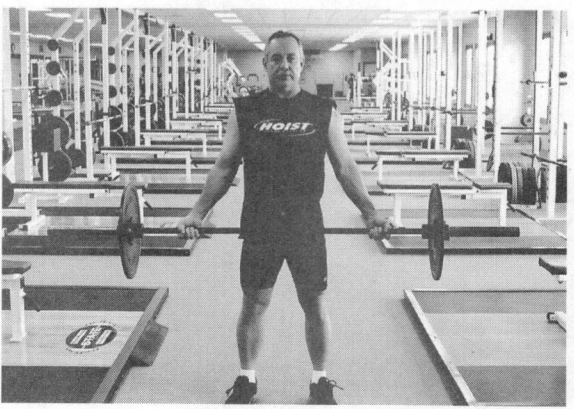

EZ Curls: Work the bicep, brachioradialis, and the brachialis.

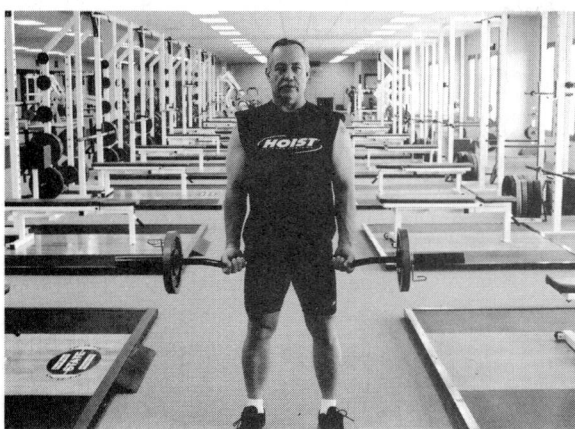 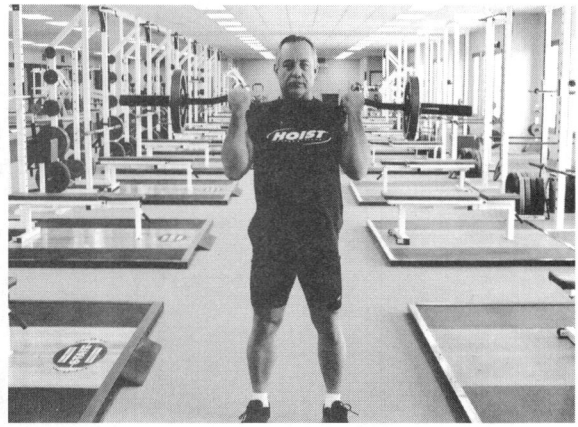

Reverse Grip Barbell Curls: Work the extensors of the wrist and fingers along with the brachioradialis, brachialis and the biceps.*

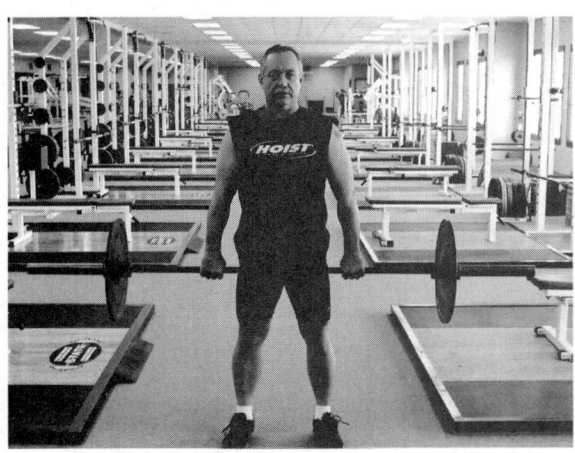 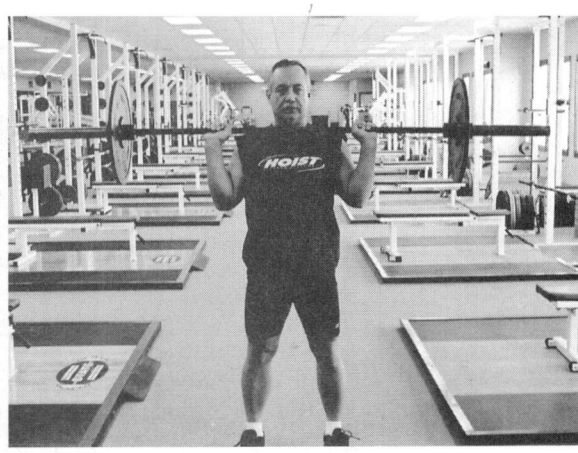

Dumbbell Exercises

Dumbbell Curls: Work the biceps, brachioradialis, brachialis, and anterior deltoids.

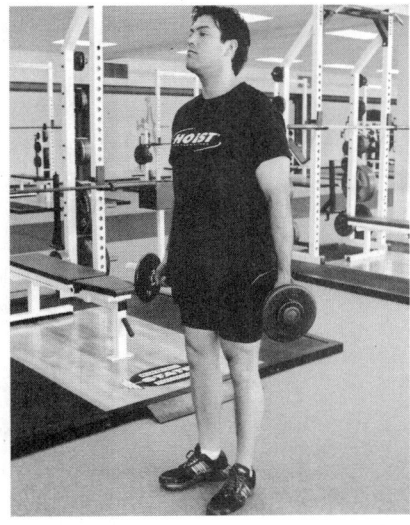 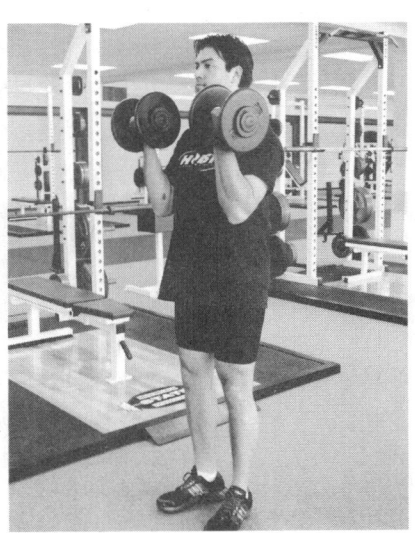

Standing

Alternate Dumbbell Curls:
Work the same way as
dumbbell curls only you
alternate raising dumbbells so
that when one dumbbell is at
the completion of the
exercise, the other one is at
the beginning of the exercise.

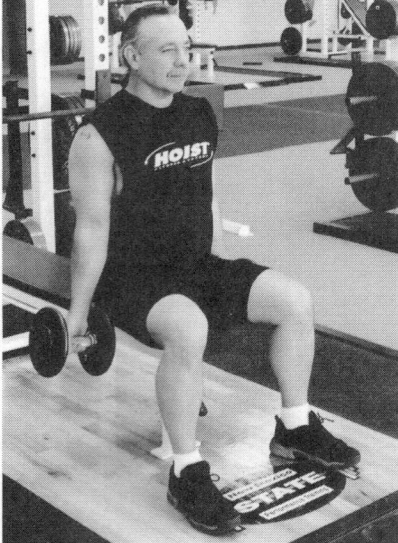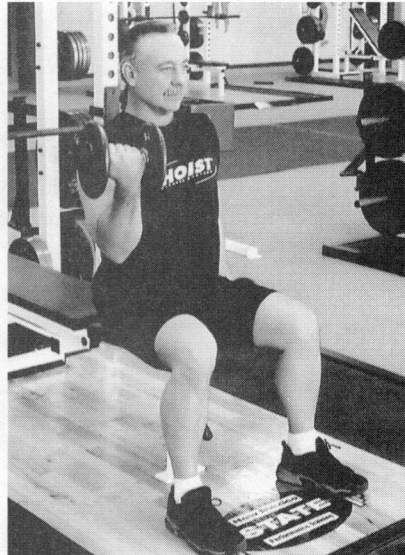

Seated Alternating

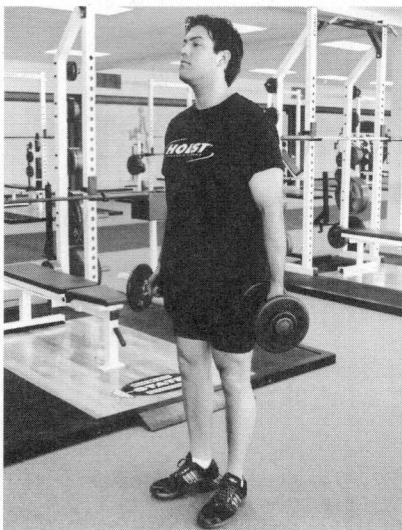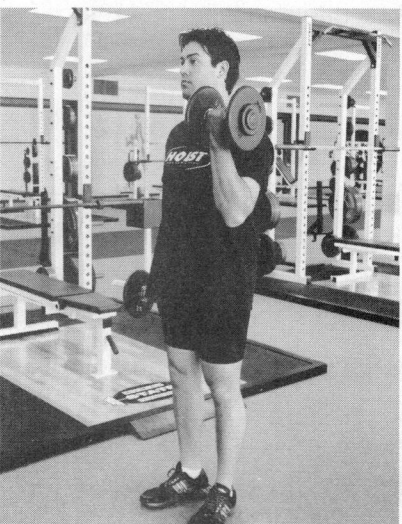

Standing Alternating

Hammer Curls and Alternate Hammer Curls: Work the brachioradialis, biceps, and brachialis.
The alternating style is described above.

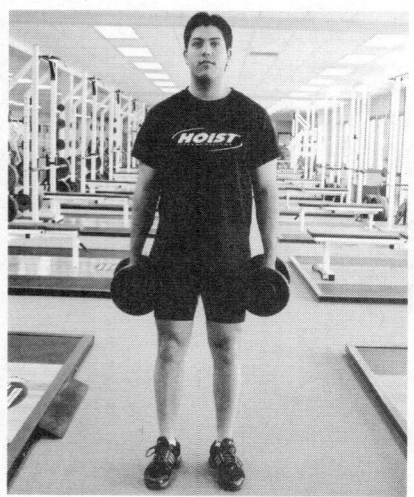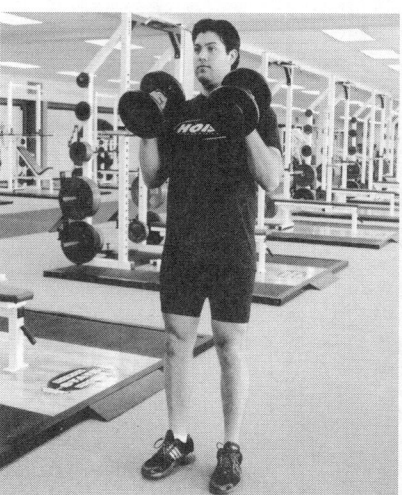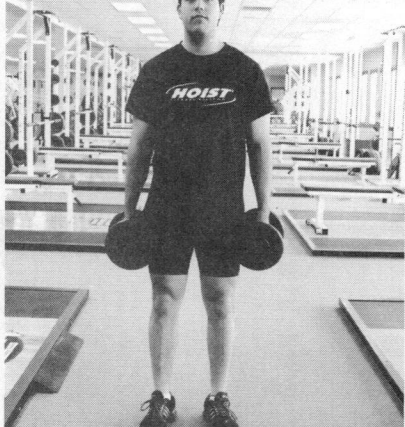

Standing

Standing Alternating

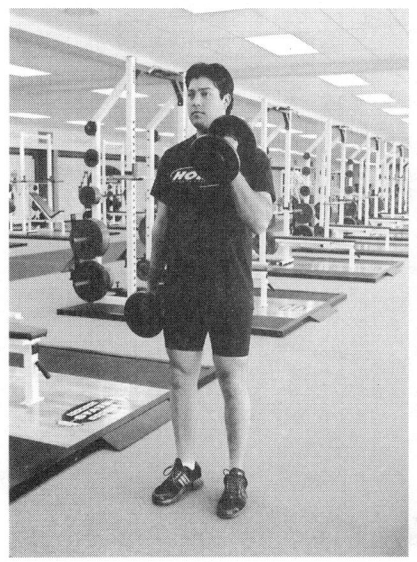
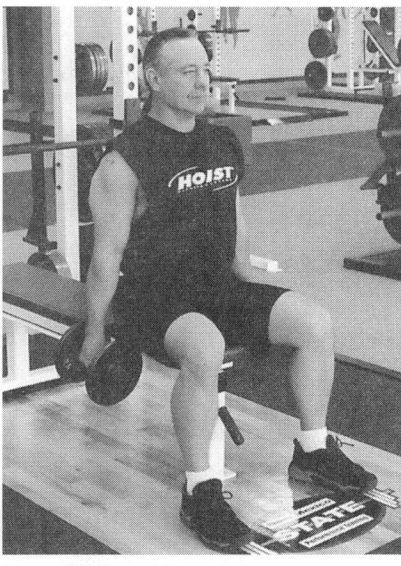
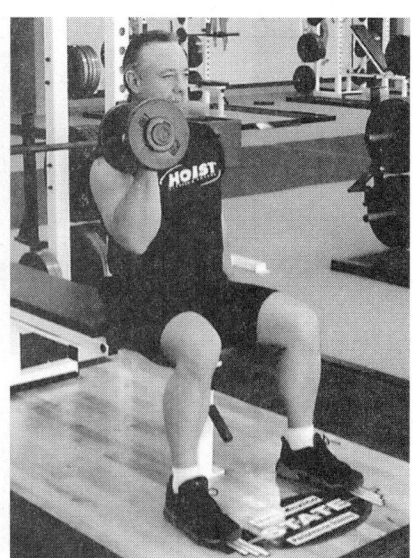

Standing Alternating, cont'd   Seated Alternating

Concentration Curls: Isolate the biceps, brachialis, and brachioradialis.

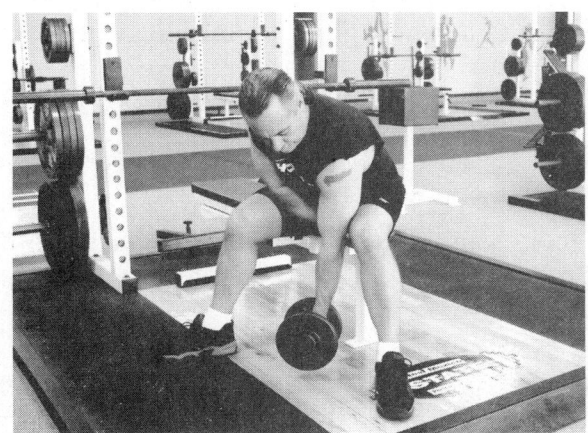
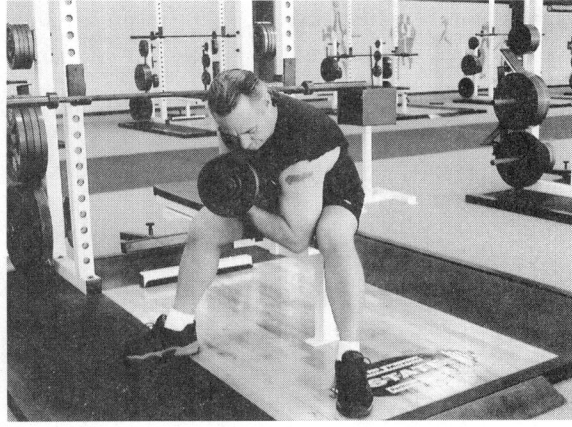

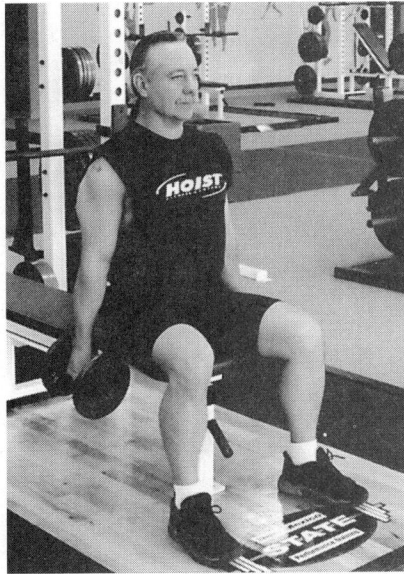
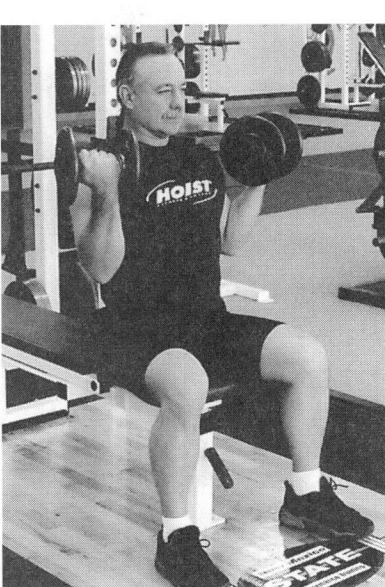

Seated Dumbbell Curls: Work the same as standing only there you are seated. Hand positions and their influence remain the same.

Neutral to Supinated Grip

Incline Dumbbell Curls: Great for pre-stretching the bicep muscle.

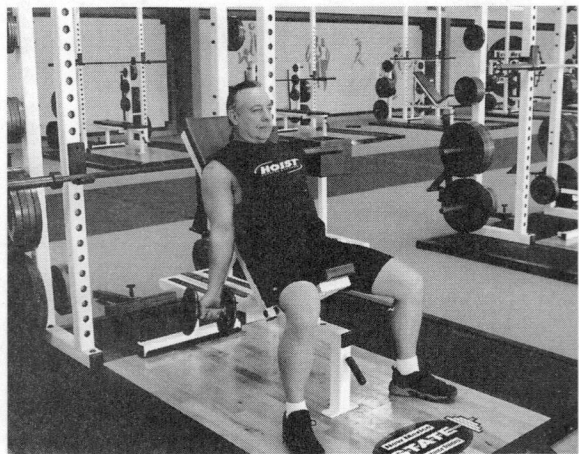 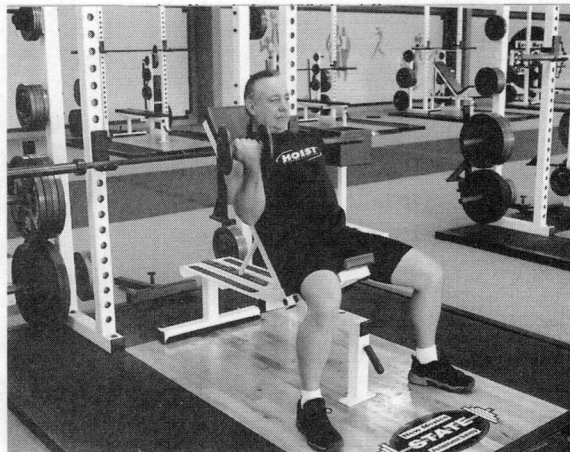

Alternating

Note: The muscles worked when doing curls will depend on the hand position. When using a supinated grip and curling the weight up, the bicep is the main part worked. Using a neutral grip and curling the weight up will work the brachioradialis. Starting with a neutral grip and finishing with a supinated grip will work the biceps and brachialis.

Machine Exercises

Machine Curls: Work on the biceps, brachialis, and brachioradialis. These curls isolate the muscles and generally are done on machines containing weight stacks.

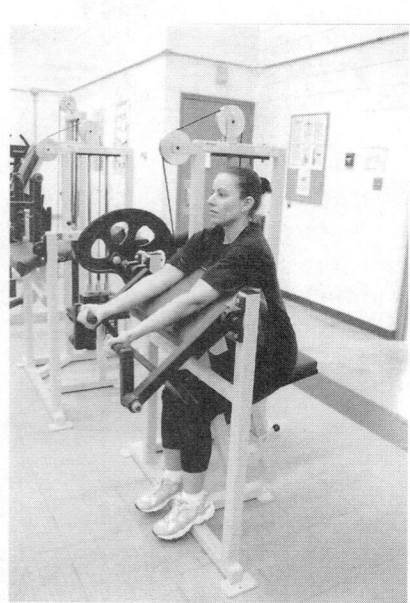 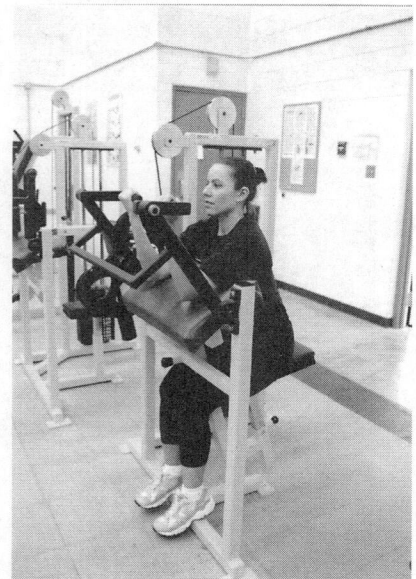

Cable Curls: Work the biceps, brachioradialis, and brachialis. They are done using either a straight bar, handle, or rope attached to the cable going to a weight stack.

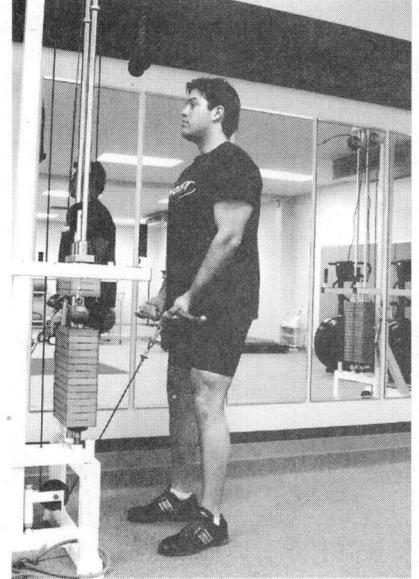 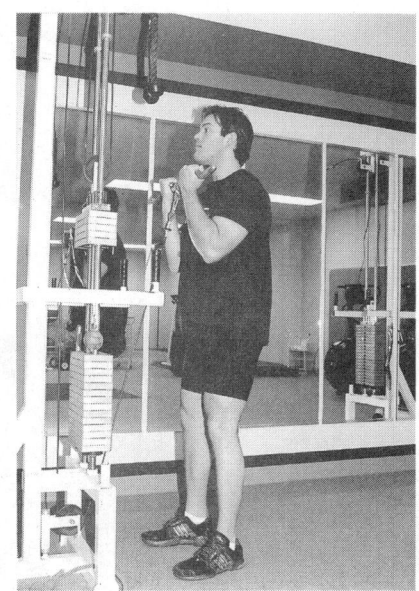

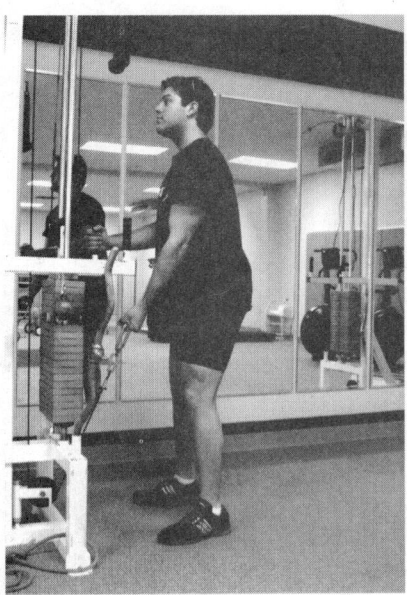 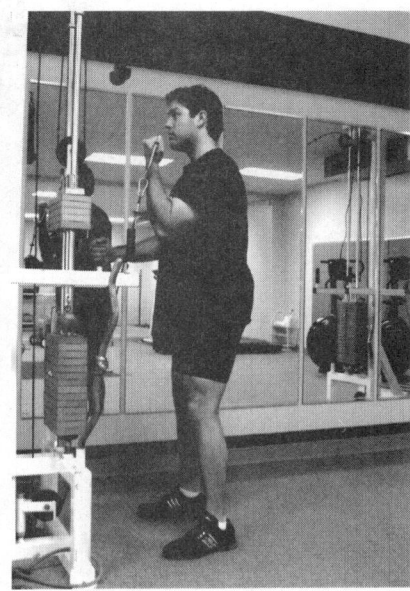

One-Arm Cable Curls

Hint: On all bicep exercises, keep your arms firmly to your sides and "squeeze" the weight at the completion of the movement.

Note: Preacher curls and exercises using the preacher bench have been intentionally left out. This is because of the unusually high shear forces generated in the elbow joint and the potential for pain and/or injury. If you do these exercises and experience any pain in the elbow joint, cease the exercise immediately and seek professional advice.

Free Weight Exercises for the Triceps

To maximally work the triceps, especially the "workhorse" or medial head, do the following reps for each muscle part: Medial head, 10–12 reps at 60–70% of 1 rep max; lateral head, 8–10 reps at 70–80% of 1 rep max; long head, 4–6 reps at 80–90% of 1 rep max.

Barbell Tricep Exercises

Standing or Seated Overhead Barbell Extensions: Using a Straight Bar and EZ Curl Bar, these exercises will work all three heads of the triceps: the long, lateral, and medial heads. Try to keep the elbows in to execute these movements correctly.

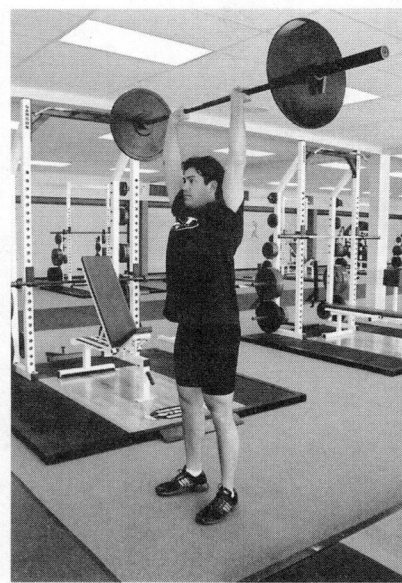 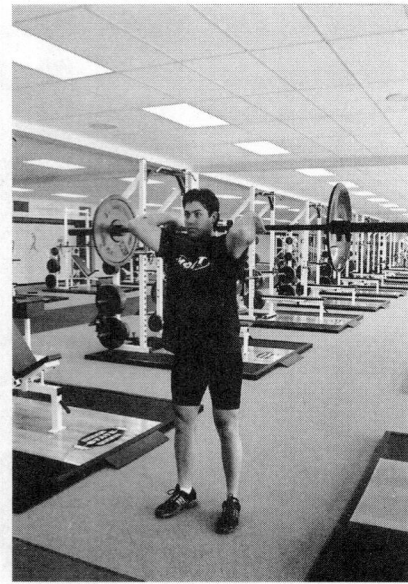

French Press: Using a Straight Bar and EZ Curl Bar, these exercises will work the entire triceps as described above.

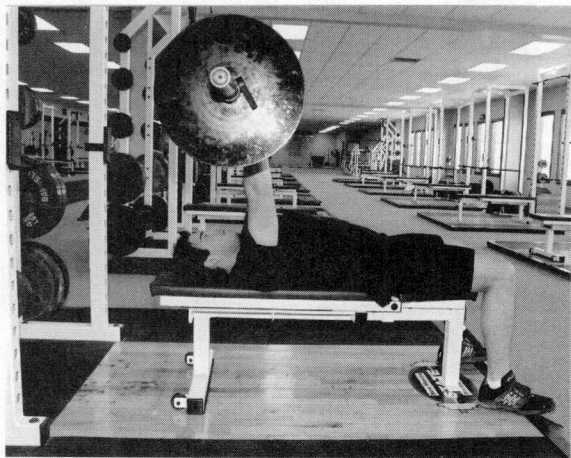 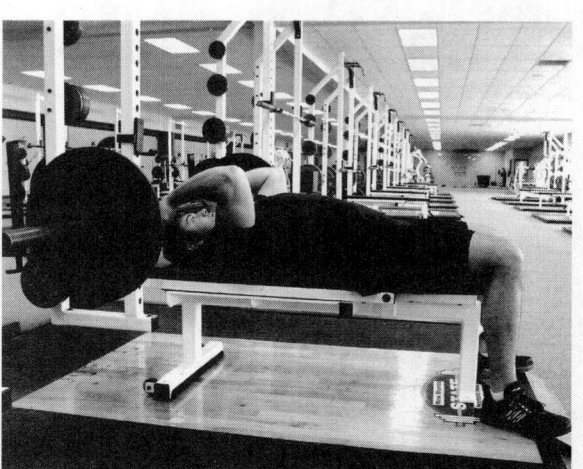

Straight Bar

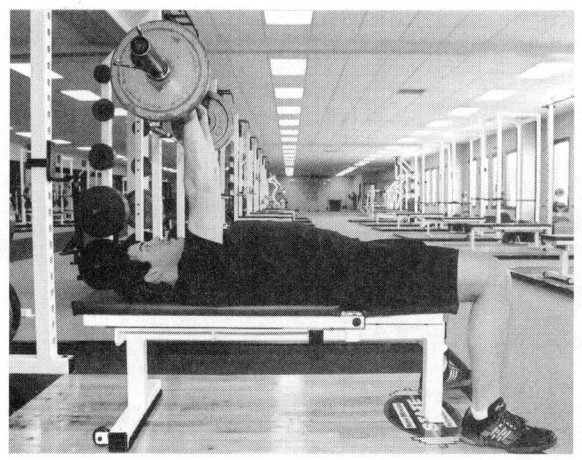 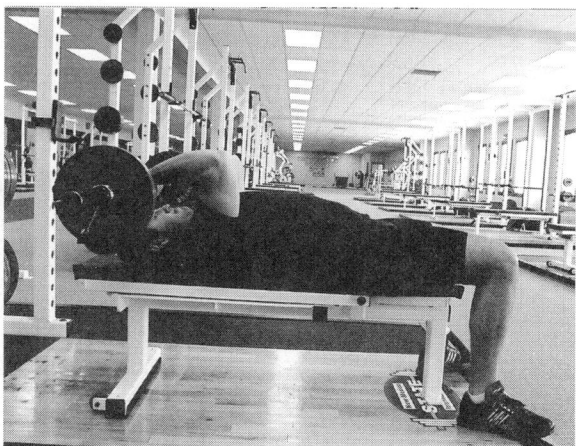

EZ Curl Bar

Bench Dips: With or without a weight-plate, will work the triceps, pectorals, and anterior deltoid. This is an excellent exercise for strengthening and developing the triceps. Adding weight-plates will increase the resistance and make these muscles work harder.

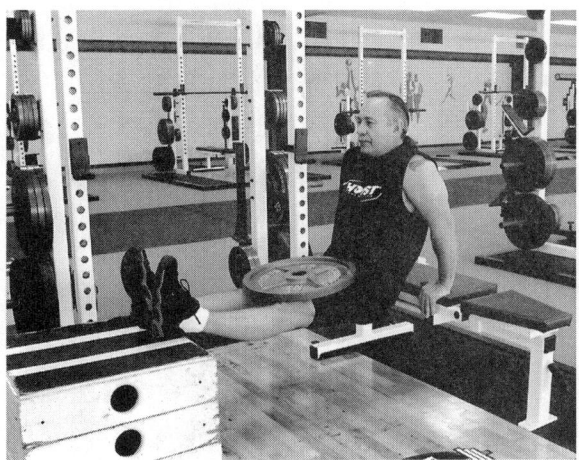 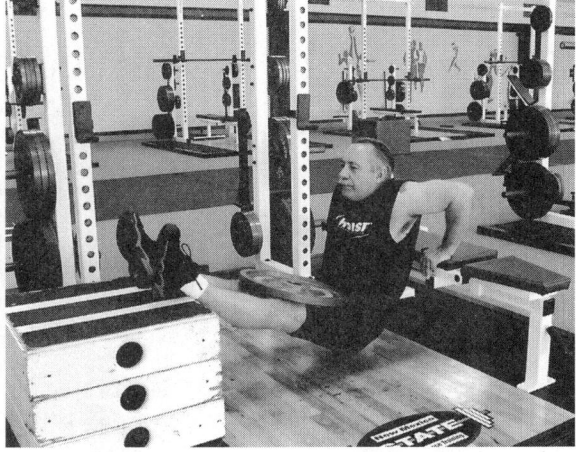

With Weight Plate

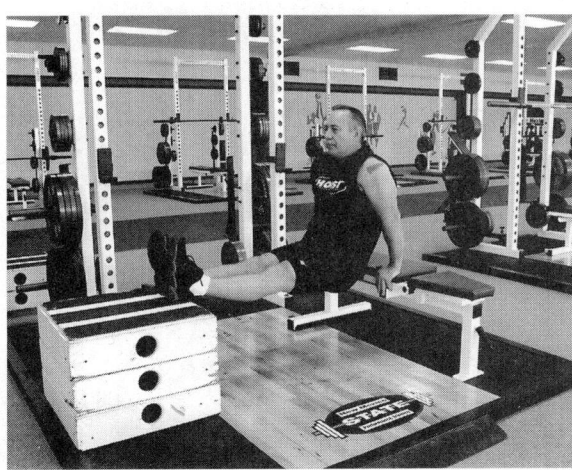 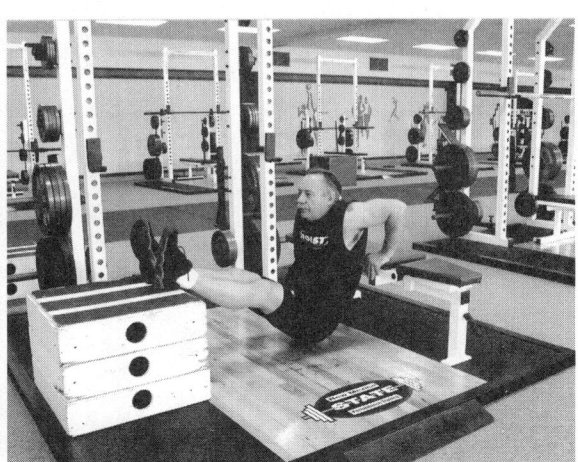

Without Weight Plate

Dumbbell Exercises for the Triceps

Dumbbell Overhead Extensions: Work all three heads of the triceps. It can be done standing or seated.

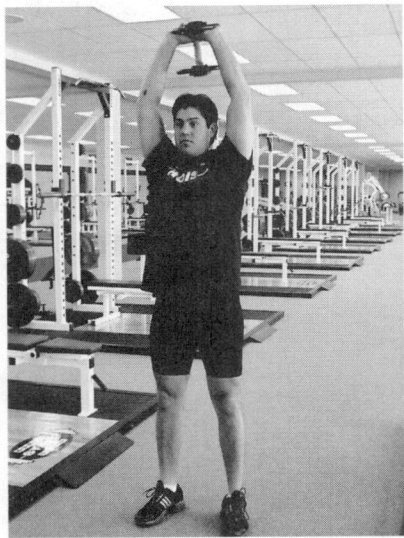 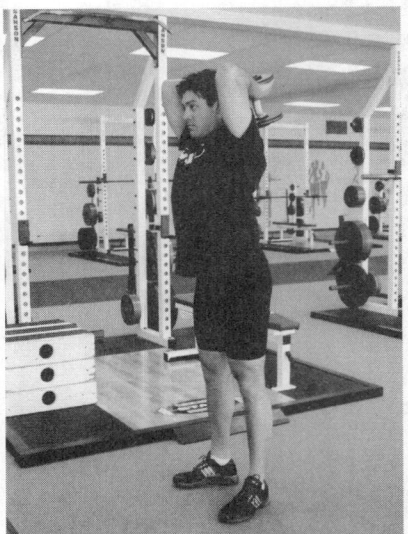

Dumbbell Kickbacks: Work all three heads of the triceps. Try to keep your elbow high at your side and kick the weight up using only the forearm.

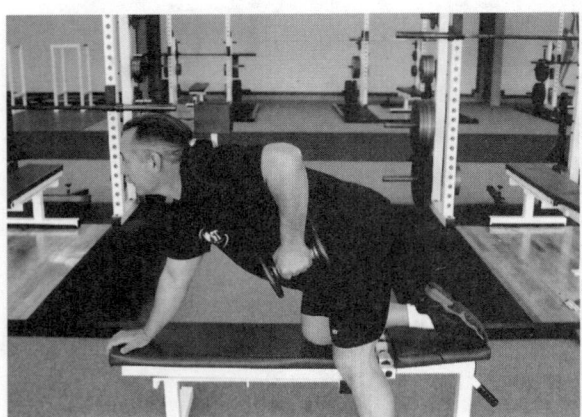 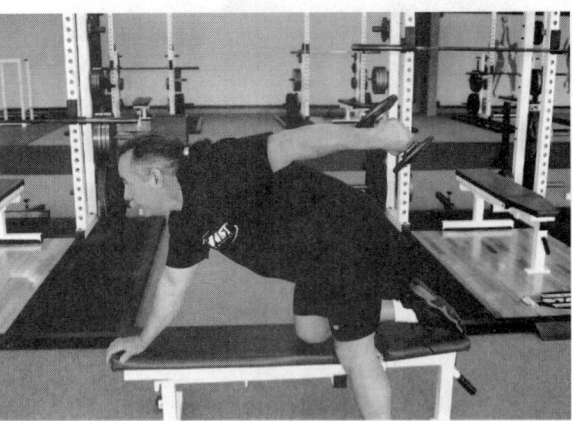

Neutral Grip

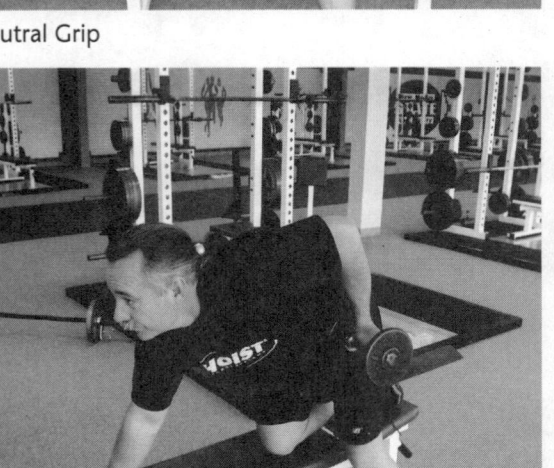 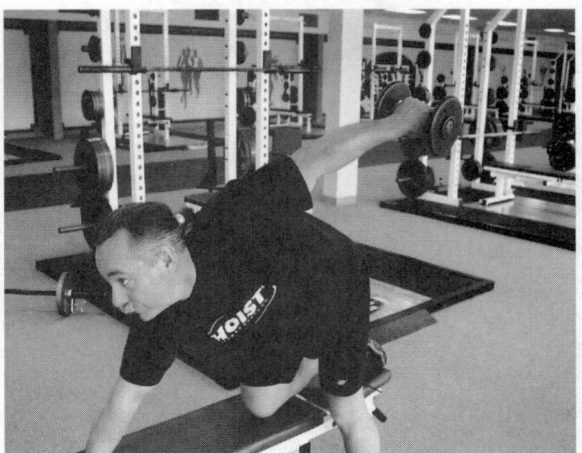

Supinated Grip

Dumbbell Single Arm Extensions: Can be done seated or standing because of the position, stretches the long head of the triceps.*

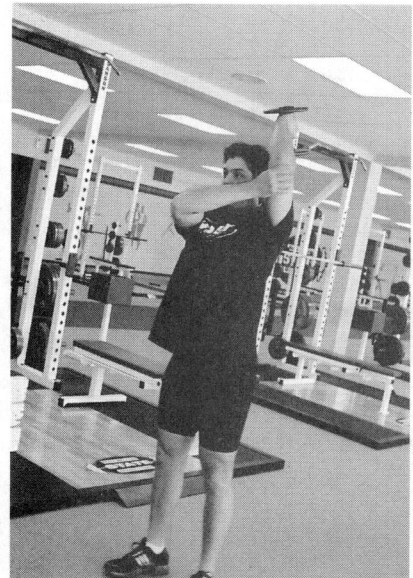 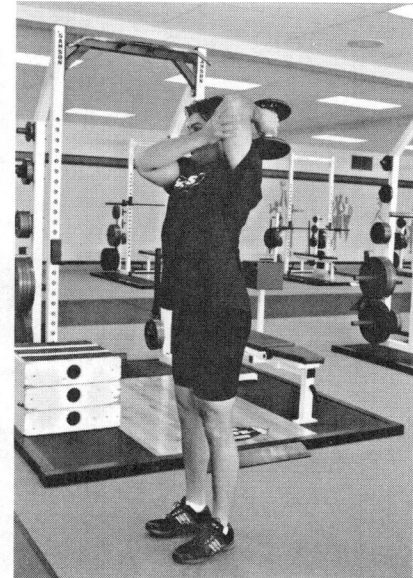

Machine Tricep Extensions

Cable Pushdowns: Work the triceps in an isolation fashion by keeping the arms tucked into the sides. This exercise can be done using either a bar, handle, or rope. Using a supinated grip will work the medial head of the triceps more.

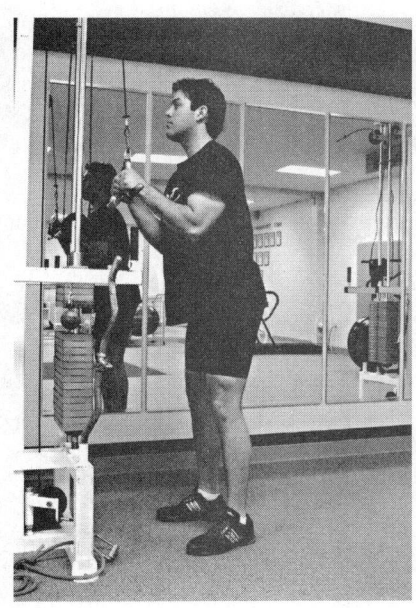 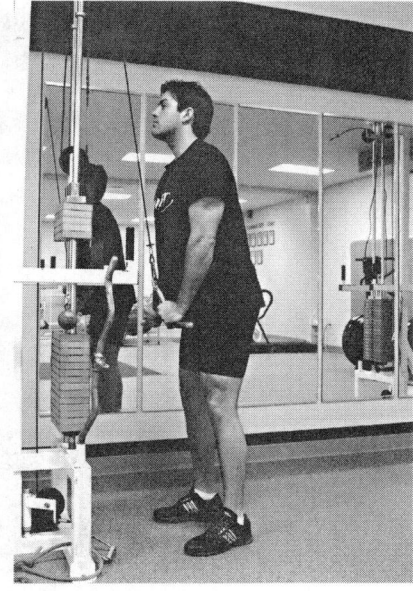

Cable Overhead Extensions:
Done in the same fashion as above, but facing away from the exercise machine. Works the three heads of the triceps

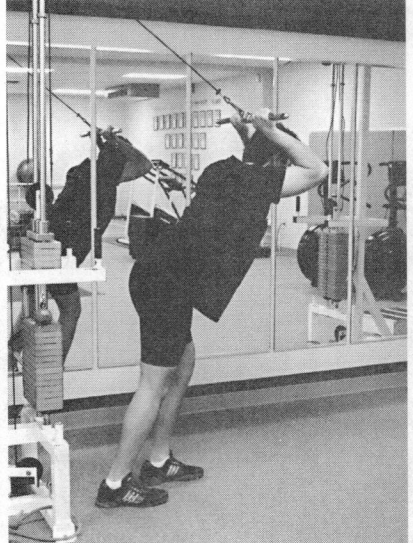 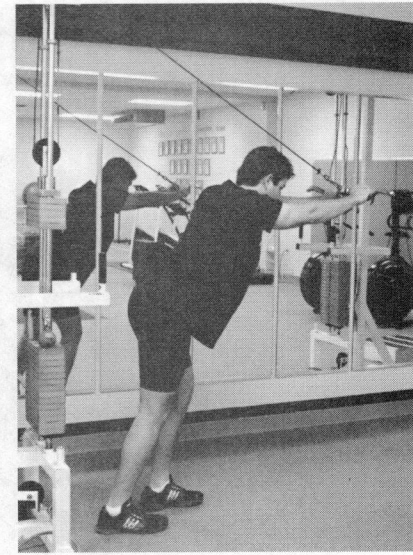

One-Arm Cable Tricep Pushdowns: Works the triceps overall.

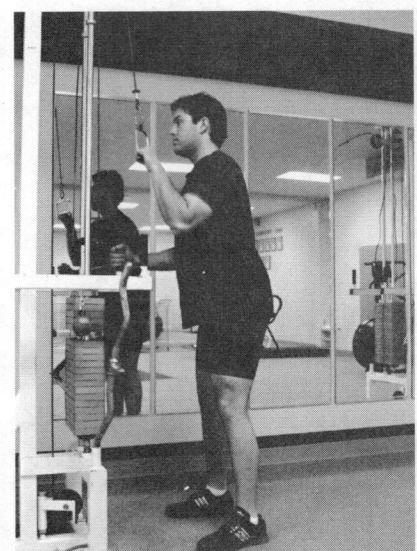 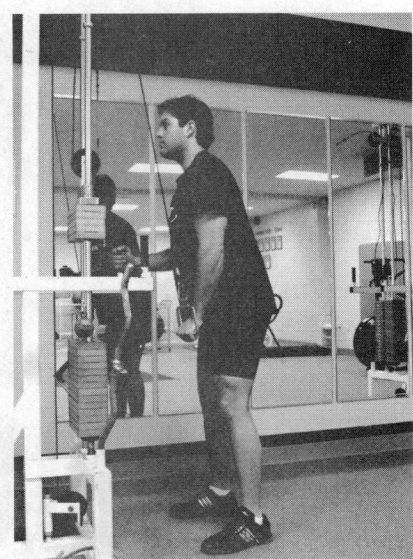

Reverse Pushdowns: Work the triceps and especially the medial head.

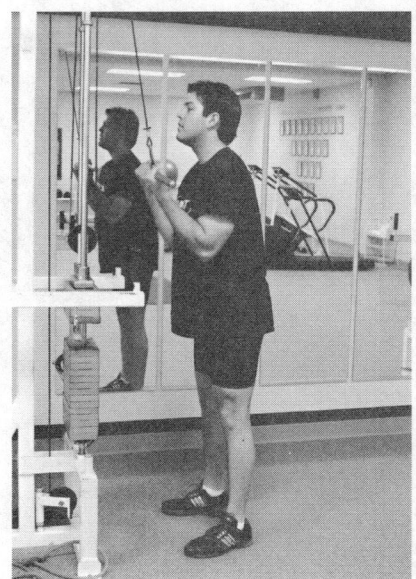 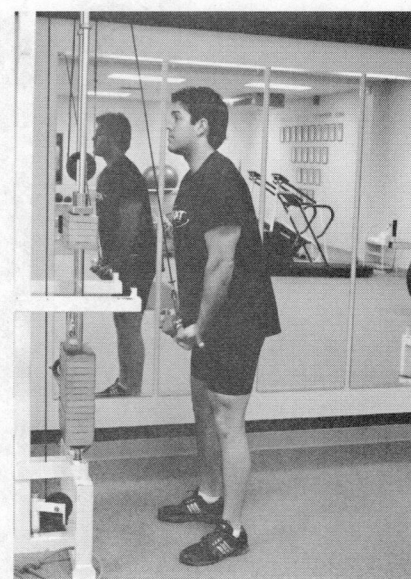

Rope Extensions: Work the triceps and changes the grip position from neutral at the beginning of the movement to pronated at the completion of the movement. Does not change the involvement of the triceps.

Hint: On all triceps exercises, try to keep the elbows in. Do not let the elbows flair out away from your sides.

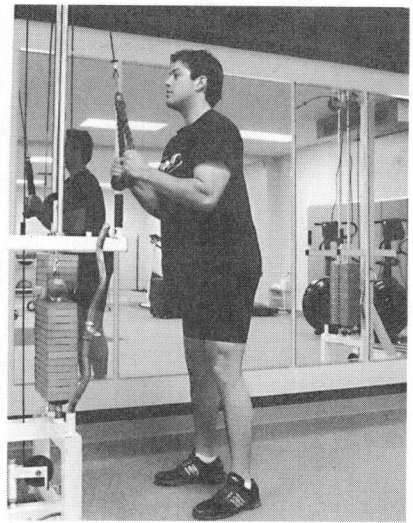 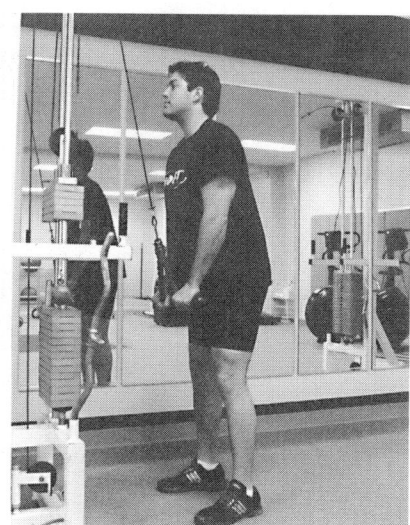

Forearm Exercises

Barbell Wrist Curls: Work the flexors—flexor carpi radialis, palmaris longus, flexor digitorum superficialis, flexor digitorum profundus, and the flexor carpi ulnaris.

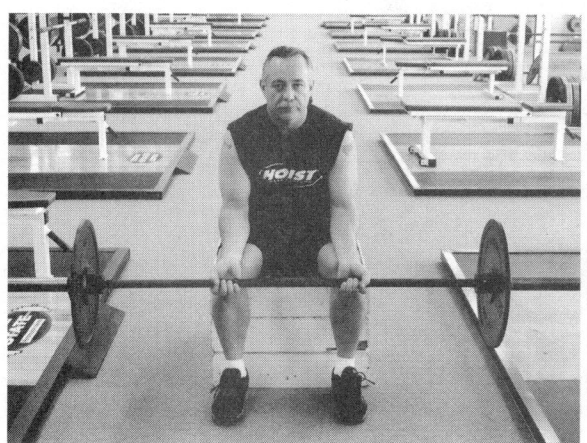 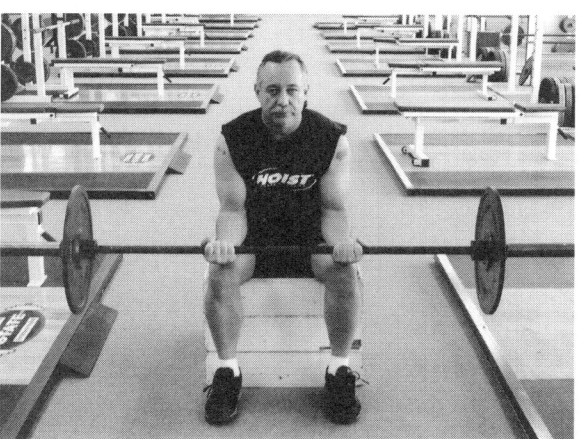

Barbell Wrist Extensions: Work the extensors—extensor digitorum, extensor digiti minimis, extensor carpi ulnaris, extensor carpi radialis longus, and extensor carpi radialis brevis.

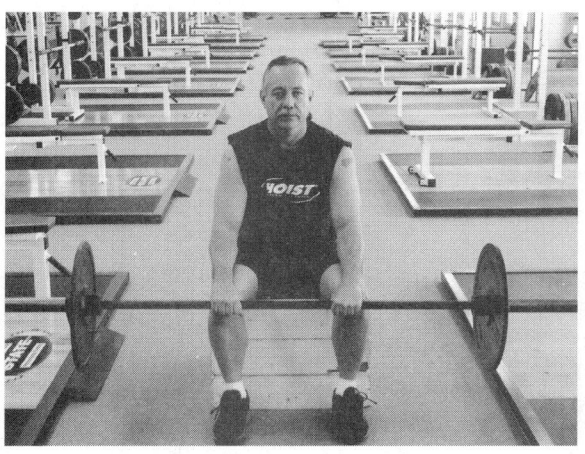 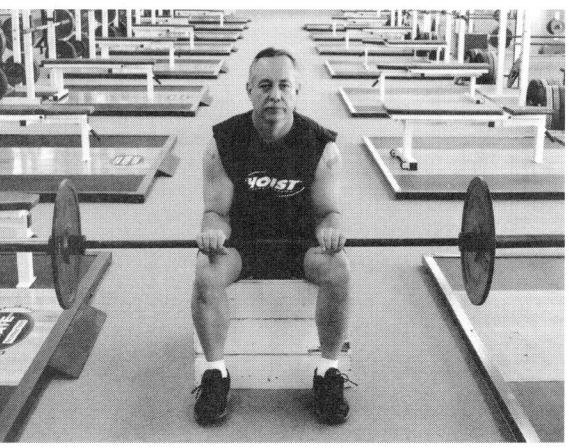

Wrist Rolls-Flexion: Work the same muscles as barbell wrist curls.

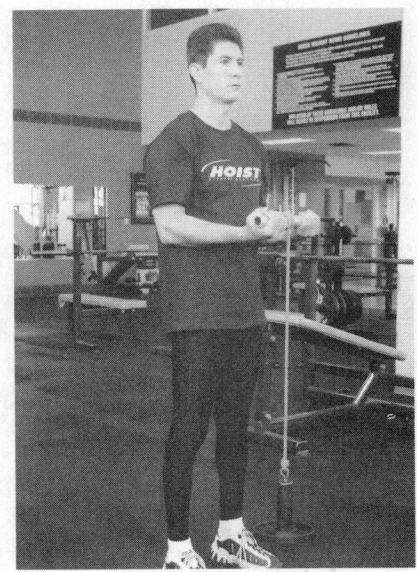

Wrist Rolls-Extension: Work the same muscles as barbell wrist extensions.

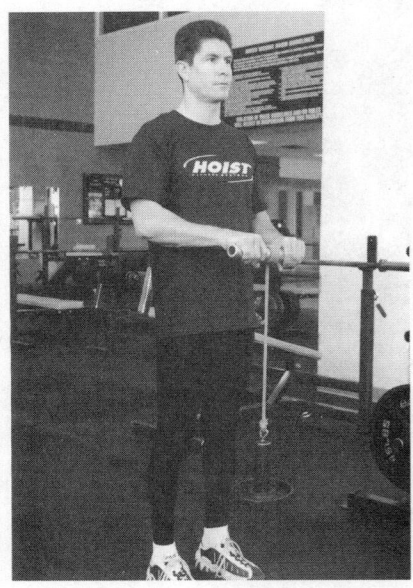

Frank and Ernest

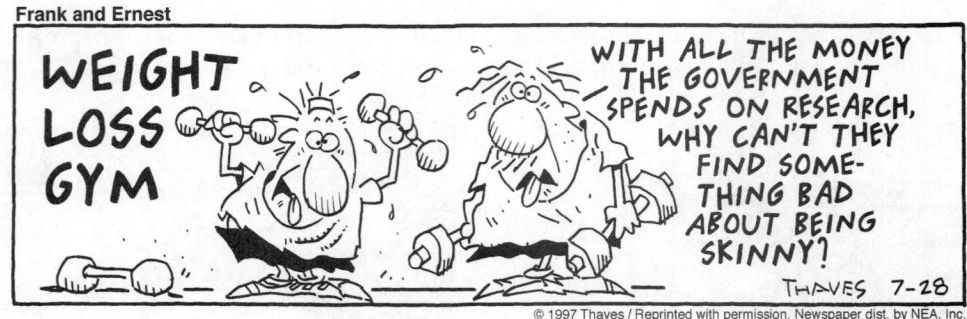

© 1997 Thaves / Reprinted with permission. Newspaper dist. by NEA, Inc.

(*Asterisk indicates information from, "Strength Training Anatomy" by Frederic Delavier, Human Kinetics. This information is used as reference material.)

1. Andrews, G. (September 2002). Angles, Positions and Variations. A thorough study of strength training. *Personal Fitness Professional.* 30–38.

CHAPTER 5 SELF TEST

Please feel free to write on this page

True or False

1. _____ Narrow grip barbell curls work the long head of the bicep.
2. _____ Dumbbell kickbacks work all three heads of the triceps.
3. _____ Reverse pushdowns will work the triceps and especially the long head.

Multiple Choice

4. _____ What are the two parts of the upper limbs?
   a. arm and forearm
   b. biceps and triceps
   c. arm and biceps
   d. forearm and deltoids

5. _____ Concentration curls isolate what three muscles?
   a. biceps, brachialis, triceps
   b. biceps, brachialis, brachioradialis
   c. biceps, brachioradialis, forearms
   d. biceps, brachialis, forearms

6. _____ Using what grip will work the brachioradialis muscle?
   a. supinatd grip
   b. natural grip
   c. neutral grip
   d. reverse grip

7. _____ What is the largest muscle in the upper part of your arm?
   a. biceps
   b. triceps
   c. deltiods
   d. forearms

8. _____ Which is not a major muscle in the forearm?
   a. extensor carpi radialis longus
   b. extensor carpi ulnaris
   c. flexor carpi radialis
   d. flexor minimis ulnaris

9. _____ Why is it important to keep your elbows high at the side of your head when you are doing overhead triceps extensions?
   a. keeps the attention on the triceps
   b. prevents injuries
   c. keeps the attention on the biceps
   d. so you don't hit yourself with a dumbbell

10. _____ Which one of the answers is not a muscle of the triceps?
    a. triceps brachii medial head
    b. triceps brachii lateral head
    c. triceps brachii short head
    d. triceps brachii long head

NOTES

Please feel free to write on this page

Thigh/Leg Muscles and Exercises

Frank and Ernest

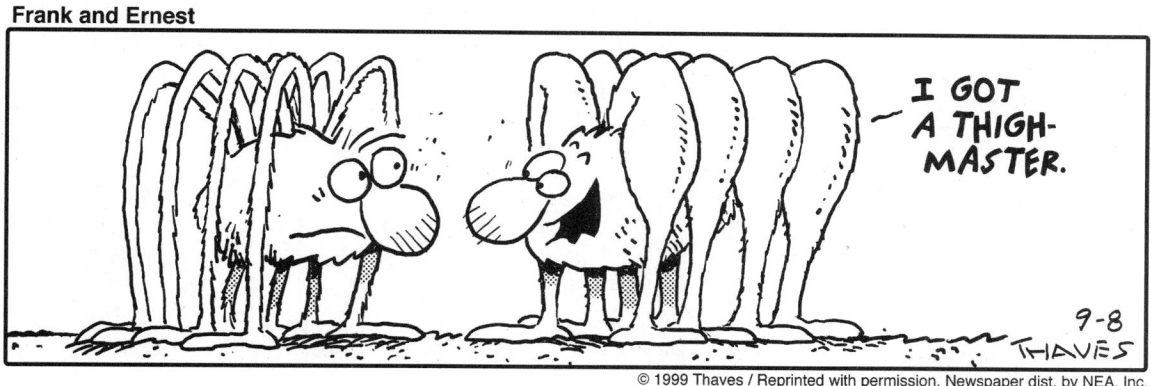

© 1999 Thaves / Reprinted with permission. Newspaper dist. by NEA, Inc.

Thigh and Leg Muscles

The muscles of the lower limbs can be divided into the thigh muscles and leg muscles. The major thigh muscles are the vastus medialis, vastus intermedius, vastus lateralis, and the rectus femoris (quadriceps or quad's); the biceps femoris-long head, biceps femoris-short head, semimembranosus, and semitendinosus (hamstrings or hams); gluteus medius and gluteus maximus (gluteals or glutes); adductor longus, adductor magnus, pectineus, and gracilis (adductors); gluteus medius, gluteus maximus, and tensor fasciae latae (abductors). The leg muscles are the gastrocnemius-lateral head and gastrocnemius-short head (calves), the soleus, and the tibialis anterior. Also in the leg are the extensor digitorum longus, extensor hallucis longus, peroneus longus, peroneus brevis, flexor digitorum longus, and the flexor hallucis longus.

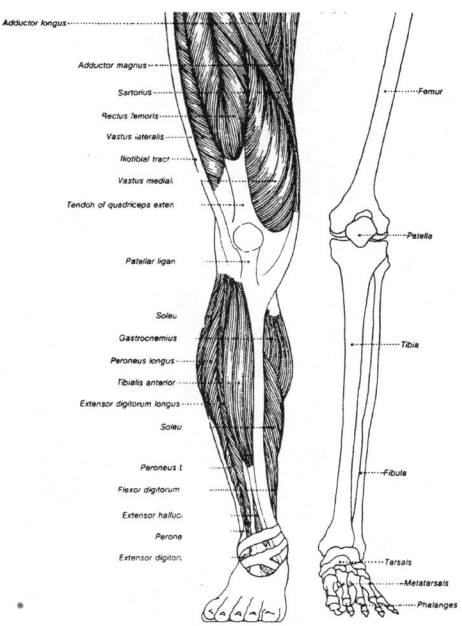

The action of the quadriceps is the extension of the lower leg. The hamstrings are responsible for knee joint flexion. The adductors are responsible for pulling one leg or both in toward the centerline of the body. The abductors are responsible for movement of the legs away from the centerline of the body. In the lower leg, the calves are responsible for plantar flexion. This action allows the heel to rise while the ball of the foot remains on the floor. Conversely, when the heel remains on the floor and the toes rise off the floor, we have dorsi flexion. The muscles involved in this action are the anterior tibialis, with help from the extensor digitorum longus, and the peroneus tertius. The calves are responsible for movement of the ankle and foot. The gastrocnemius, soleus, peroneus longus, and peroneus brevis, plantar flex or move the foot in a downward direction. The gastrocnemius muscles also assist in knee flexion.

Free Weight Exercises for the Legs

Barbell Exercises

Squats: Work the quadriceps, gluteals, adductors, erectors, abdominals, and hamstrings. They can be done as either regular or full squats (Olympic squats). Regular squats require the thighs to be parallel to the floor at the conclusion of the squat, while full squats require the thighs to be considerably below parallel to the floor. Sometimes full squats are called "butt to ankle" squats.*

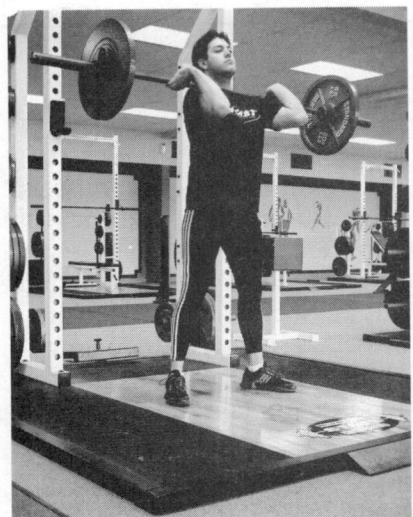
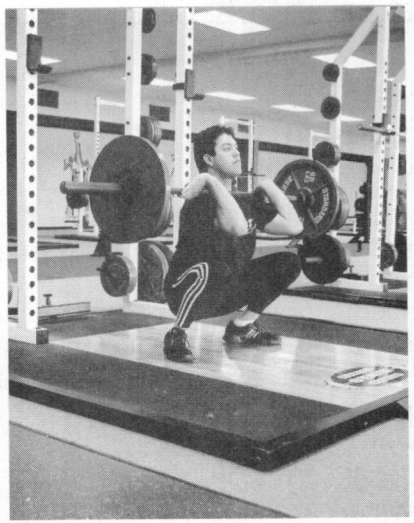

Front Squats

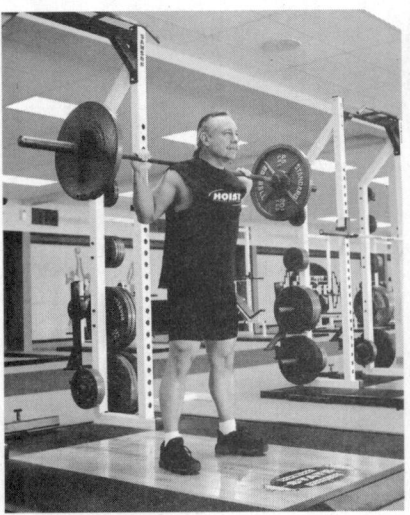
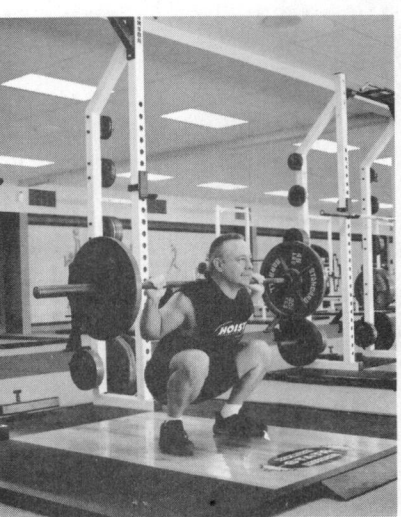

Olympic Back Squats

Front Squats: Work the above-mentioned muscles but place more of a work load on the quadriceps than do back squats.*

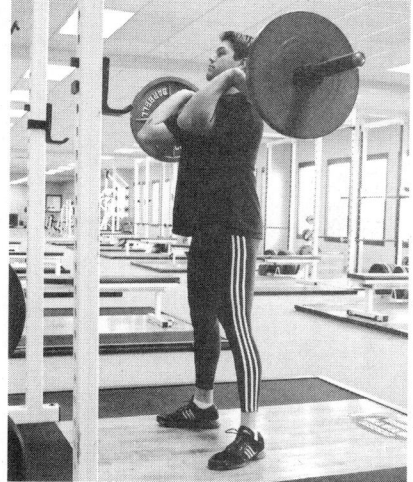

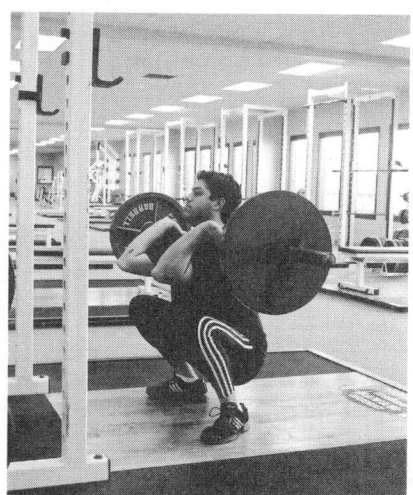

Olympic Front Squats

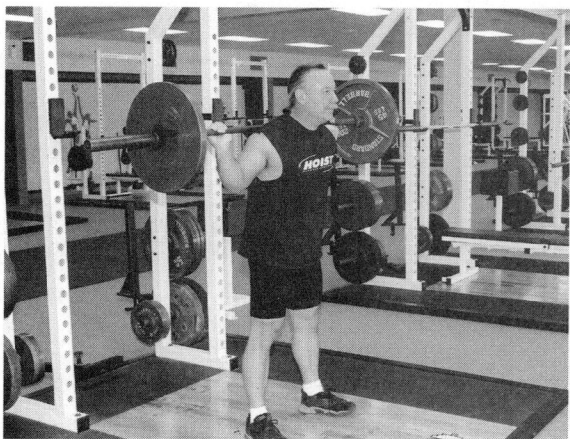

Regular Back Squats

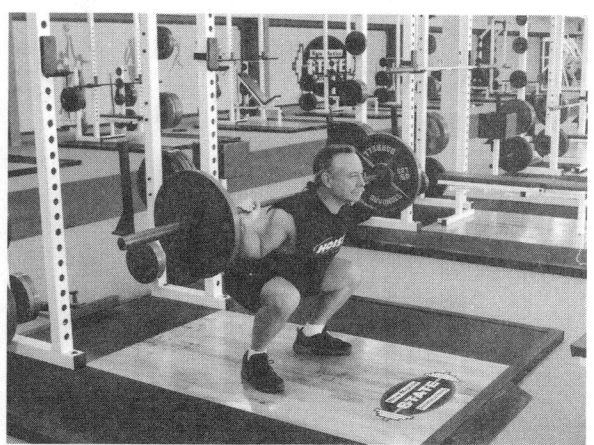

High Bar vs. Low Bar Squats: High bar squats are typically done by Olympic weight lifters, while low bar squats are done by powerlifters. High bar squats will distribute the weight of the bar equally between the hip and knee joint. Low bar squats will place more load on the the hip joint. Because of the bar position, powerlifters will be able to squat with more weight due to the use of hip and back musculature.

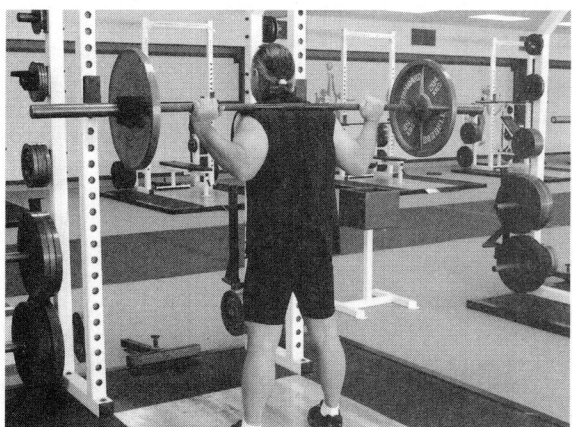

High Bar Squats

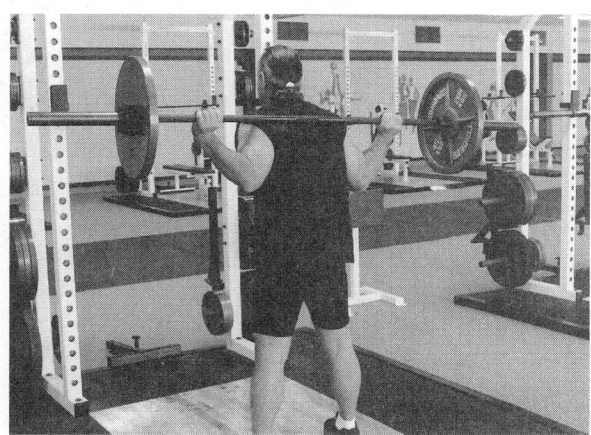

Low Bar Squats

Lunges: Work the gluteals and quadriceps. By taking a larger step forward, more work will be placed on the hamstrings. When in the lunge position, keep the knee over the ankle to reduce the chance of injury to the patella. When lunging to the front, the leg that is lunging is the working leg; however, when lunging to the rear, it is the stationary leg that is working. Walking lunges are another variation, and are an advanced exercise because of the constantly changing center of gravity and balance that is required.*[1]

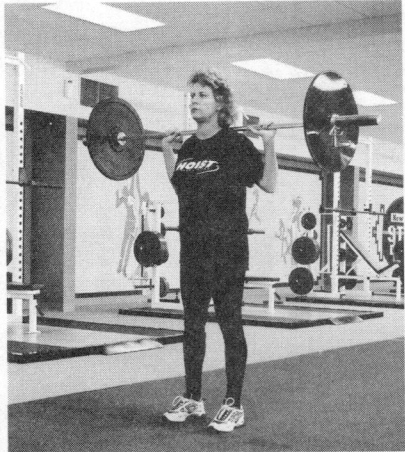 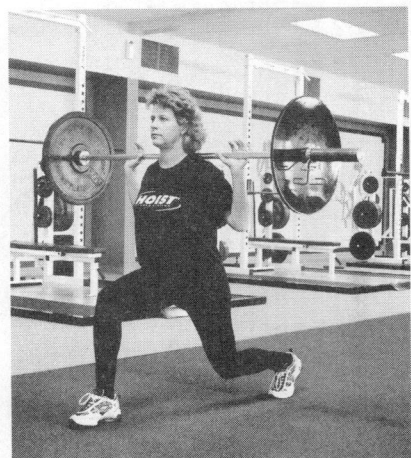

Stationary Barbell Lunges

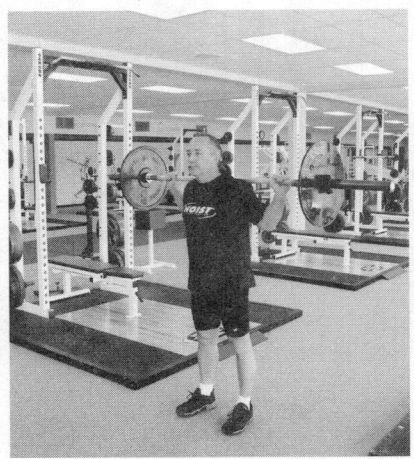 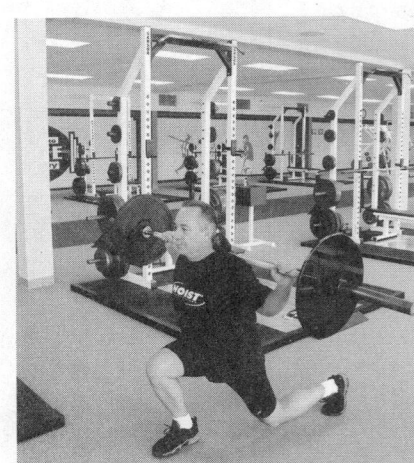

Walking Barbell Lunges #1   #2

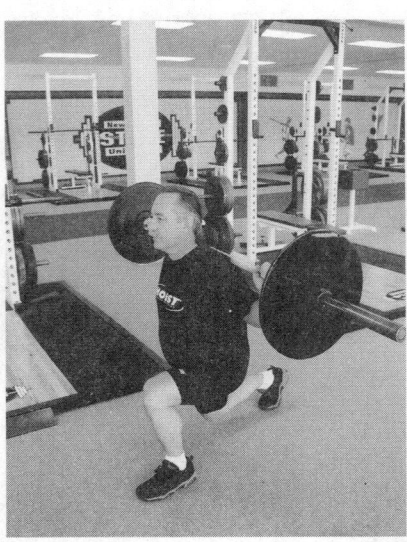 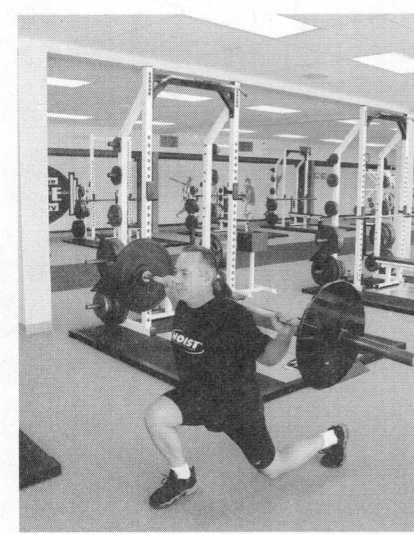

#3   #4

Romanian Deadlifts: Work the gluteals and hamstrings.

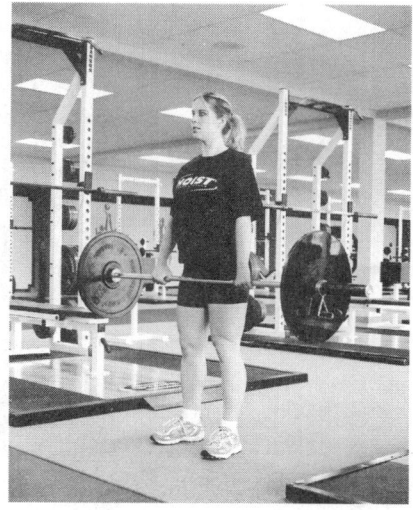 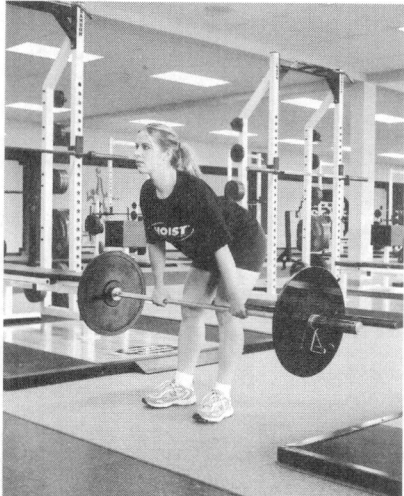

Lunge-Squat Combo: Works the quadriceps, gluteals, hamstrings, adductors, abdominals, and erectors.

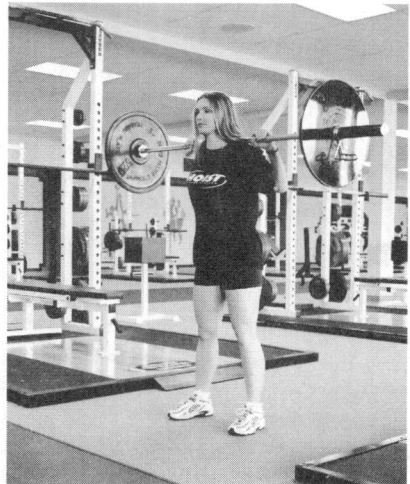 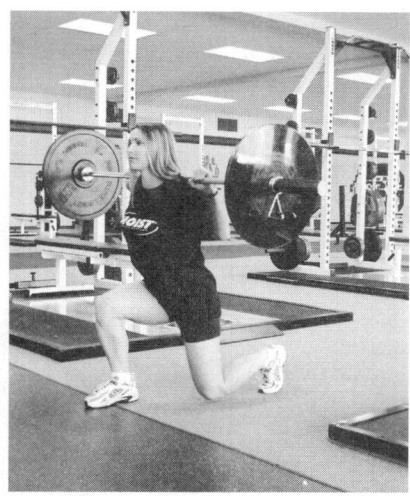

Start Position Lunge   Step out with one leg and then the other

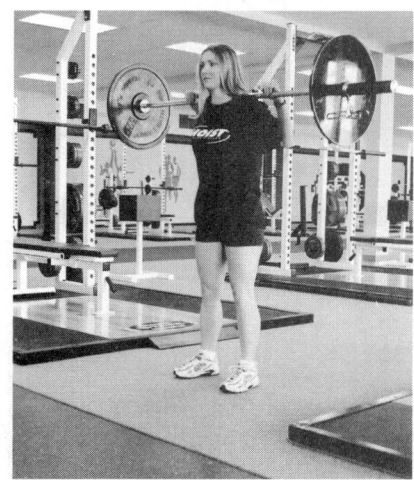 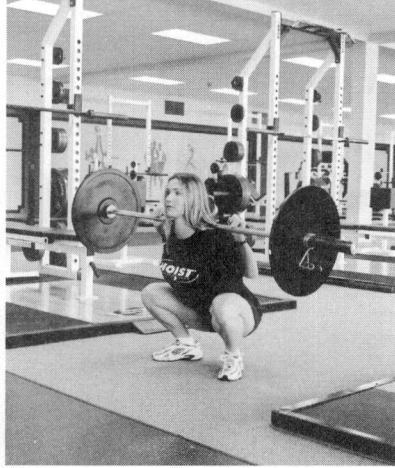 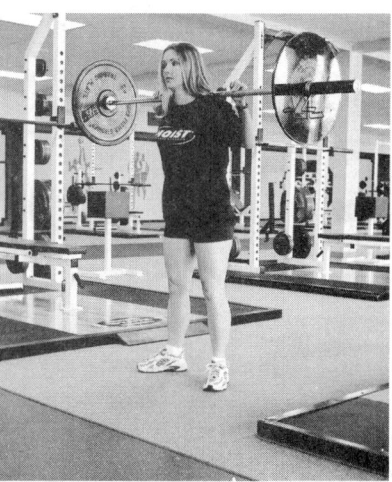

Start Position Squat   Squat   Finish

Dumbbell Exercises

Dumbbell Squats: Work the quadriceps and gluteals.*

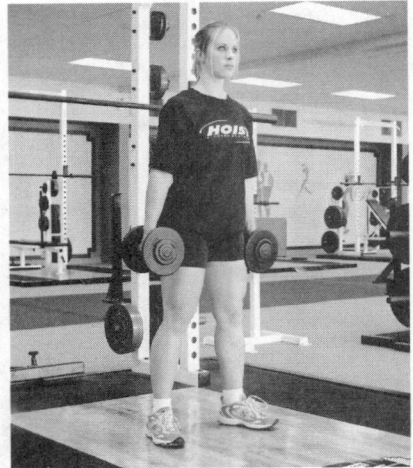 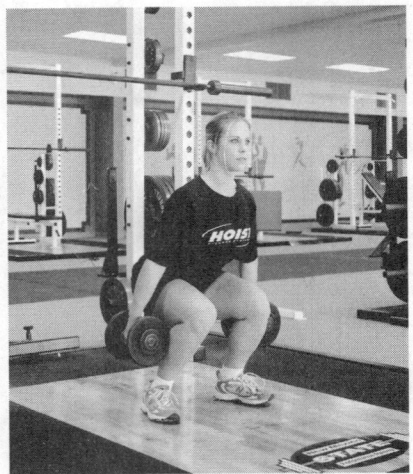

Dumbbell Lunges: Work the gluteals and quadriceps. By taking a larger step forward, more work will be placed on the hamstrings. When in the lunge position, keep the knee over the ankle to reduce the chance of injury to the patella. When lunging to the front, the leg that is lunging is the working lead; however, when lunging to the rear, it is the stationary leg that is working. Walking lunges are another variation, and are an advanced exercise because of the constantly changing center of gravity and balance that is required.*[1]

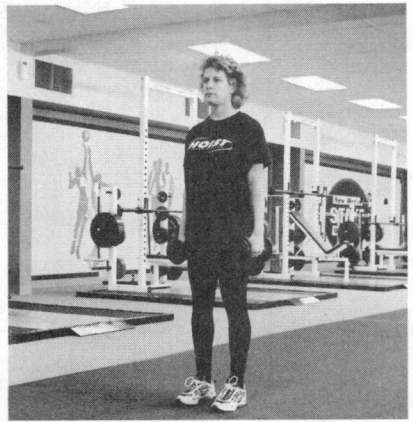 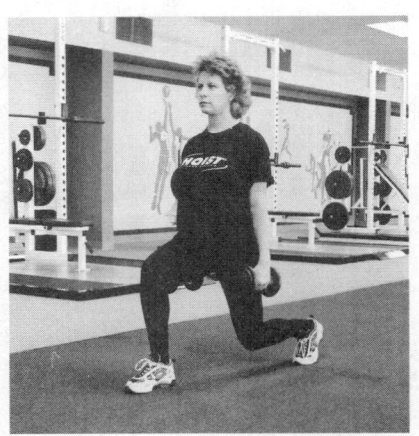

Stationary – Alternating Legs

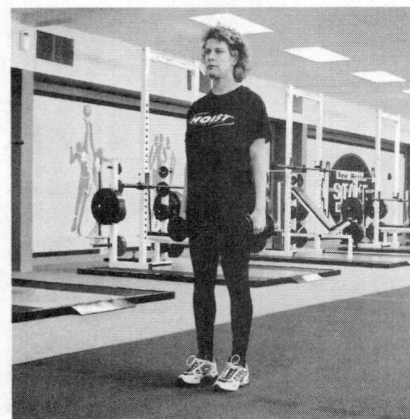 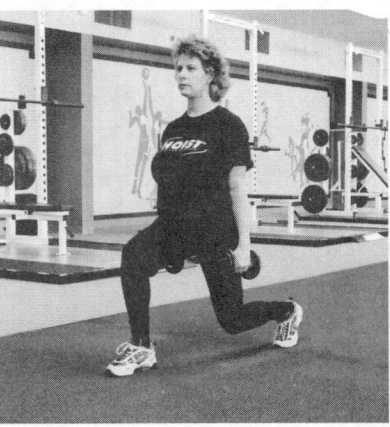 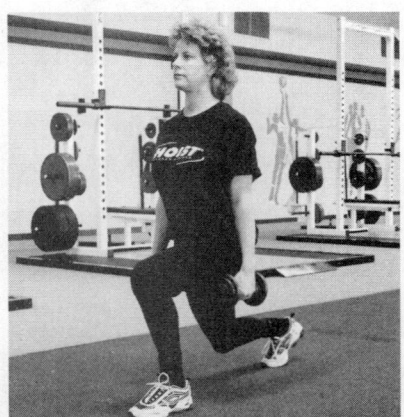

Dumbbell Walking Lunges

Machine Exercises

Smith Machine Squats: Work the quadriceps and gluteals.

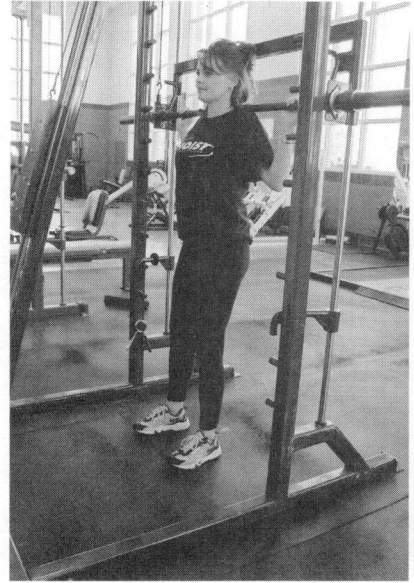 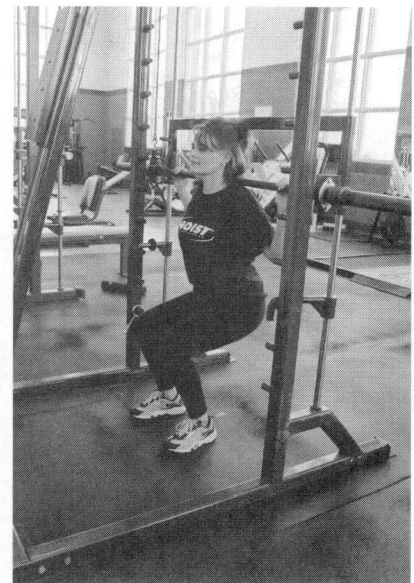

Smith Machine Lunges: Work the gluteals and quadriceps.

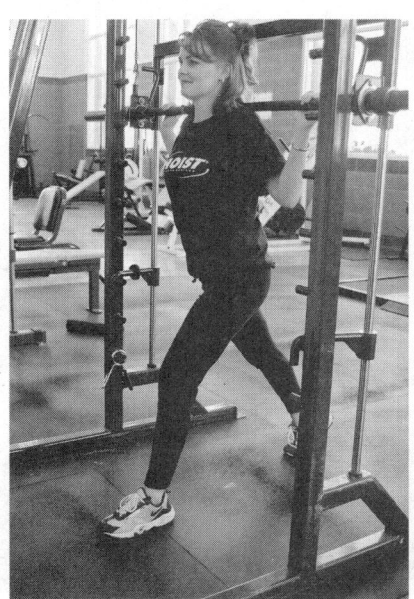 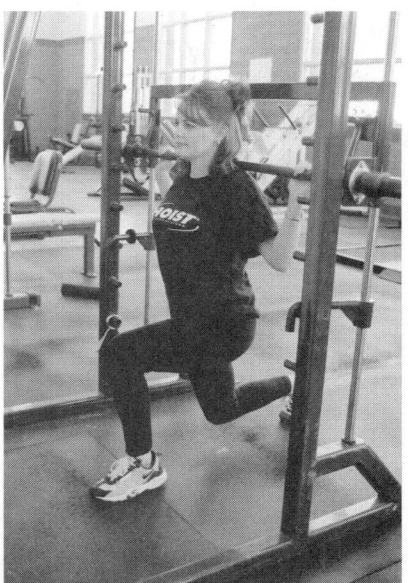

45 Degree Leg Press: Works the quadriceps and gluteals. Foot position makes a difference in using the 45-Degree Leg Press. With the feet high on the footplate, more work will be done by the gluteals and hamstrings. With the feet low on the footplate, more work will be done by the quadriceps. When the feet are spread apart, the adductors will do more work. When the feet are close together, more work will be done by the quadriceps.*

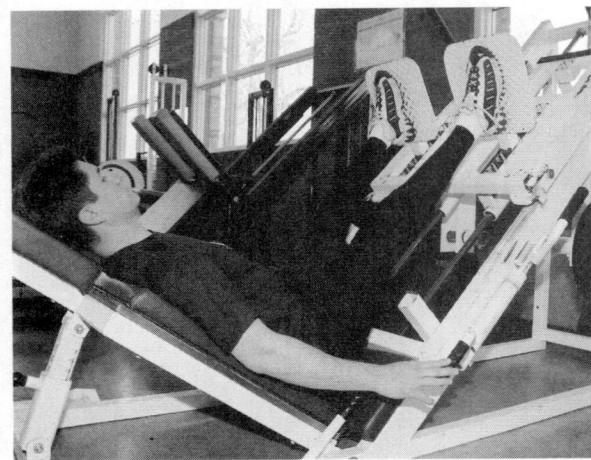 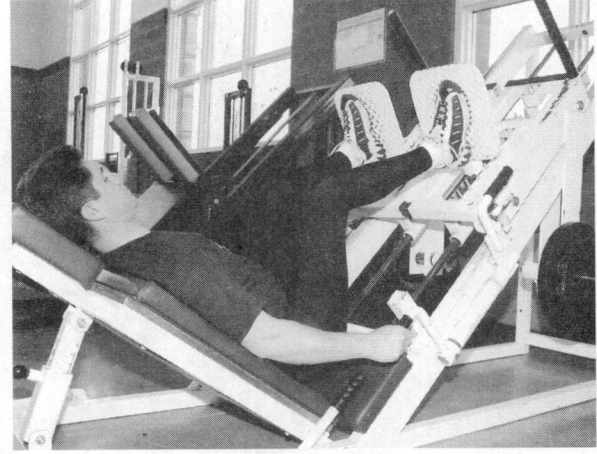

Horizontal Leg Press: Works the quadriceps and gluteals.

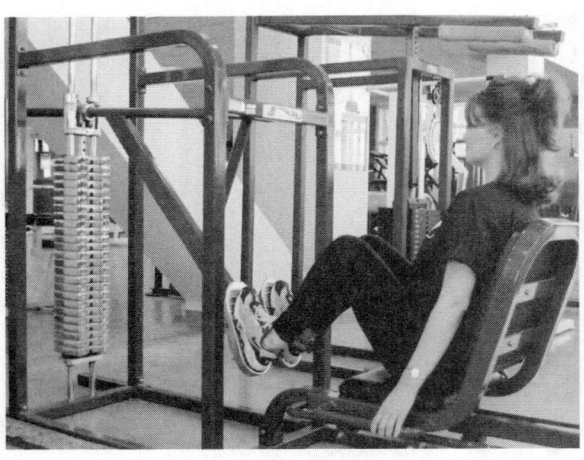 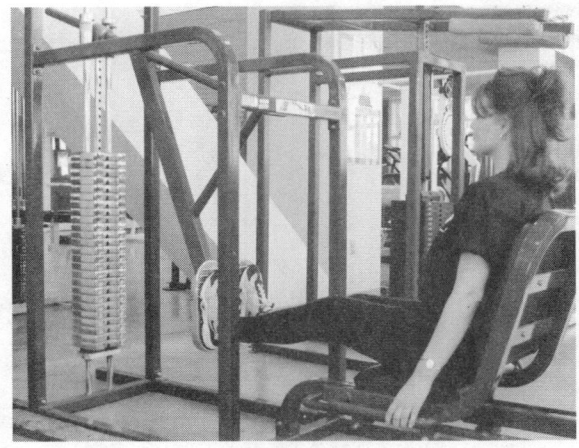

Hack Squat: Works the quadriceps. The foot placement is the same as the 45-Degree Leg Press.*

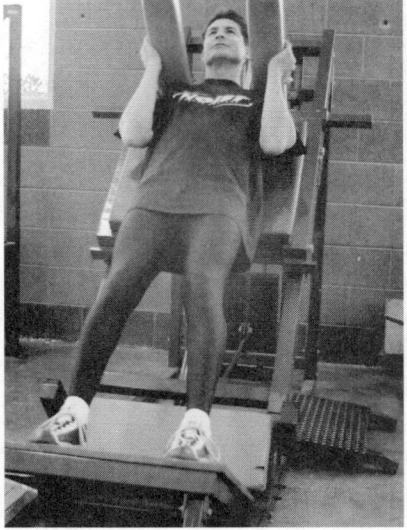 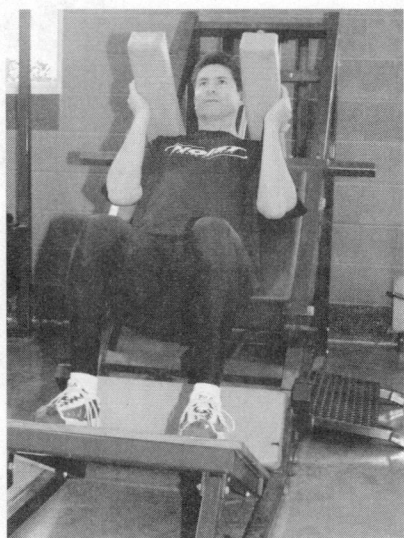

Glute Blaster: Works the gluteals.

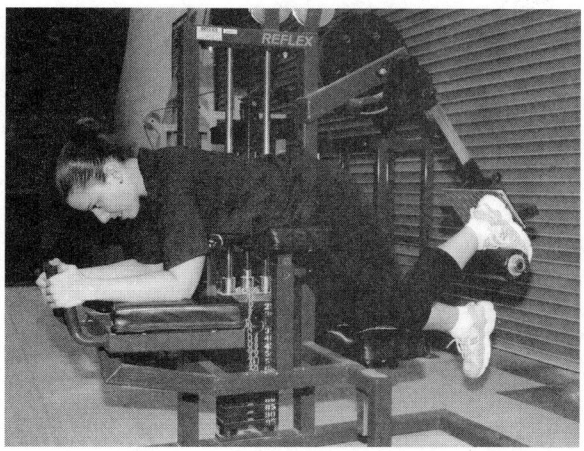 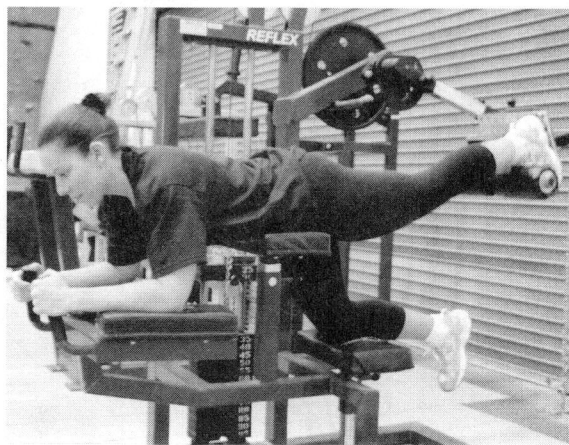

Seated Leg Curls: Work the hamstrings and gastrocnemius.* This is the most effective way to work the hamstrings because of the pre-stretch.

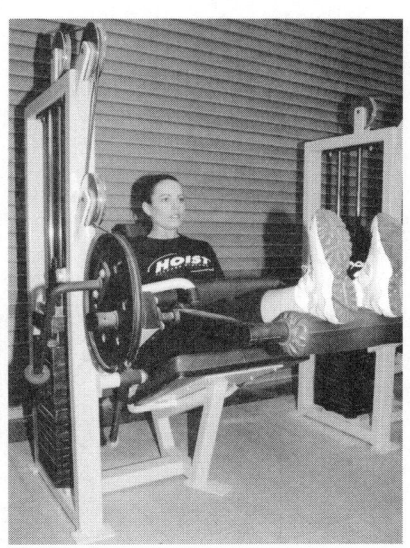 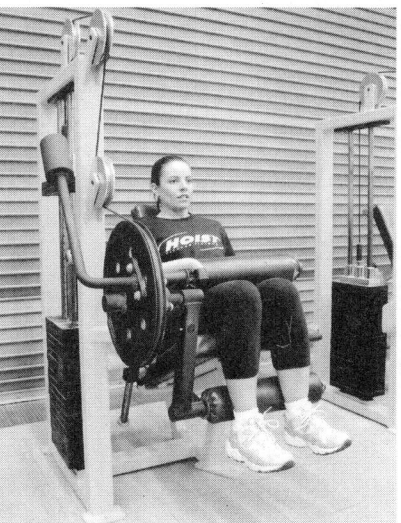

Lying Leg Curls: Work the hamstrings and gastrocnemius.* If you point your toes straight when doing this movement, you will remove the gastrocnemius from the exercise and concentrate on the hamstrings.

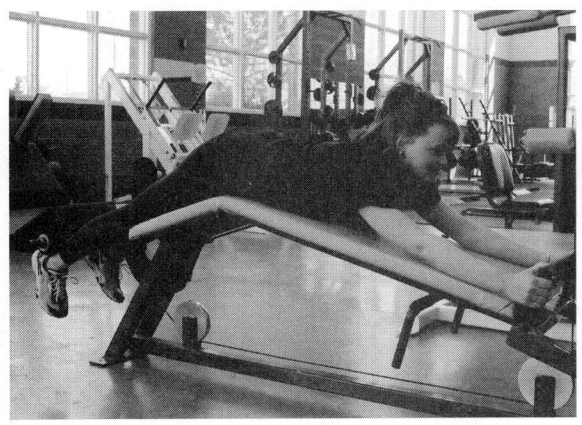 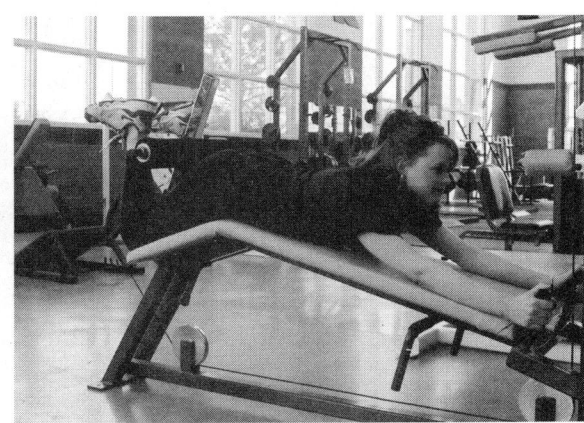

Seated Leg Extension: Works the quadriceps as an isolation exercise. If this exercise hurts the knee, try placing a rolled up towel between the thighs and squeeze as you perform the movement. This will put more emphasis on the vastus medialis and hip adductors and take some of the pressure off of the patella. Because of the shear forces placed on the knee joint, I do not recommend this exercise, however, if you must do it, use light weight and avoid an extreme starting position. Personally, I would prefer to do front squats to develop the "Tear Drop" of the quadriceps muscle.

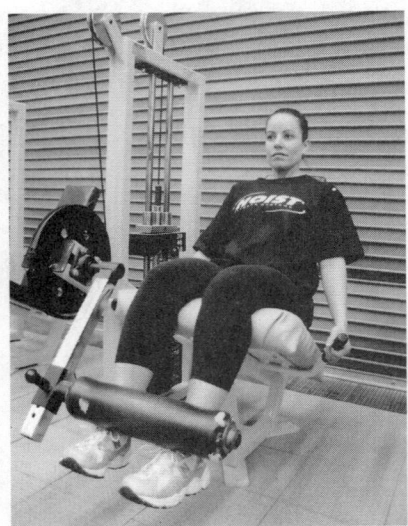 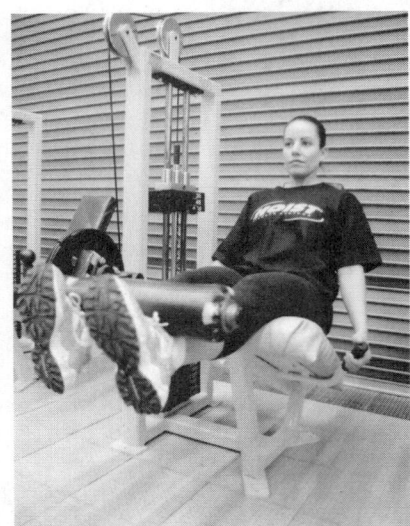

4-Way Multi-Hip

Abduction: Work the gluteus maximus, gluteus medius, and tensor fascia latae (abductors).*

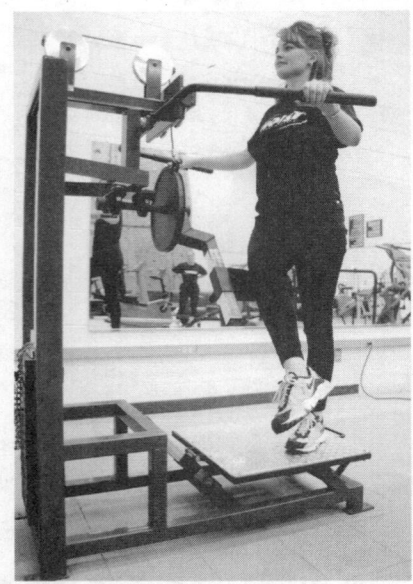 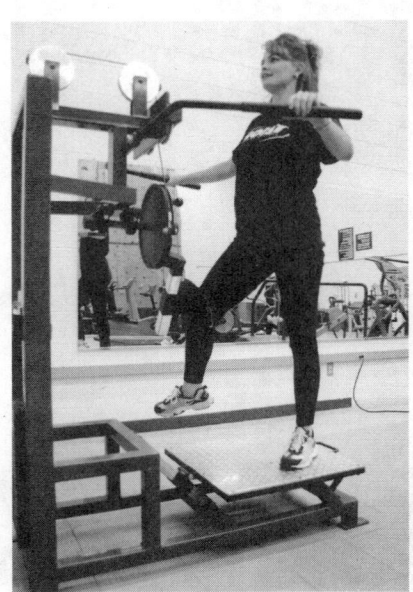

Start

Finish

Adduction: Work the pectineus, adductor longus, adductor magnus, and gracilis (adductors).*

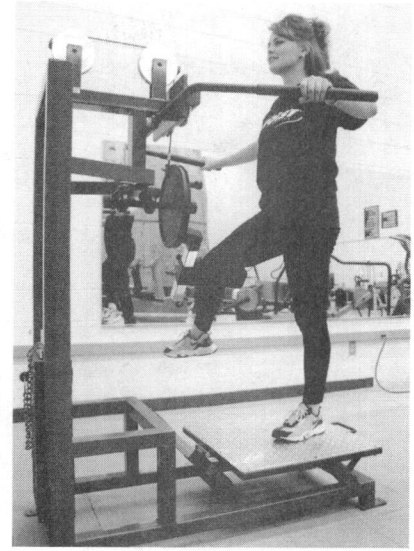
Start

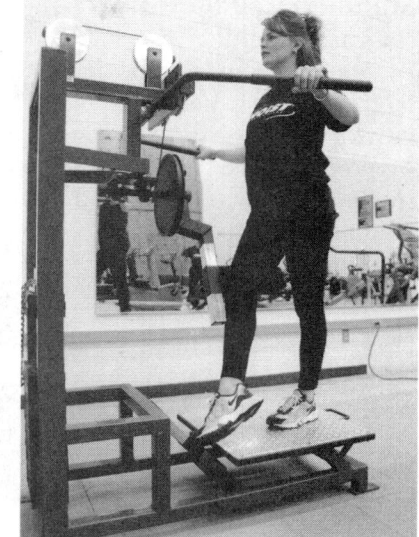
Finish

Hip Flexion: Works the rectus femoris, sartorius, and iliopsoas primarily and tensor fasciae latae secondarily.

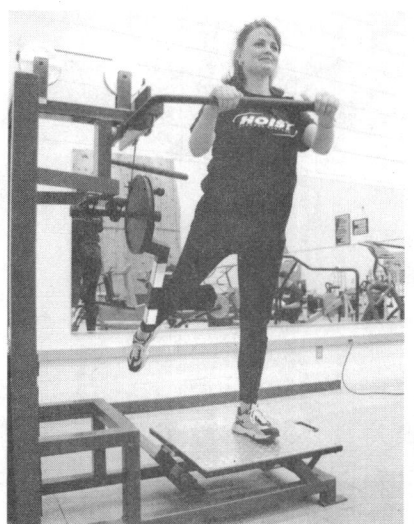
Start

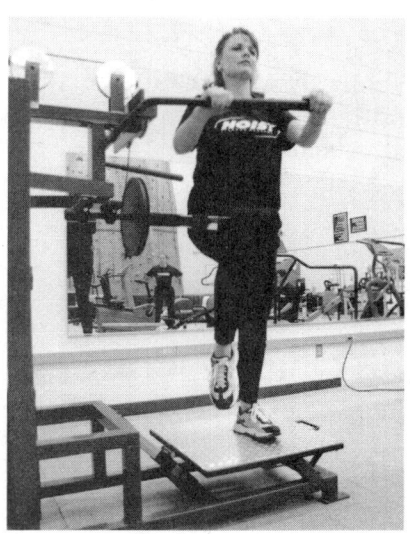
Finish

Hip Extension: Works primarily the gluteus maximus, and to a lesser degree, the semitendinosus, semimembranosus, and biceps femoris, long head.

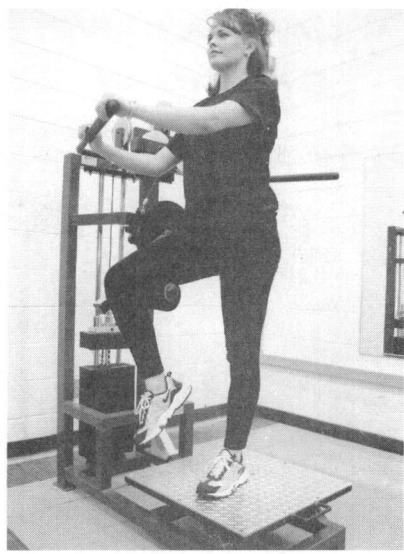
Start

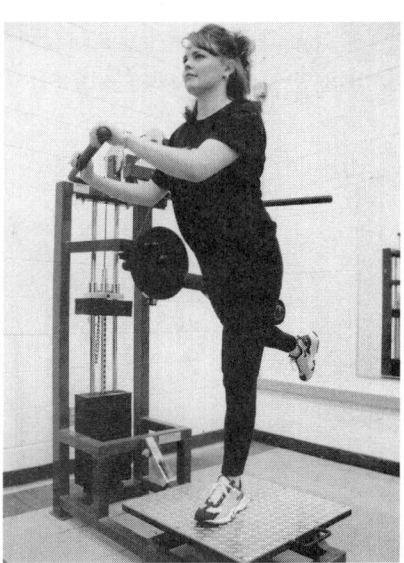
Finish

Standing Calf Raises: Work the gastrocnemius and soleus. By pointing the toes in, the lateral head of the gastrocnemius will be worked; by pointing the toes out, the medial head will be worked. Changing the toe position changes the stress on the muscle.*

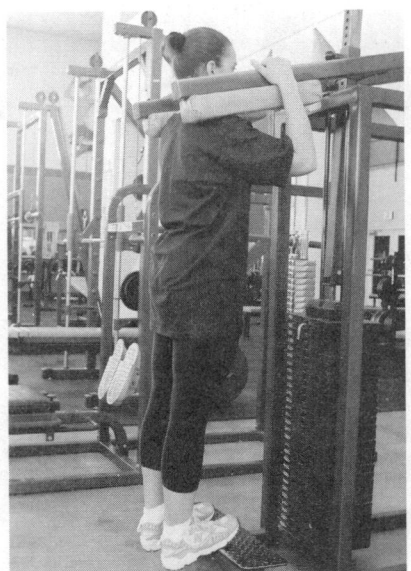 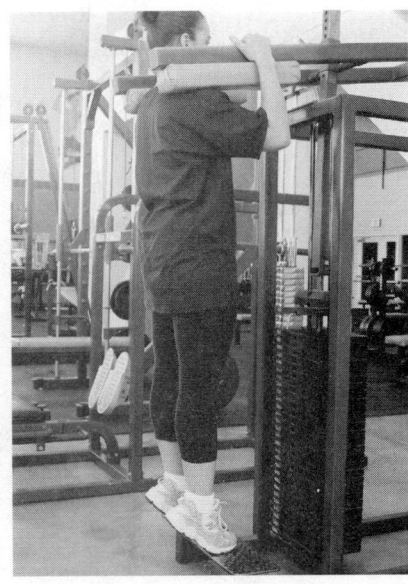

Seated Calf Raises: Primarily work the soleus, with some gastrocnemius involvement.*

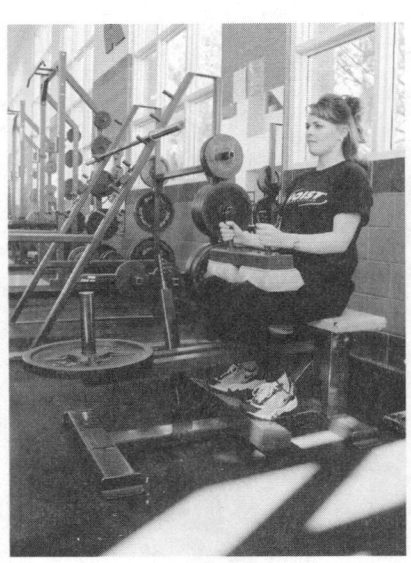 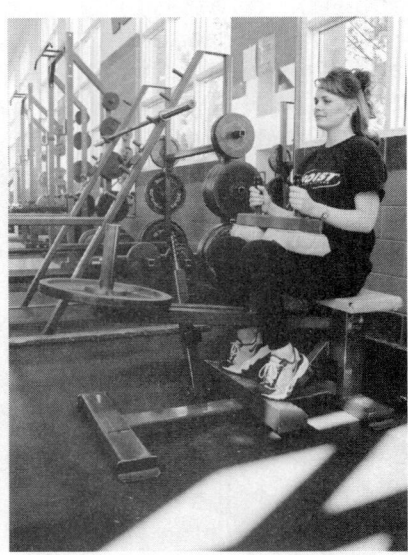

Donkey Calf Raises: Work the gastrocnemius and the soleus.*

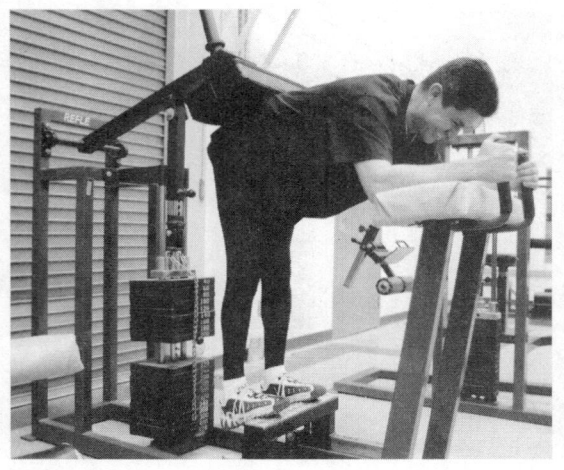 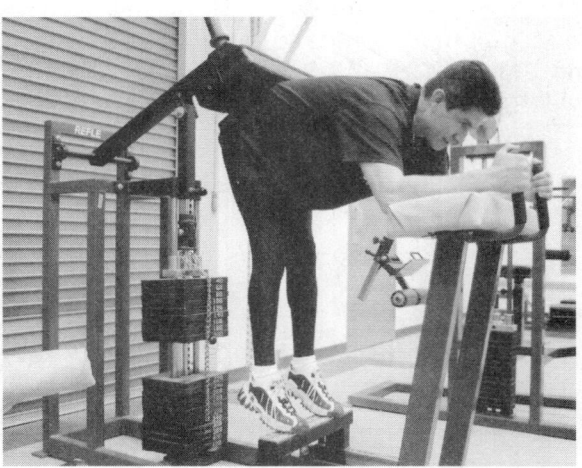

Calf Machine Foot Positions

Toes Straight: Works the medial and lateral head of the gastrocnemius equally.

Toes In: Places more emphasis on the lateral head of the gastrocnemius.

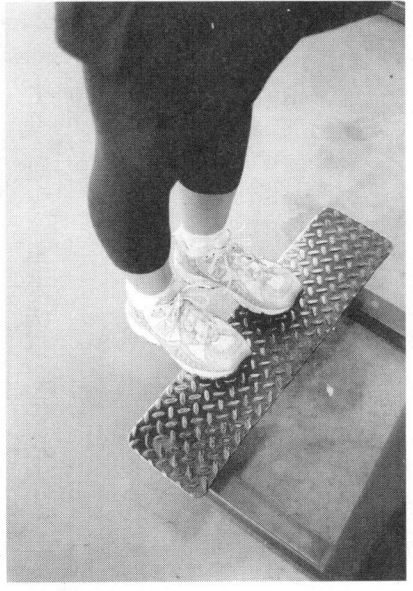

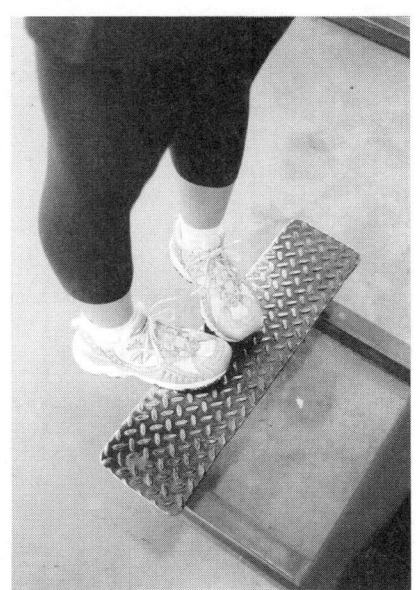

Toes Out: Places more emphasis on the medial head of the gastrocnemius.

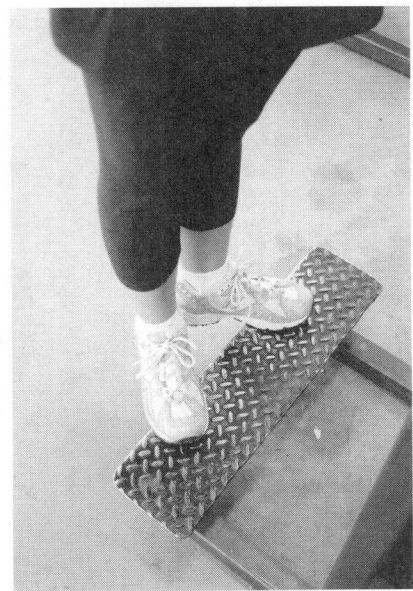

Cable Exercises

Cable Abduction: Works the gluteus maximus, gluteus medius, and tensor fascia latae (abductors).*

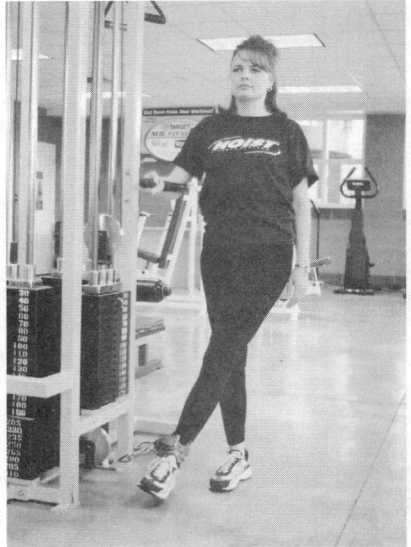 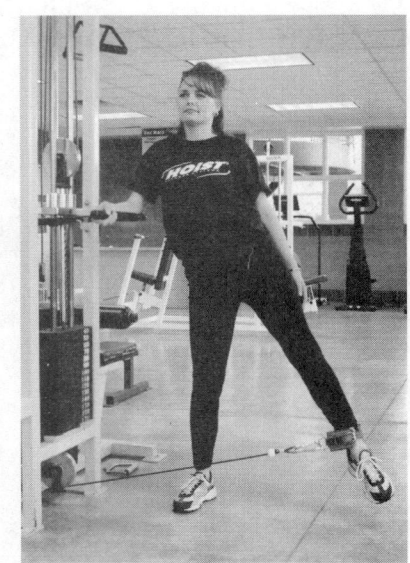

Cable Adduction: Works the pectineus, adductor longus, adductor magnus, and the gracilis (adductors).*

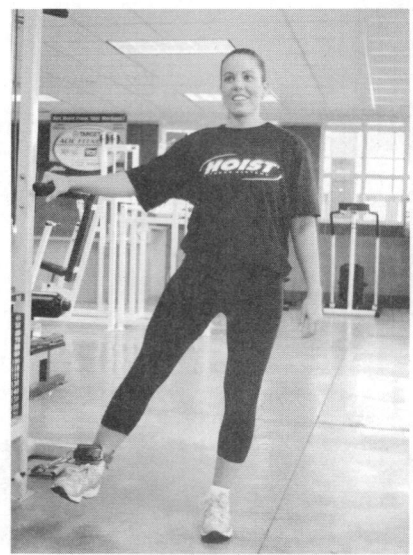 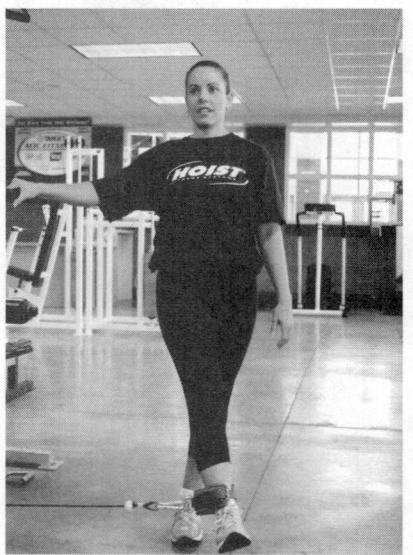

Cable Hip Extension: Works the gluteus maximus and the hamstrings.*

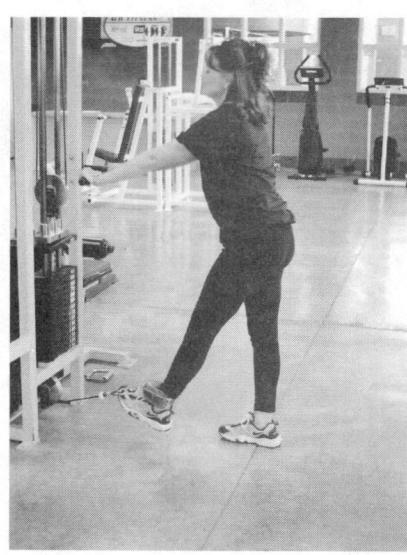 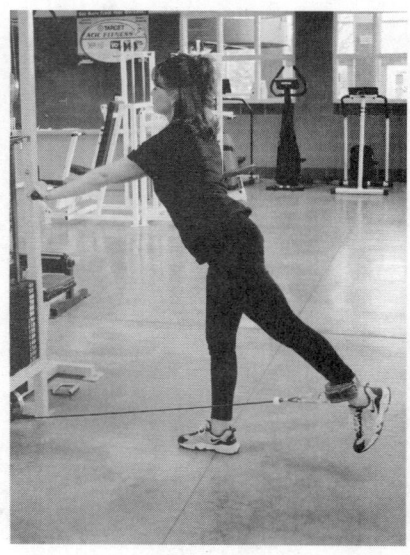

Cable Hip Flexion: Works the hip flexors.

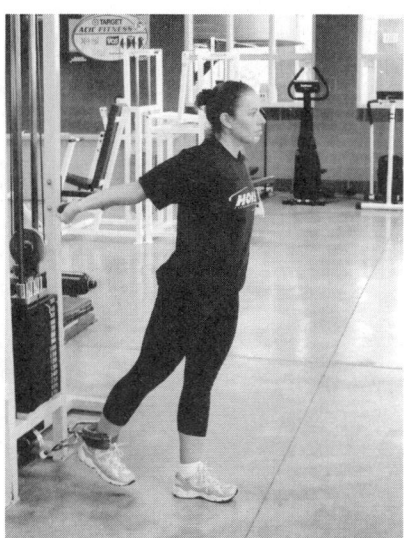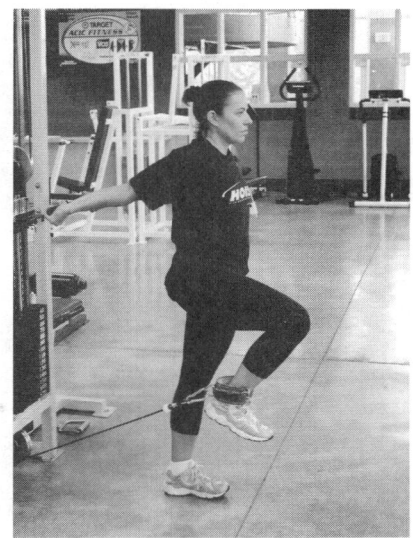

To Squat or Not

To squat or not, that is the question. With all of the available machines in a gym, why should anyone squat; especially since machines are so convenient and easy to use? The answer to this question lies in the word "function." If the training you do is going to apply to everyday life, then the training must be functional to the demands of life. While many leg machines may isolate the muscles, as in the leg extension or leg curl, in real life we rarely isolate muscles to any degree.

Squatting, however, is very similar to normal patterns of daily living, including picking up boxes, sitting down, and so on. It is also very sports-specific to many sporting activities that are engaged in during our spare time.

Squatting also has advantages in that it does not produce the shear forces at the knee that the leg extension and leg curl do.[2]

How to Squat

1. Insure that the bar is loaded evenly, with the correct amount of weight and collars holding the weight-plates on.
2. Place the hands evenly on the bar with a shoulder-width or slightly wider grip, and thumbs around the bar. The hands will be in a pronated position.
3. Step under the bar with both feet. The bar should be approximately mid-back high for powerlifting squats, or higher for Olympic weightlifting squats.
4. Hold chest up and pinch shoulder blades together.
5. Position the bar and weight, centered on the back, resting across the posterior deltoids and middle to upper trapezius.
6. Straighten both legs to lift the bar from the rack.
7. Use a hip-width or slightly wider stance with toes pointed out slightly.
8. Keep feet flat on the floor.
9. Head and eyes remain level.
10. Hold the breath from the start of the movement to past the sticking point on the ascent.
11. Descend in a slow and controlled manner until the thighs are parallel to the floor for a regular squat, or further for a full squat.

12. Avoid bouncing or twisting from the bottom position.

13. The hips and shoulders should rise at the same rate, with the torso remaining in an upright position.

14. Exhale on the exertion phase of the lift as you stand up.

15. Do not allow the knees to come together during the ascent and *never round the back*.

16. Upon completion of the set, put the bar back in the rack.[4] (Modified slightly by Doug Briggs)

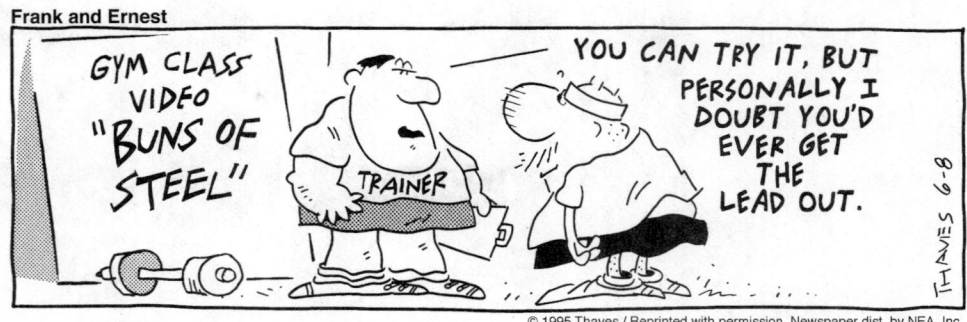

Frank and Ernest

GYM CLASS VIDEO "BUNS OF STEEL"

TRAINER

YOU CAN TRY IT, BUT PERSONALLY I DOUBT YOU'D EVER GET THE LEAD OUT.

THAVES 6-8

© 1995 Thaves / Reprinted with permission. Newspaper dist. by NEA, Inc.

(*Asterisk indicates information from, "Strength Training Anatomy" by Frederic Delavier, Human Kinetics. This information is used as reference material.)

1. Andrews, G. (September 2002). Angles, Positions and Variations. A thorough study of strength training. *Personal Fitness Professional.* 30-38.

2. Palmittier, R. A., Kani-nan, A., Scott, S. G. and Chao, E. Y. S. (1991). Kinetic chain exercise in knee rehabilitation. *Sports Medicine.* 11(6): 402:413.

3. Wretenberg, P., Y. Feng, and U.P. Arborelius. High-and-low-bar squatting techniques during weight training. Med. Sci. Sports Exerc. 28(2):218-224. 1996.

4. A Position Statement and Literature Review of the Squat Exercise in Athletic Conditioning. (1992). Colorado Springs, CO: National Strength and Conditioning Association.

CHAPTER 6 SELF TEST

Please feel free to write on this page

Multiple Choice

1. _____ Name the different types of exercises (listed in the chapter) used for the thigh and leg muscles.
   a. Cable
   b. Machine
   c. Dumbbell
   d. Barbell
   e. All of the above
   f. None of the above

2. _____ When performing a squat, which statement is *incorrect*?
   a. Hold chest out and pinch shoulder blades together.?
   b. Avoid bouncing or twisting from the bottom position.
   c. Keep heels on board or slightly raised area.
   d. Head and eyes remain level.

3. _____ What is the movement of the leg away from the center of the body?
   a. Abduction
   b. Adduction

4. _____ What are the hamstring muscles responsible for?
   a. Knee extension
   b. Knee flexion
   c. Hip flexion
   d. Hip extension

5. _____ What muscles do lunges work?
   a. Gluteals
   b. Quadriceps
   c. Hamstrings
   d. A & C
   e. A & B
   f. None of the above

6. _____ Cable adduction does not work the _____ ?
   a. Pectineus
   b. Adductor longus
   c. Adductor magnus
   d. Tensor fascia latae

True or False

7. _____ The Rectus femoris is one of the names of the muscles for the quadriceps.

8. _____ Vastus intermedialis is the scientific name for the hamstring.

9. _____ Gastrocnemius is the scientific name for the calf muscle.

10. _____ Seated leg curls work the hamstring.

NOTES

Please feel free to write on this page

CHAPTER 7

Abdominal/Low Back Muscles and Exercises

Frank and Ernest

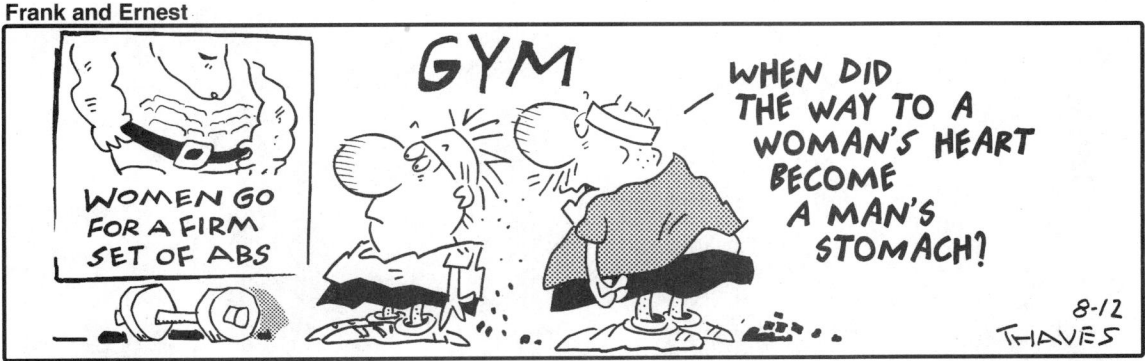

Abdominal and Low Back Muscles

The muscles of the abdominal area (trunk) can be divided into three major groups. The major abdominal muscle is the rectus abdominus (abs). The "six pack" is a result of the tendinous intersections of the rectus abdominis. The obliques are comprised of the internal and external obliques. The erector spinae consist of three muscles: the iliocostalis, longissimus, and the spinalis, and are commonly referred to as the "erectors."

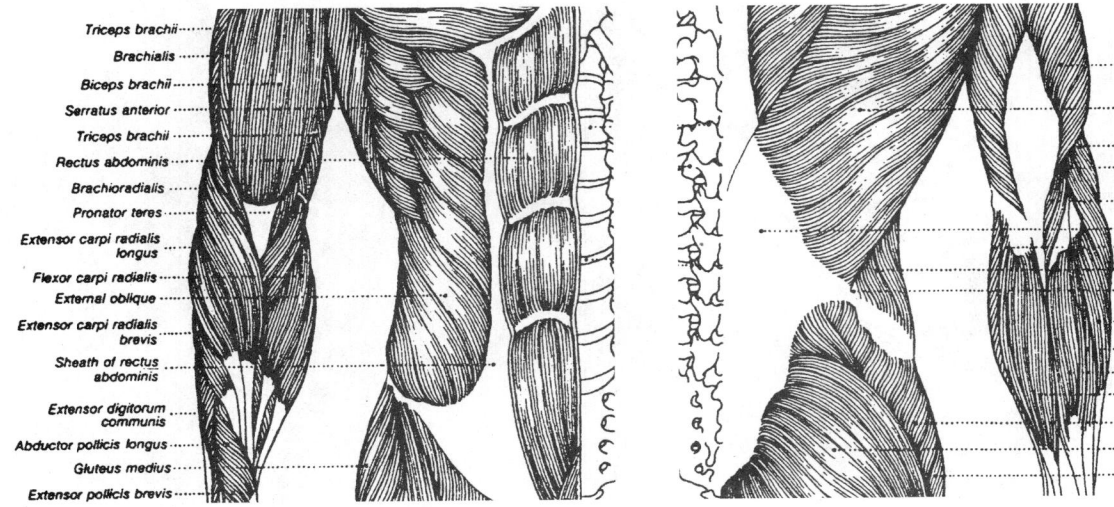

The action of the abdominal muscles is the flexion of the trunk. The obliques are responsible for trunk rotation and lateral flexion. The erector spinae muscles are responsible for spinal (trunk) extension. These muscles run from the skull to the sacrum, and are considered deep back muscles.

Free Weight Exercises for the Abdominals

When working the abdominal muscles, it is essential to keep the muscle tight throughout each type of strengthening exercise to properly and effectively work the muscle.

Sit-ups and Incline Bench Sit-ups: Work the rectus abdominus, hip flexors, and obliques. By using an incline board for sit-ups, it is possible to add more resistance.* This can also be accomplished by holding a weight-plate to the chest or behind the head.

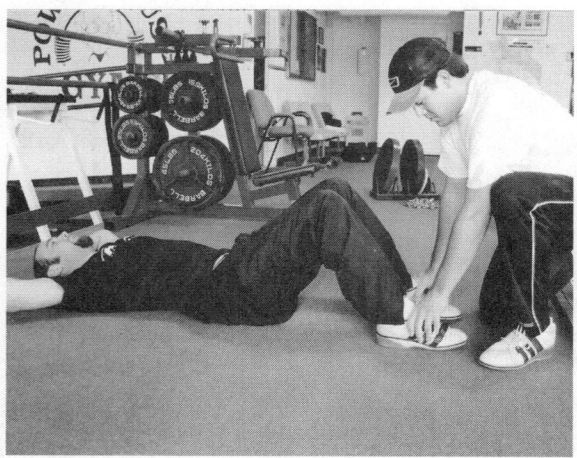 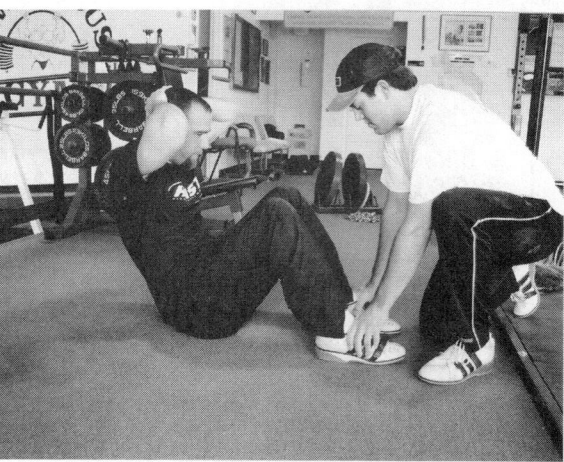

Crunches: Work the rectus abdominus. To involve more of the obliques, touch the right elbow to the left knee, and vice-versa, when doing the crunch.* Crunches can be done with the feet placed on a wall.

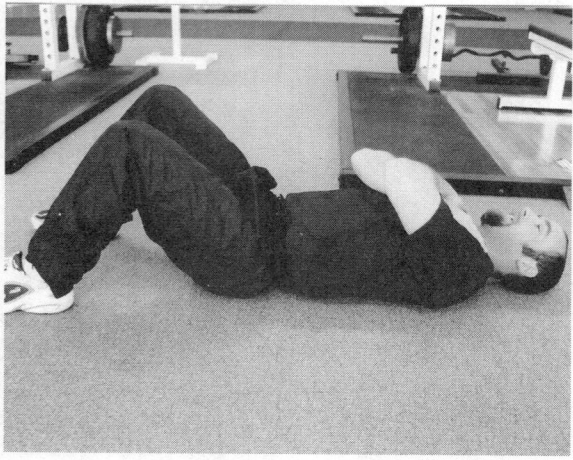 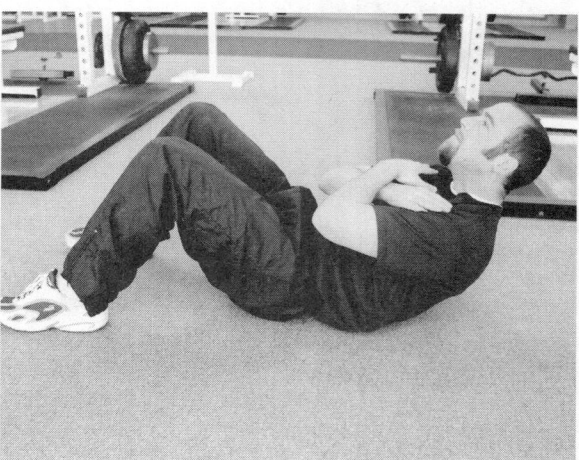

Captain's Chair Leg Raises: Work the hip flexors and the rectus abdominus. In order to isolate the abs, do not let the knees drop below horizontal. Keeping the legs straight will increase the difficulty of the exercise.* By adding lower trunk rotation, as the legs are raised, the obliques are worked.

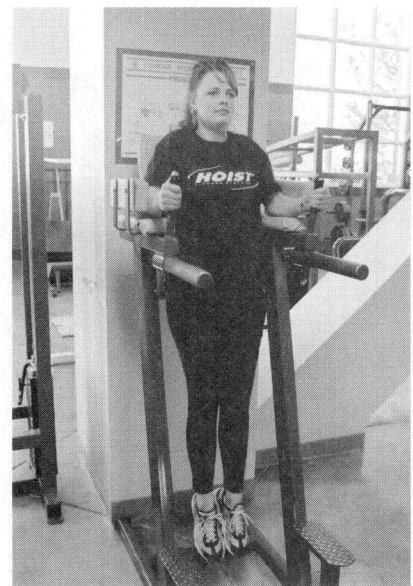 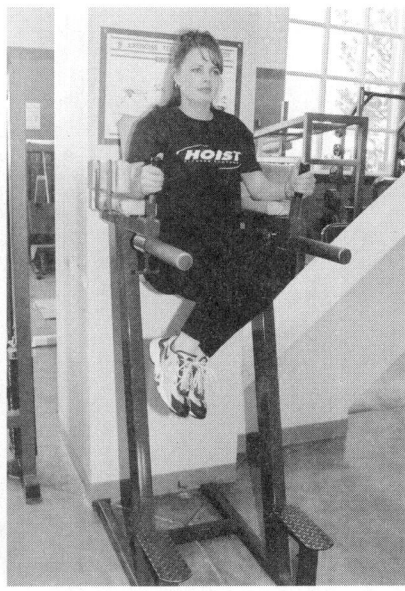 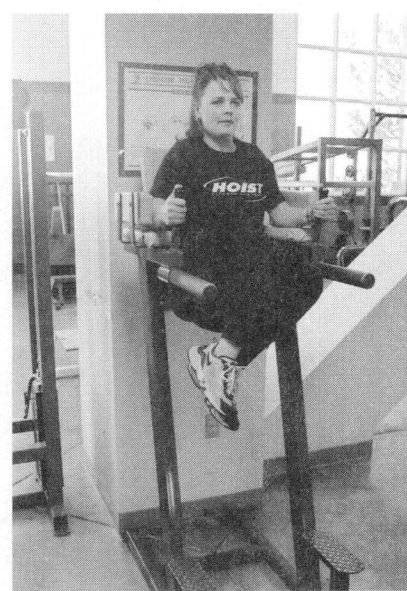

Bicycles: Work primarily the rectus abdominus, and internal and external obliques.

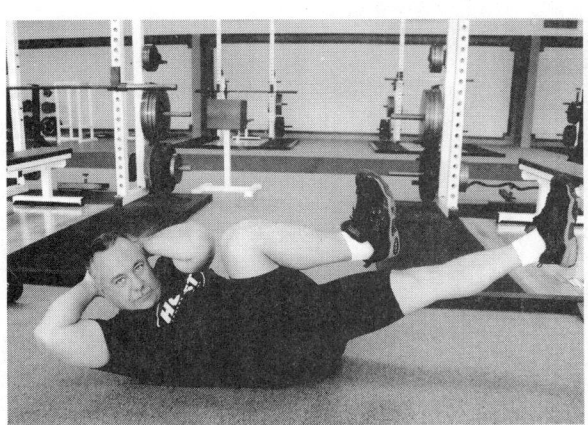 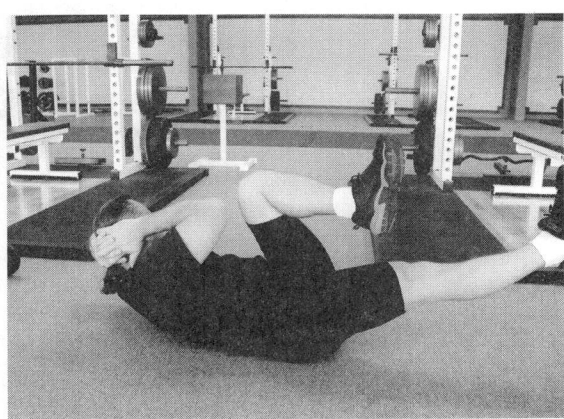

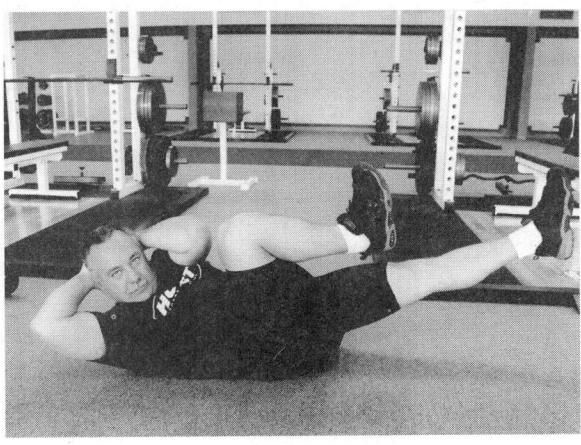

Leg Raises: Lying on the floor will work the hip flexors and the rectus abdominus. Keep the abdominal muscle tight and do not allow the low back to arch more than its normal range. Single leg raises are recommended if you cannot keep the abdominal muscle tight and maintain the normal low back curvature throughout the exercise. Keeping the legs straight will increase the difficulty of the exercise.*

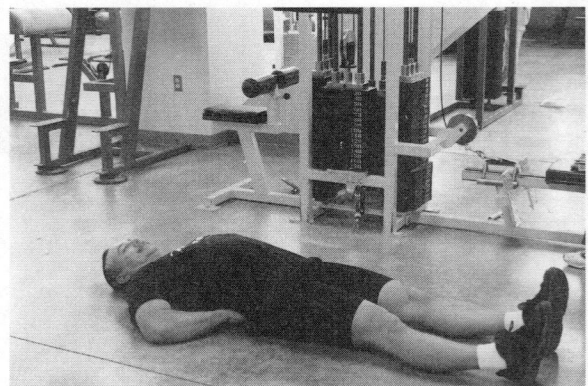 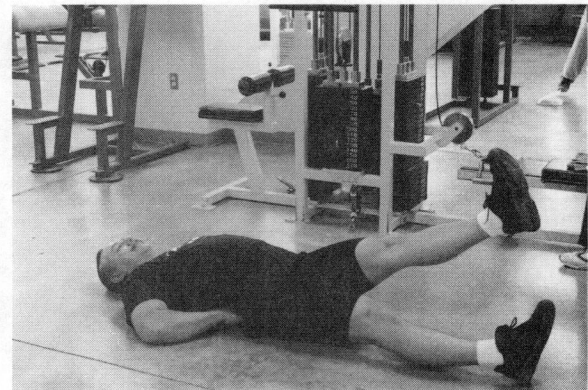

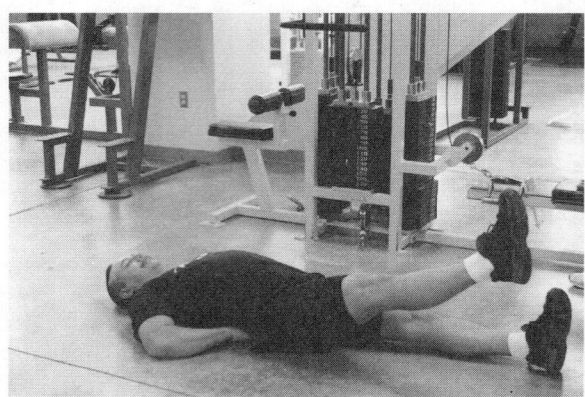

Leg Press Ups: Work the rectus abdominus and internal obliques.

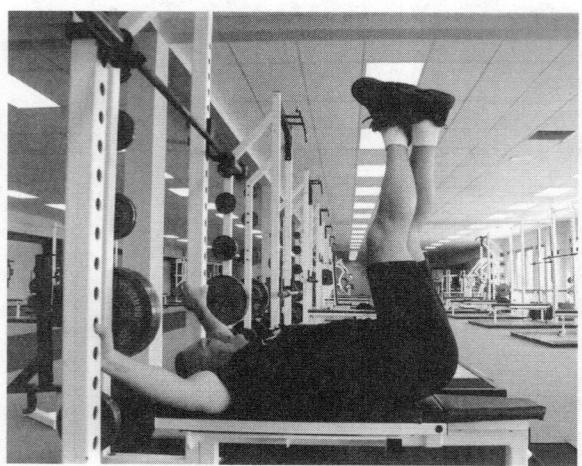 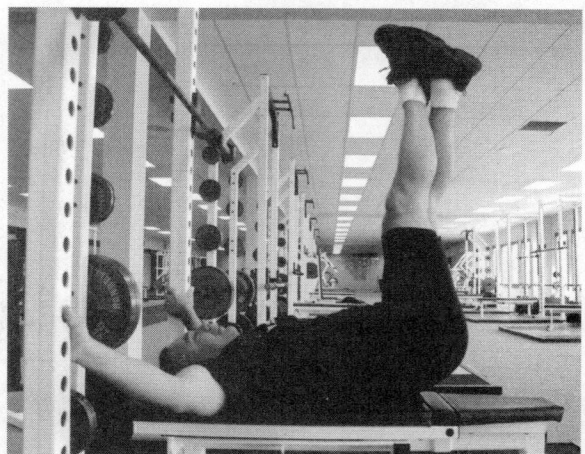

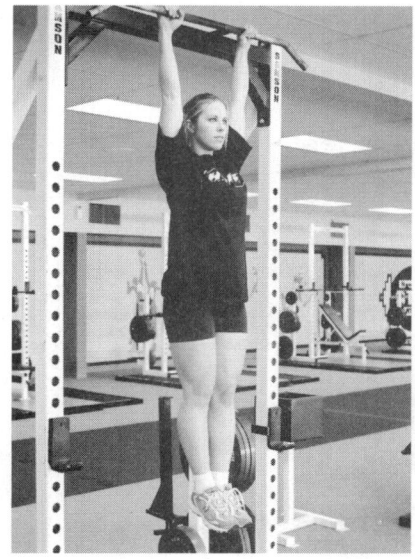 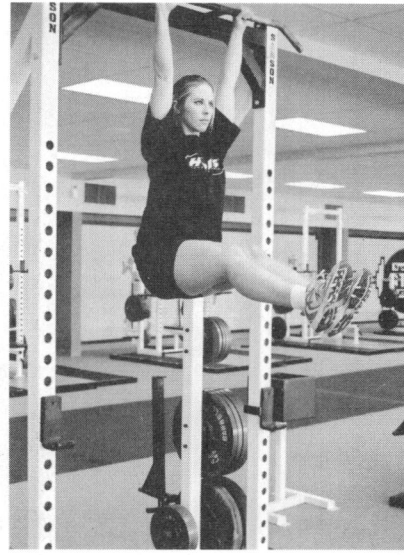

Hanging Leg Raises: With the knees at horizontal, this works the rectus abdominus and hip flexors.

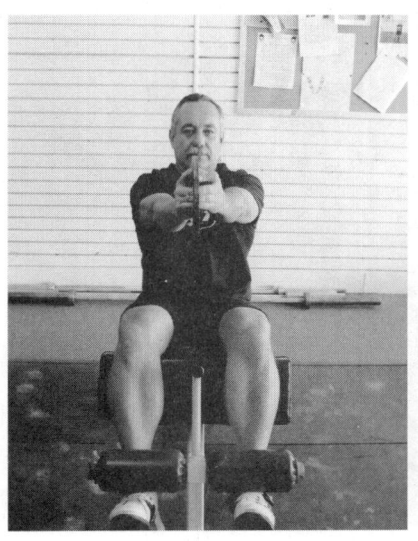

Start

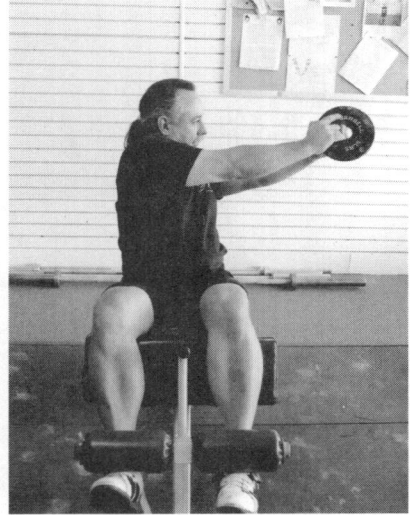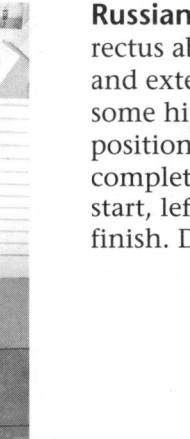

Left

Russian Twists: Works the rectus abdominus, internal and external obliques, and some hip flexors. Hold each position for 10 seconds. One complete rep would include start, left, center, right, and finish. Do 20 reps.

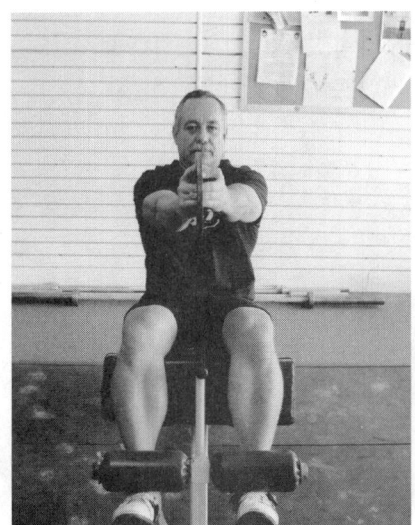

Center

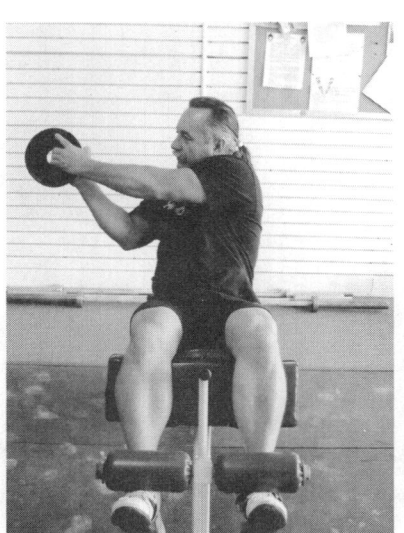

Right

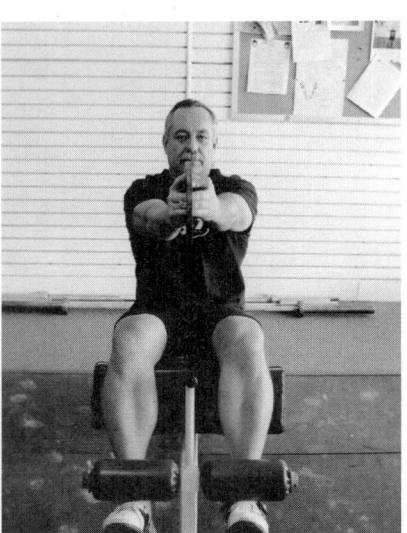

Finish

Obliques

Flexion Twists with a Stick: Work the external and internal obliques and some rectus abdominus. This exercise may be done either sitting or standing.

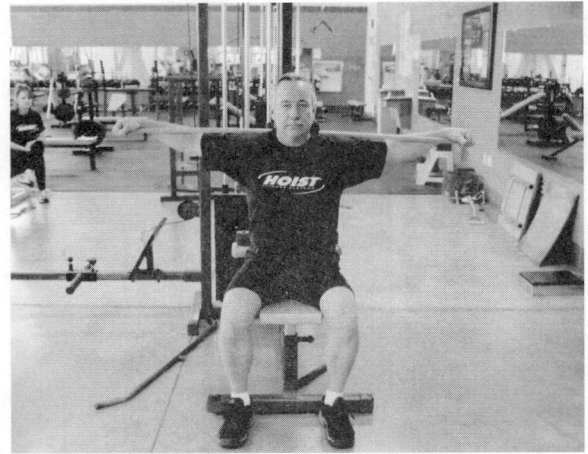
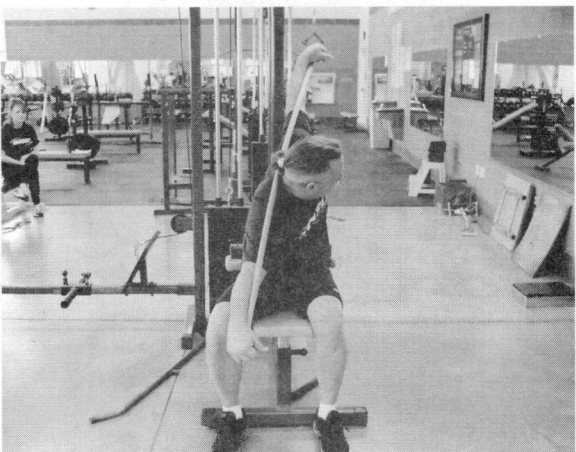

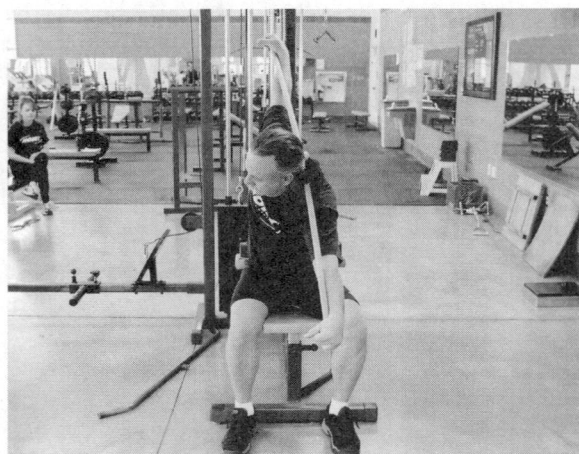
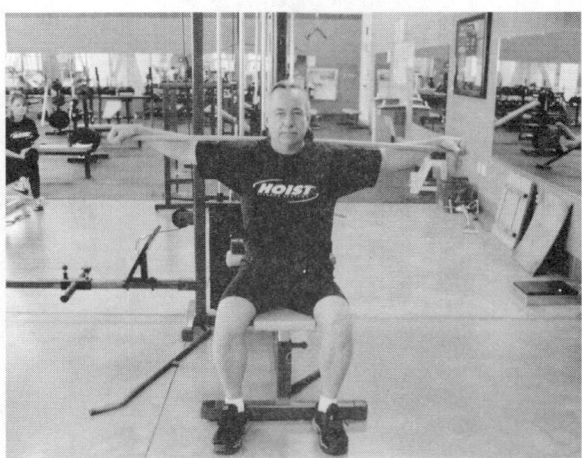

Dumbbell Side Bends: Work the obliques, some rectus abdominus, and quadratus lumborum. The muscles of the side bending are the muscles working and responsible for lateral flexion.

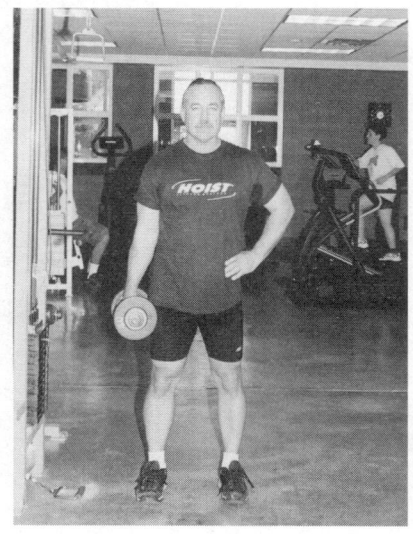
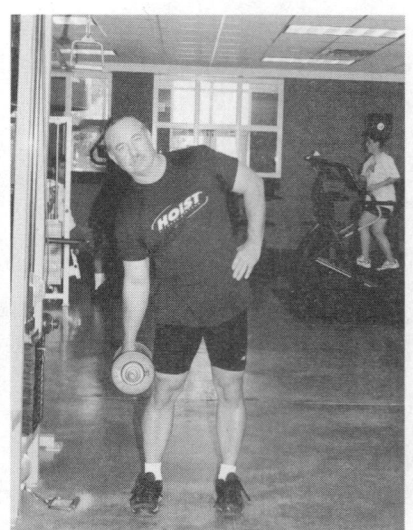

Cable Side Bends: Work the obliques, some rectus abdominus, and, quadratus lumborum.

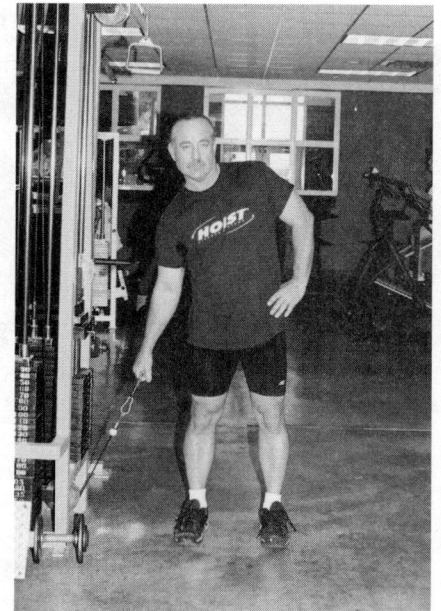 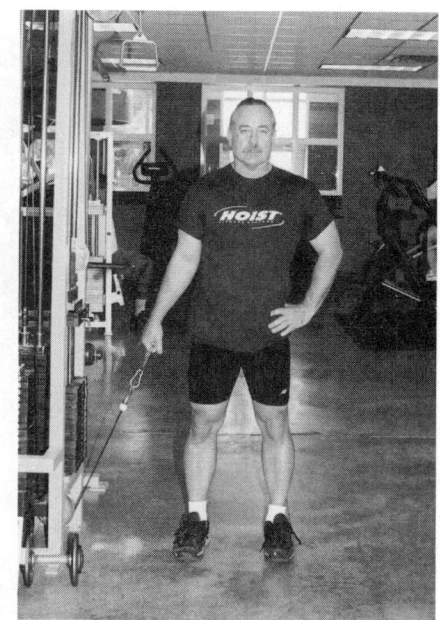

Machine Exercises

Machine Crunches: Work the rectus abdominus, obliques, and hip flexors.

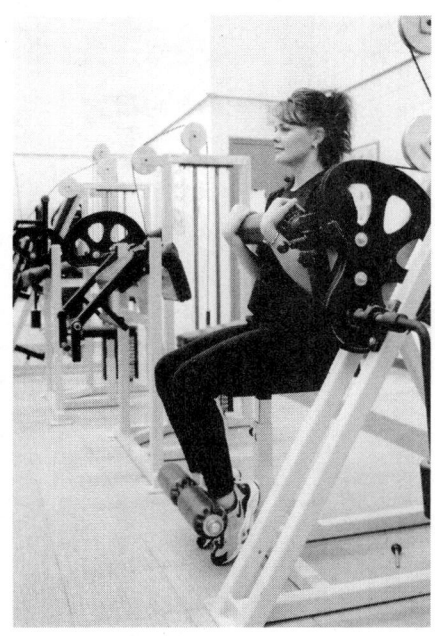 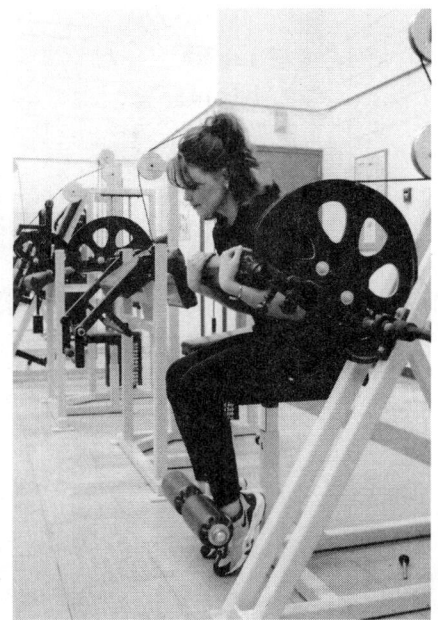

Cable Crunches: Work the rectus abdominus and obliques.

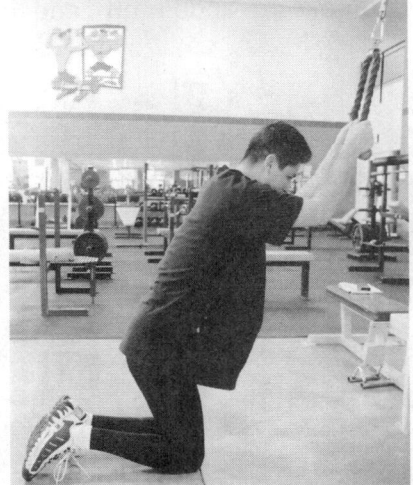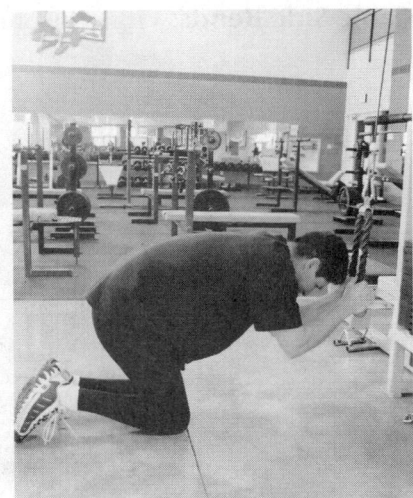

Cable Obliques: Work the internal and external obliques.

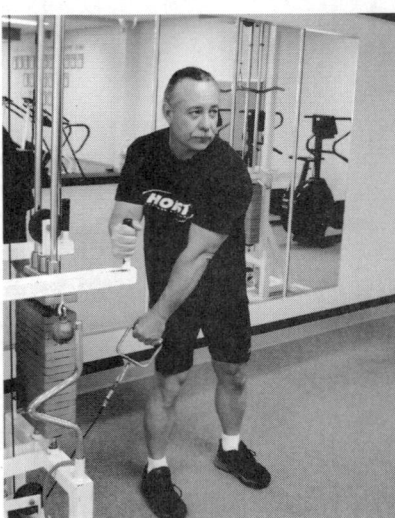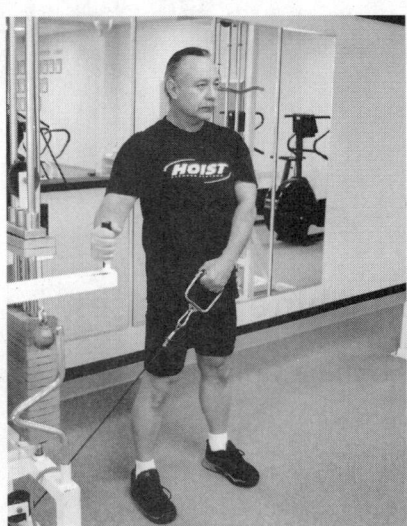

Low Back Exercises

Hyperextensions: Work the gluteus maximus, semitendinosus, semimembranosus, biceps femoris, (hamstrings) and erectors.*

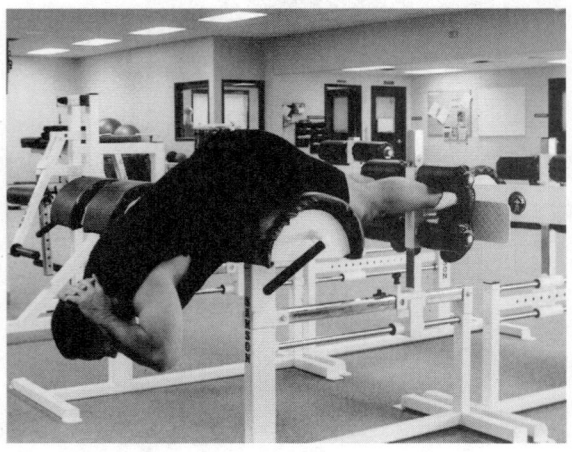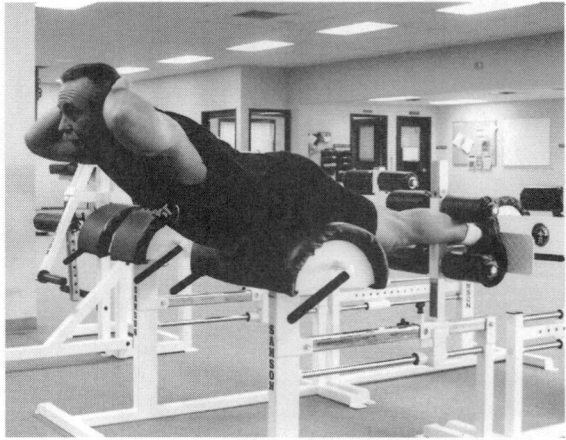

Reverse Hyperextensions: Work the gluteal, erectors, and the hamstrings.

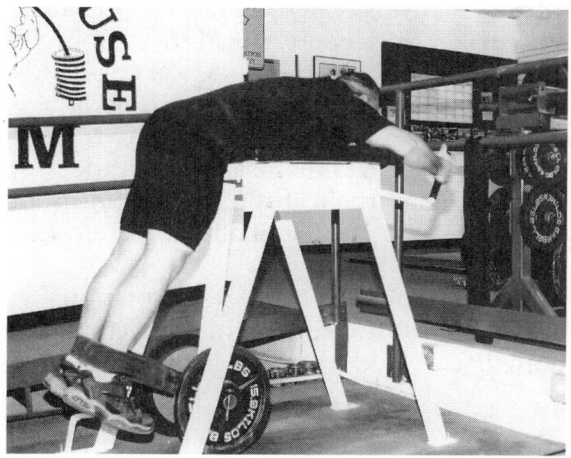 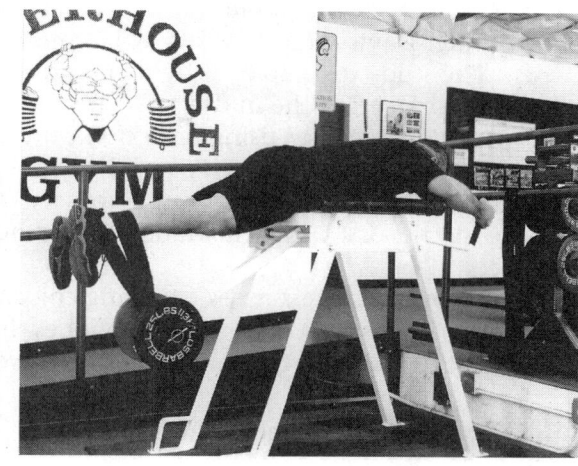

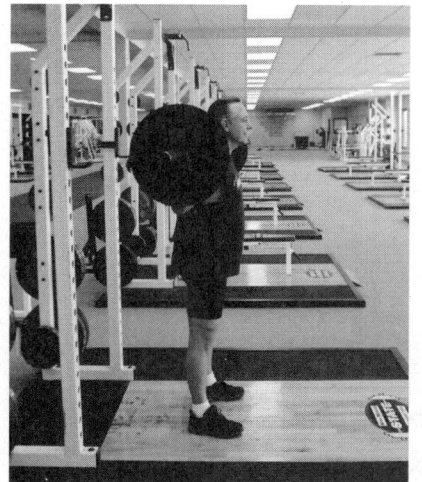 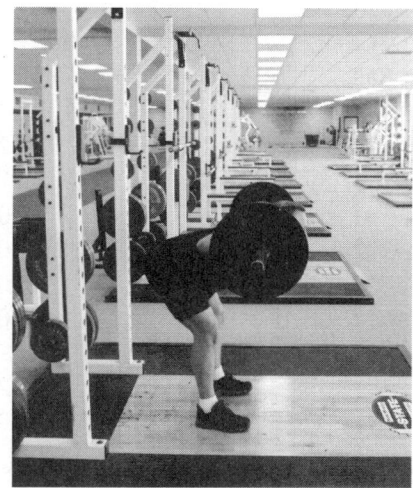

Good Mornings: Work the gluteals, erector spinae, and the hamstrings.

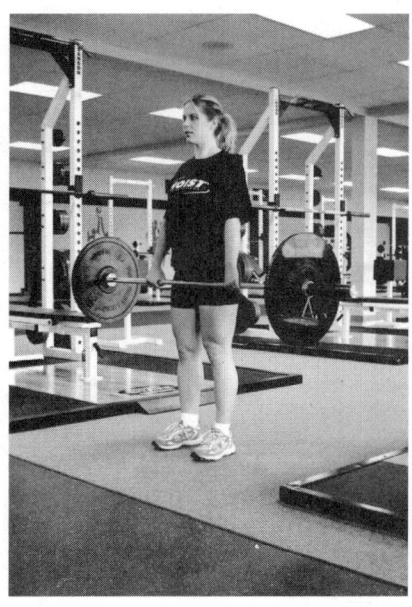 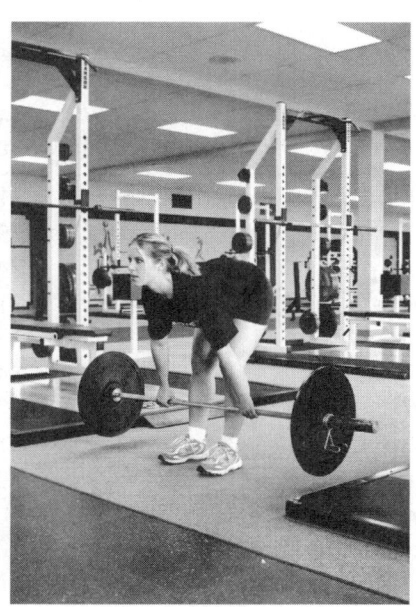

Stiff-Legged Deadlifts: Works the erectors, gluteus maximus, biceps femoris, semitendinosus, and the semimembranosus (hamstrings).

Which Ab Exercise Is the Best?

In a recent study done at the Biomechanics Lab at San Diego State University, researchers Peter Francis, Ph.D., and Jennifer Davis, M.A.,[1] looked at 13 common abdominal exercises and ranked them from best to worst. The study used 30 healthy men and women ranging in age from 20 to 45 years old, and included exercises targeting the midsection. Traditional crunches, modified crunches, partial body weight exercises, and exercises using both home and commercial gym equipment were explored.

Using electromyography (EMG) equipment, the researchers monitored muscle activity in the upper and lower rectus abdominus. Muscle activity was also measured in the rectus femoris to measure activity of the hip flexors. Using the traditional crunch as a baseline with a value of 100, the exercises were compared.

What was found is that exercises requiring constant abdominal stabilization and body rotation generated the most muscle activity in the obliques. In looking at the muscle activity in the rectus abdominus and the obliques, the following results were reported:

TABLE 7.1 Activity in Rectus Abdominus

Ranking	Exercise	Mean % of Activity
1	Bicycle Maneuver	248
2	Captain's Chair	212
3	Exercise Ball	139
4	Vertical Leg Crunch	129
5	Torso Track	127
6	Long Arm Crunch	119
7	Reverse Crunch	109
8	Crunch with Heel Push	107
9	Ab Roller	105
10	Traditional Crunch	100
11	Exercise Tubing Pull	92
12	Ab Rocker	21

Based on this study, the top three exercises for working the rectus abdominus (abs) are:

1. Bicycle Maneuver
2. Captain's Chair
3. Exercise Ball

TABLE 7.2 Obliques

Ranking	Exercise	Mean % of Activity
1	Captain's Chair	310
2	Bicycle Maneuver	290
3	Reverse Crunch	240
4	Vertical Leg Crunch	216
5	Exercise Ball	147
6	Torso Track	145
7	Crunch with Heel Push	126
8	Long Arm Crunch	118
9	Ab Roller	101
10	Traditional Crunch	100
11	Exercise Tubing Pull	77
12	Ab Rocker	74

As with any exercise routine, it is a good idea to vary the exercises that are done, to avoid stagnation and to train a muscle in all possible ways. Dr. Francis recommended that several exercises from the top third be chosen and done for approximately five minutes per day. Abdominal exercises are important because they help the abs maintain good posture and often alleviate low back pain.

Upper versus Lower Abs

Based on the EMG activity during the study on abs as reported above, Dr. Francis has concluded that most exercisers are unable to independently recruit the upper and lower abdominal muscles. The data from the study indicates that the upper and lower rectus abdominus act as one large muscle group, and not two independent muscle groups. Personal trainers and other fitness professionals have held that it is possible to work the upper and lower abs independently, although this does not appear to be true.

The "Six Pack"

As mentioned in the first paragraph, the six pack is a result of the tendinous intersections of the rectus abdominis, and is the result of genetics. The depth can be altered to a degree by increasing the thickness of the abdominal wall. This is done using heavy weights and low reps to stimulate the growth of the rectus abdominus muscle.

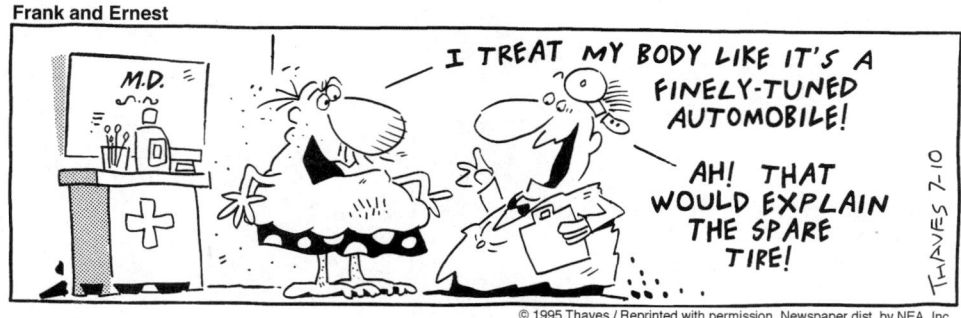

Frank and Ernest

© 1995 Thaves / Reprinted with permission. Newspaper dist. by NEA, Inc.

(*Asterisk indicates information from, "Strength Training Anatomy" by Frederic Delavier, Human Kinetics. This information is used as reference material.)

1. Francis, P., Davis, J., (2000?). *New Study Puts the Crunch on Ineffective Ab Exercises*, ACE FITNESS MATTERS, May/June 2001.

Please feel free to write on this page

True or False

1. _____ When working with the abdominal muscles, it is essential to let the muscles relax throughout each type of strengthening exercise.

2. _____ The erector spinae muscles run from the skull to the sacrum and are considered deep back muscles.

3. _____ The upper and lower rectus abdominus act as two independent muscle groups.

4. _____ Bending the legs will make leg raises more difficult to do during exercise.

5. _____ Exercises requiring constant abdominal stabilization and body rotation have been found to generate the least muscle activity in the obliques.

Multiple Choice

6. _____ The muscles of the abdominal area (trunk) and lower back can be divided into how many major muscle groups?
   a. 2
   b. 3
   c. 6
   d. 7

7. _____ Which muscle is not included in the erector spinae?
   a. Spinalis
   b. Latissimus dorsi
   c. Iliocostalis
   d. Longissimus

8. _____ Hanging leg raises with the knees horizontal work which muscle(s)?
   a. Rectus abdominus
   b. Hip flexors
   c. Internal obliques
   d. Both a and b
   e. Both a and c

9. _____ The top exercise for working the rectus abdominus is
   a. Sergeant's sit-ups
   b. Captain's chair
   c. Lieutenant's lunges
   d. Constable's crunches

10. _____ To involve more of the obliques during crunches, you should touch the
   a. right elbow to the left knee
   b. right elbow to the right knee
   c. left elbow to the left knee
   d. both b and c

NOTES

Please feel free to write on this page

Answers: 1. False   2. True   3. False   4. False   5. False   6. b   7. b   8. d   9. b   10. a

CHAPTER 8

Olympic-Style Weightlifting

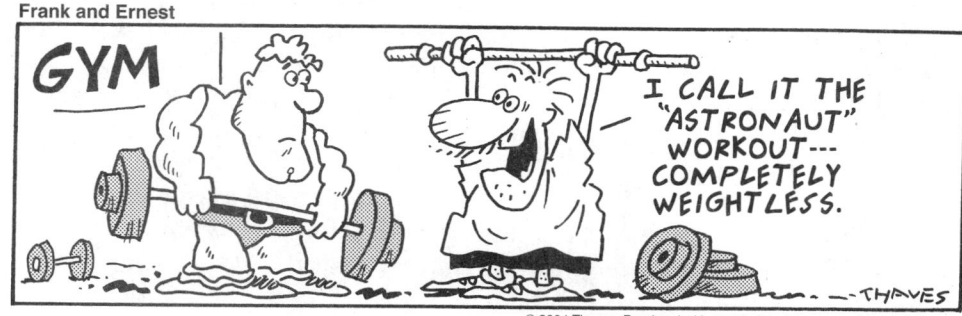

Frank and Ernest

© 2001 Thaves. Reprinted with permission. Newspaper dist. by NEA, Inc.

Olympic-Style Weightlifting

Olympic-style weightlifting is one of the best ways to get in shape, whether for competition or as an adjunct to regular weight training. Not only is it functional in that it works almost every muscle in the body, but it works for both men and women. The results you feel and see will be almost immediate.

Competitive Olympic Weightlifting

In Olympic weightlifting, two lifts are contested. The first is the snatch, in which a bar with weights is lifted overhead from a platform in one continuous motion. As the weight is lifted overhead, the weightlifter drops underneath the weight to catch it in a squat position and then stands up with the weight to listen for the referees signal to return the weight to the platform. The clean & jerk is the second lift contested; in this lift the bar and weight are lifted from the platform to an overhead position using two motions. The first motion is known as the clean; in this motion the bar and weight are lifted to the shoulders before the second motion or the jerk is attempted. In the jerk, the bar and weight are thrust overhead in a continuous motion and caught by extended arms. Again, the weightlifter must wait for the referee to give a "down signal," where the weight is returned to the platform in a controlled manner. Three referees judge both lifts, each giving a good lift signal (white light) or a no lift signal (red light). For a lift to be counted as good, the lifter must receive a minimum of two white lights. This is truly a sport for men and women.

Weightlifting History[1]

As a basic athletic activity and a natural means to measure strength and power, the lifting of weights was present in both the ancient Egyptian and Greek societies. Boosting its international importance chiefly in the 19th century, weightlifting was among those few sports (alongside athletics, swimming, gymnastics, fencing, wrestling, shooting, and cycling), that appeared on the program of the first Modern Olympic Games in 1896 in Athens, Greece. The first World Championships in this sport had been staged five years earlier, on March 28, 1891, in London, with seven athletes representing six countries.

Weightlifting is one of the only sports whose history in worldwide competitions spans three centuries—from 1891 through the 20th century and into the 21st century.

At the beginning of the century, Austria, Germany and France used to be the most successful nations. Later on, Egypt, then the United States of America, reigned. In the 1950s and the following three decades, the Soviet Union's weightlifters played the protagonists' role, with Bulgaria becoming a main challenger. Since the mid-90s however, Turkey, Greece and China have catapulted to the lead. The most recent world power in weightlifting is Greece among the men, and China among the women. Other Asian countries are emerging as strong contenders for the championship titles. Overall, however, Europe is the most powerful continent in competitions of both genders.

The International Weightlifting Federation (IWF) today comprises 167 affiliated nations. Approximately ten thousand weightlifters participate annually in official competitions; weight training, however, is an indispensable tool for strength development for all sports, and billions of people all over the world work out with the barbell for the sake of fitness. Entry numbers into the World Championships have increased year by year. The participation record was broken at the 1999 World Championships in Athens, Greece, with 660 athletes from 88 countries participating. Including the Olympic Games of 2000 in Sydney, the men have competed in 21 Olympic Games and 70 World Championships, and the junior men in 27 Junior World Championships. The women's first Olympic appearance was in Sydney 2000; they have participated in 13 senior and 7 Junior World Championships. The 8,000th medal in weightlifting was issued at the 2001 World Championships—to a woman in the 63 kg category—in Antalya, Turkey.

Weightlifting at the Olympic Games

Since 1896, weightlifting has been featured in 21 Olympic Games. In the sport's 21st Olympic appearance in Sydney, the program for the first time included women competitors as well as men. The most successful Olympic weightlifter of all times are Naim Süleymanoglu (Turkey), who won three Olympic Champion titles (1988, 1992, 1996); Hungarian Imre Földi is a record holder, being a five-time Olympian (1960, 1964, 1968, 1972, 1976), while American Norbert Schemansky is the only one who won medals in four Games: a silver in 1948, gold in 1952, and bronze in 1960 and 1964.

Weight Classes in Olympic Weightlifting

There are seven weight classes for women and eight weight classes for men in Olympic weightlifting. All measurements, whether body weight or weight on the bar, are measured in kilograms. The conversion factor is approximately 2.2 lbs. per 1 kilo.

The women's weight classes are 48 kg., 53, kg., 58 kg., 63 kg., 69 kg., 75 kg., and 75+ kg.

The men's weight classes are 56 kg., 62 kg., 69 kg., 77 kg., 85 kg., 94 kg., 105 kg., and 105+ kg.

Muscles Worked Using the Olympic-Style Lifts and Their Variations

Almost every muscle in the body from head to toe is worked when doing the snatch or the clean & jerk. The pectoralis major and minor, the biceps, and the extensors of the forearms will do minimal work in the execution of the Olympic-style lifts.

Coaching

If you are new to the sport of weightlifting, it is a good idea to seek out a qualified coach to teach you the correct technique. Not enough can be said about utilizing a good coach. A good coach will be one that has experience competing and coaching Olympic-style weightlifting. Coaches can be found through USA Weightlifting or the American Weightlifting Association, Inc. The USAW website (www.usaweightlifting.org,) has a section entitled "Contacts." Click on Contact and then go to USAW Local Weightlifting Committees (LWCs). There will be a list of all the LWCs in the U.S. Find your state and call the president of the local LWC to find clubs and coaches in your area, or click on the "Click Here" for USAW registered clubs. This will give you a breakdown of all the individual clubs in your state, and contact numbers of the clubs and coaches in your area.

How to Perform the Snatch

It is a good idea to perform the Olympic lifts on a platform designed for this type of weightlifting. A good platform will protect you and the equipment.

Of all the exercises in the world, the snatch is the most technically difficult exercise to perform. It is done using one continuous movement to get the weight overhead. Pulling the bar from the floor to the overhead position without a pause in between is the basis for this lift. Here is a quick checklist:

1. Make sure the bar is evenly loaded; use training plates if necessary (plywood disks, plastic disks, light Olympic size 5 lb. plates, etc.).
2. Approach the bar and position the feet hip-width or a little wider, with the bar over the balls of the feet.
3. Reach down and grab the bar with a pronated grip that is equal to the distance measured elbow to elbow when your arms are held directly out from your sides, similar to the position for a scarecrow. This is easily done with a cloth tape measure.
4. Lock the elbows and rotate the elbows forward.
5. While keeping your elbows locked and rotated, begin to enter a squatting position keeping the shoulders pulled back, not up. In the squatting position, your hips will be parallel to the floor or slightly higher. There should be an arch in the back at this point and it should be maintained throughout the beginning phases of the lift. Your shoulders should be slightly in front of the bar.
6. Keeping the body tight, the arms locked and the eyes looking straight ahead, begin to stand up forcefully out of the squatting position in one smooth and continuous motion. Insure that your hips and shoulders rise at the same rate.
7. Keep the bar close to your body throughout the movement and accelerate the bar as it begins its ascent.
8. When the bar approaches your waist, continue to pull on it, keeping the arms locked. Finish the pull and coordinate it by shrugging the shoulders at the same time that you are standing on the balls of your feet.
9. As your feet come off of the floor, shoot your feet out to the sides and begin the descent under the bar.
10. As you begin the drop under the bar, the bar should be moving up without any help from your arms. There is no pressing of the bar involved here.
11. Receive the bar in a full squatting position and catch the bar at arm's length, ensuring that the arms are locked. Once the bar is received and controlled and you are in the full squat position, stand up erect and then bring your feet back together so that the tips of the toes are in a straight line with each other.
12. Congratulations! You have just performed your first snatch. With time and practice, the movement will become fast, coordinated, and powerful.

If you are truly a beginner and have never done this exercise, it would be wise to use a stick and practice the moves. Again, nothing can replace the value of a good coach when learning the Olympic lifts.

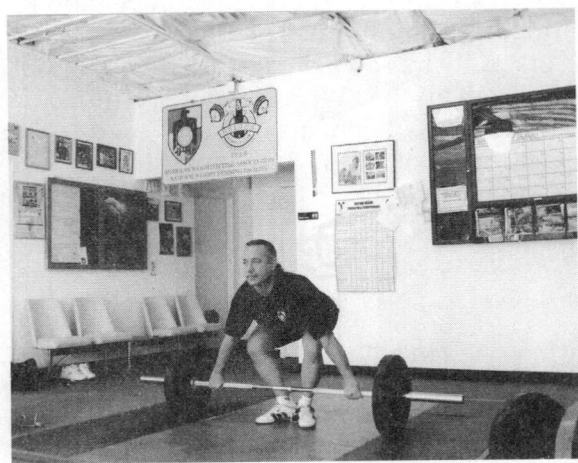
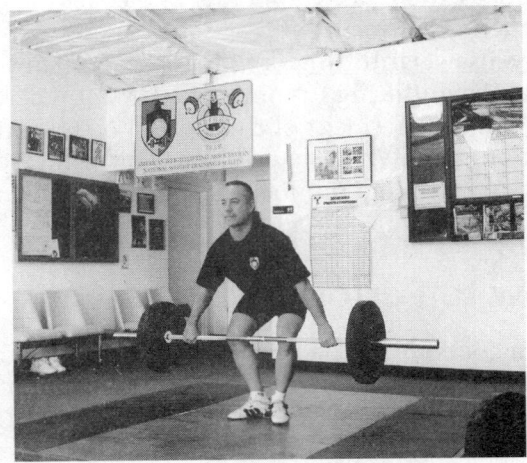

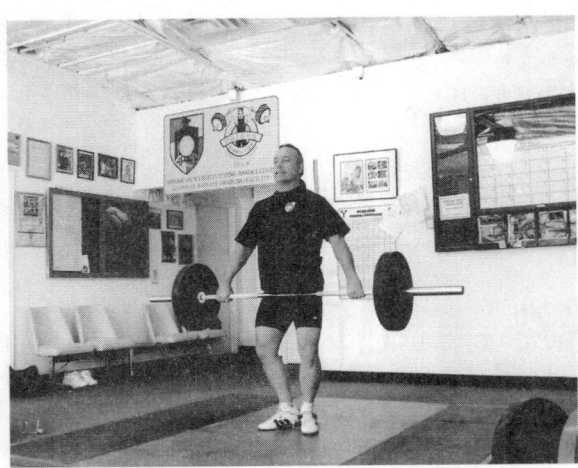
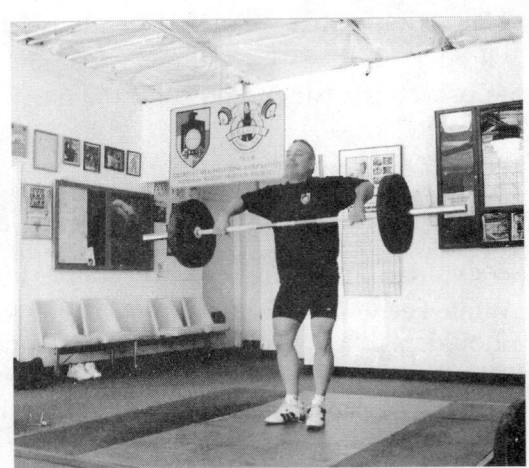

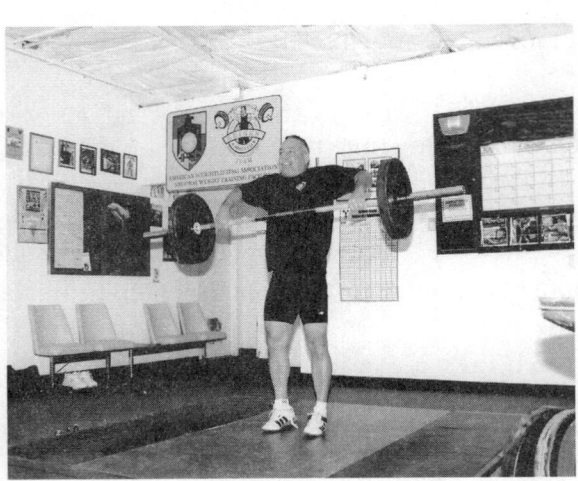
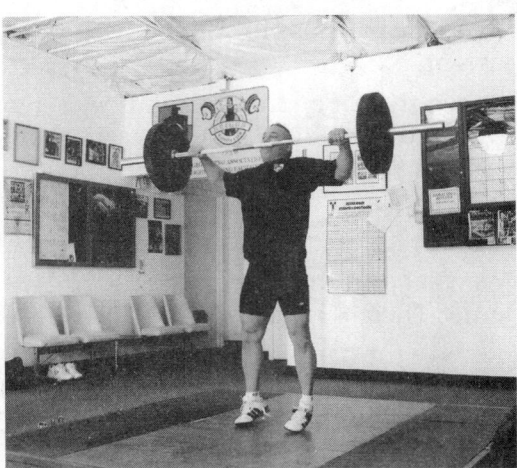

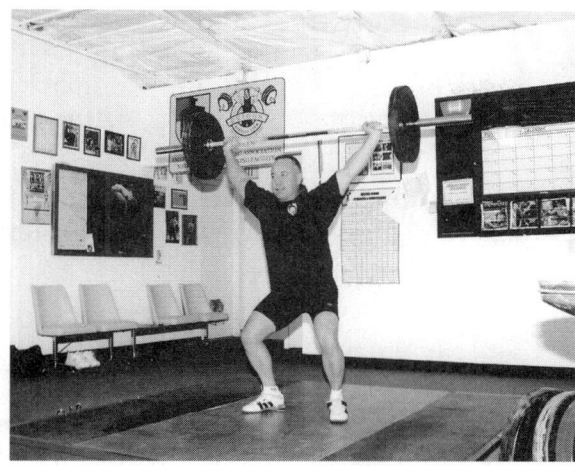
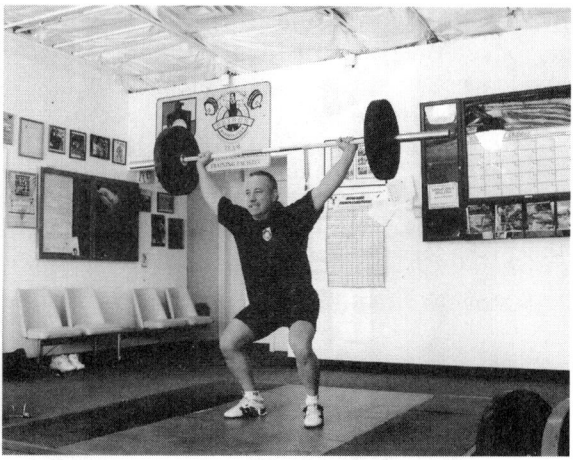

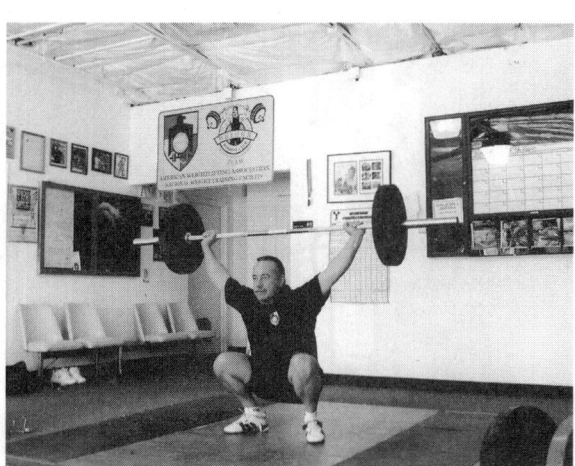
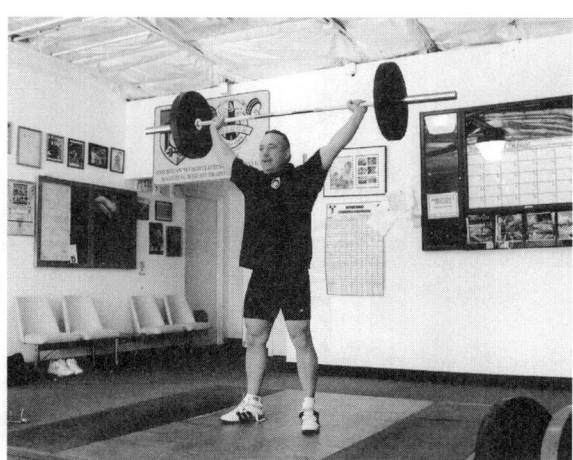

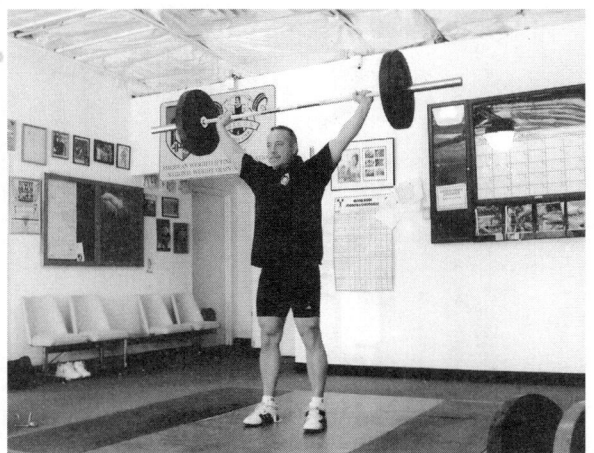

How to Clean & Jerk

The clean & jerk requires two separate movements to get the weight overhead. This lift is often referred to as the "king of all lifts," because of the amount of weight that can be lifted overhead. In the clean, the bar and weights are lifted from the platform to the shoulders in one continuous motion and received in a squatting position. After receiving the bar in the squatting position, the lifter returns to a standing position. The jerk is done from a standing position. In the jerk, the lifter bends the knees ever so slightly, resulting in a dip of the hips. The lifter then drives the bar and weight overhead in one continuous motion, using the power generated by the legs, and catches the bar and weight with the arms locked overhead, using a technique referred to as "splitting." After catching the weight, the lifter recovers or returns the legs to the starting position with the tips of the toes in line as in the snatch.

The first 10 steps of the clean are identical to the snatch, with the one difference being the width of the grip. The starting grip in the clean will be approximately shoulder width.

11. When the bar is received correctly, it will come to a rest on your clavicle and deltoids (shoulders). Your elbows will be up to the front and away from your side. There is an element of timing here so that the bar does not bang down on your body.

12. Stand up with the weight resting on your shoulders. This completes the clean.

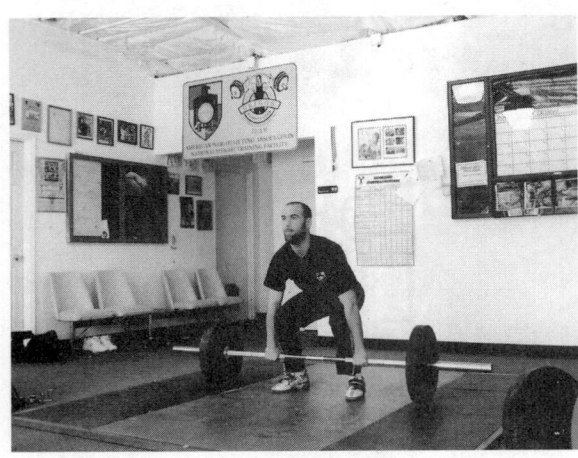
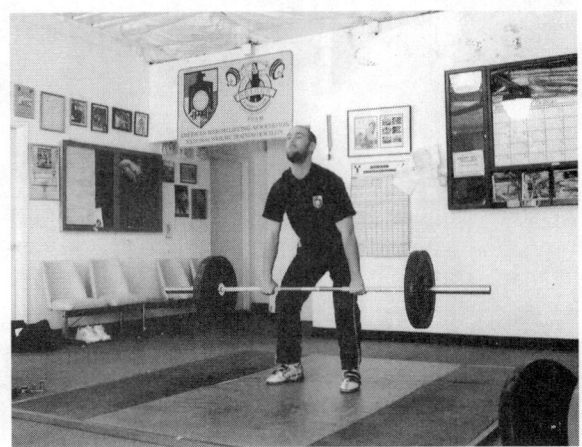
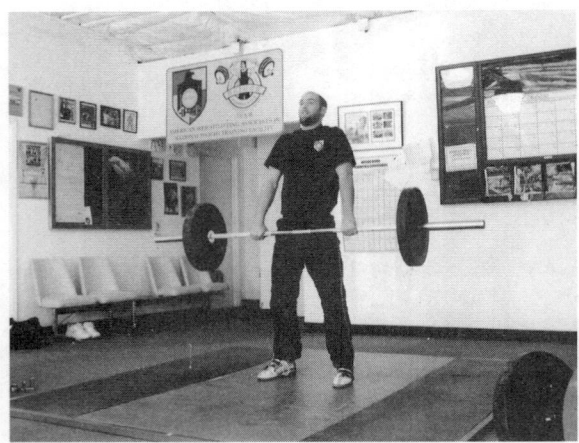
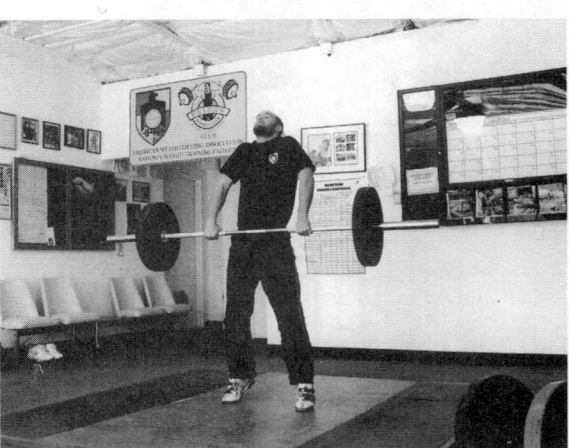
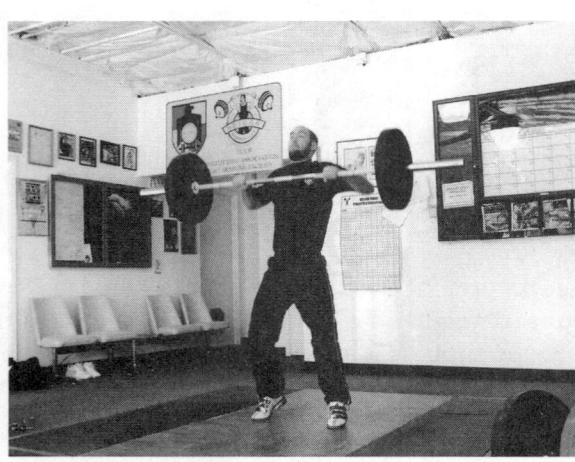
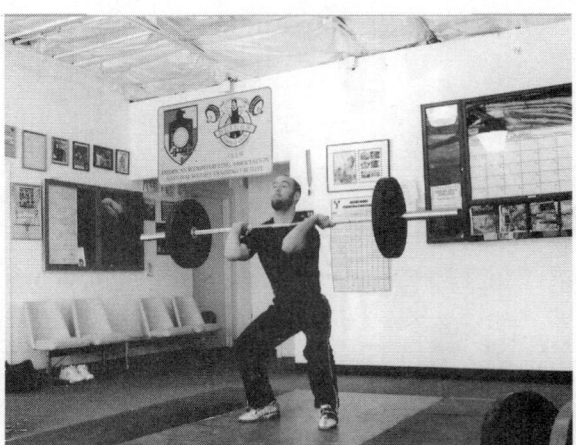

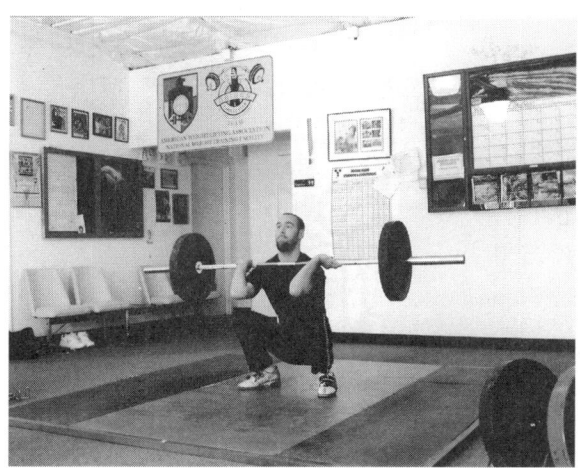
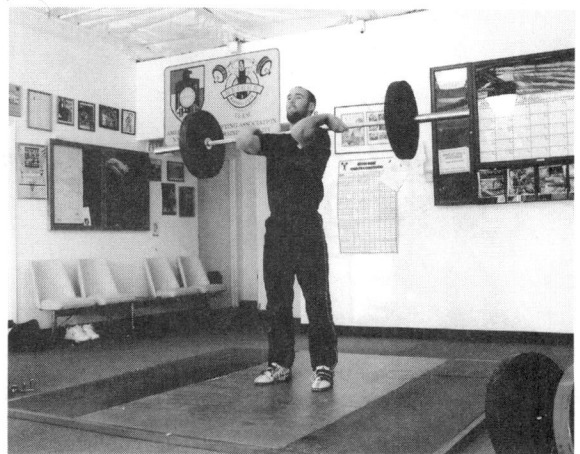

The next steps constitute the jerk.

13. With the weight racked on your shoulders and preparing for the second part of the exercise, the jerk, feel free to adjust the weight for comfort. Holding the bar lightly with a shoulder-width grip, begin to bend the knees slightly, ever so slightly, and then accelerate explosively upward, driving the weight and the bar up and off of your shoulders with your legs. The legs will provide the drive for the bar; as you rise, the bar should begin to travel upward.

14. Do not use the hands to press the bar, and do not dip into a squatting position.

15. As the bar moves upward, simultaneously drop under the bar and split the feet forward and backward, catching the bar with the arms locked out. The front foot should be pointed in slightly, and the back foot should remain straight and on the ball of the foot. The width of the stance should be such as to allow stability while holding the bar and weight overhead.

16. Recover by bringing the front foot back half of the distance from the foot to the body. Next, bring the rear foot forward and then bring the front foot backward to a point where the tips of the toes are in a straight line with each other.

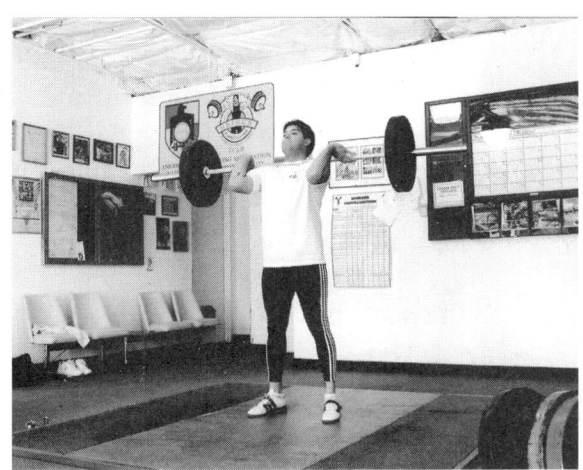
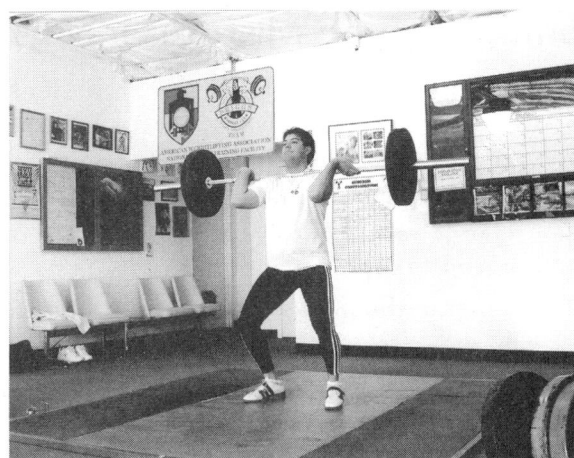

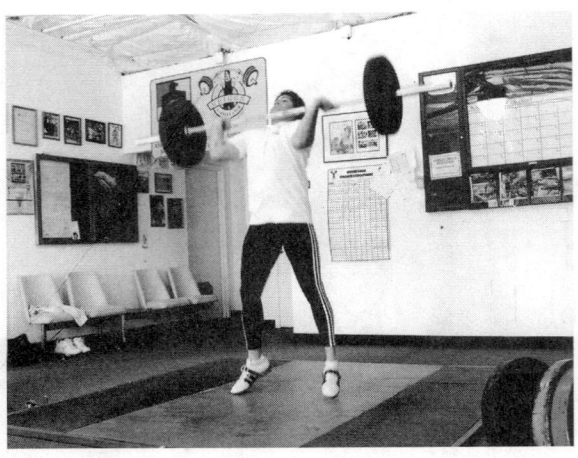 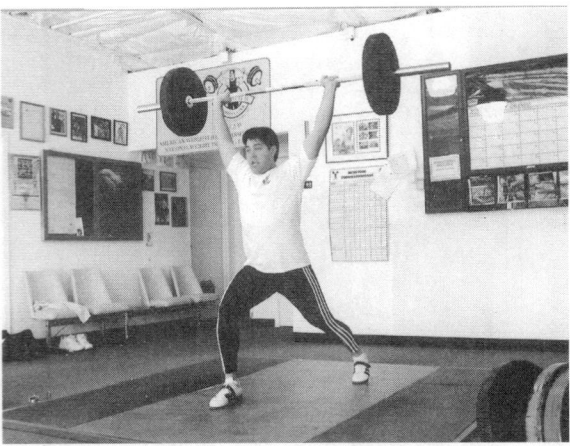

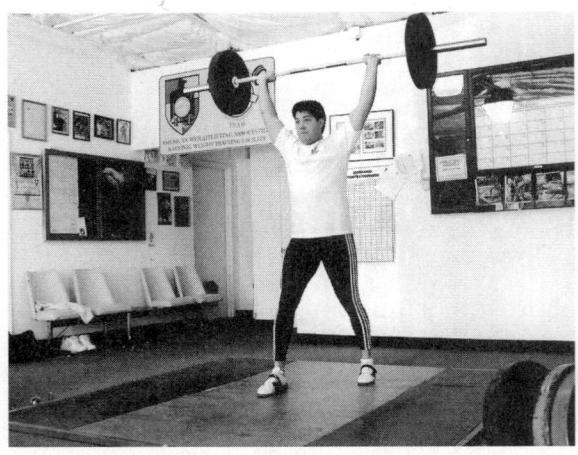 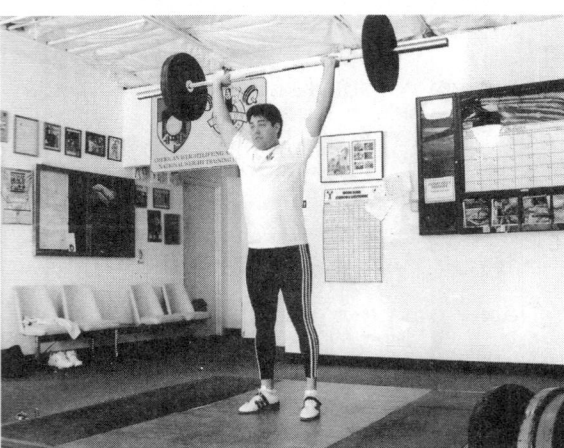

17. Congratulations! You have just performed your first clean & jerk.

Don't become discouraged, as it generally takes 5000 reps to become proficient in these two lifts.

Some Common Mistakes in Olympic Weightlifting

1. Press outs—if the athlete bends his or her arms at any time when the weight is overhead and then relocks them, it is considered a "press out."

2. Touching the arm or elbow to any part of the leg is never allowed and will result in an automatic "down" signal from the referees.

3. The weightlifter must control the weight once it is overhead, with the arms locked, until the referee gives the down signal.

4. No part of the lifter's body or uniform is allowed to touch the platform, with the exception of the feet.

5. The bar must move upward in one continuous motion in both the snatch and the clean & jerk. There cannot be any hesitation or stopping allowed.

6. After completing the lift, the weightlifter must wait for the "down" signal and, when it is received, must control the bar and weight to waist level. The bar and weight cannot be dropped from overhead.

7. The bar and weight must be returned to the platform to the front of the lifter. It cannot be dropped behind the lifter.

8. Breath normally. Always exhale on exertion. When beginning the jerk, inhale and expand the lungs. This stabilizes the bar and keeps the shoulders from dropping.

Assistance Exercises for Olympic Weightlifting

Snatch High Pulls

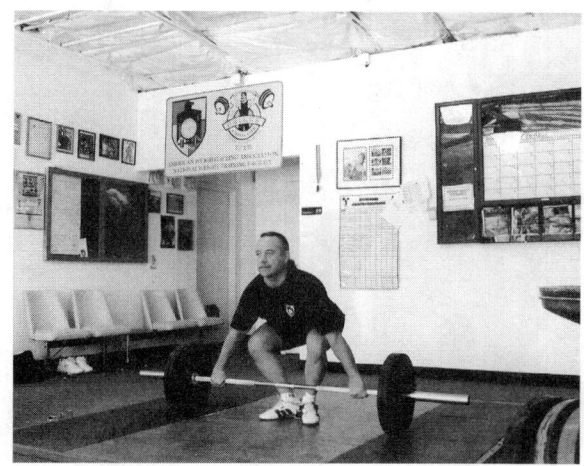
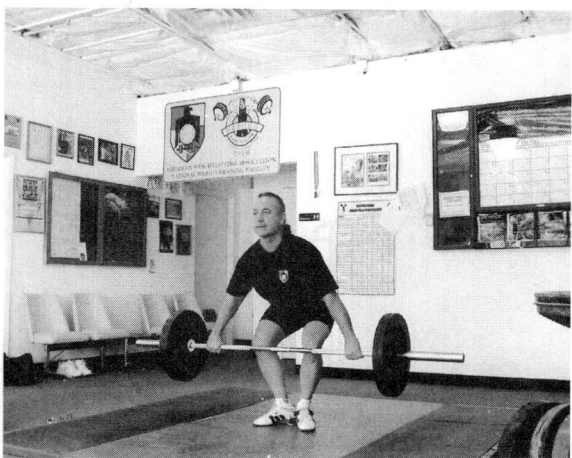

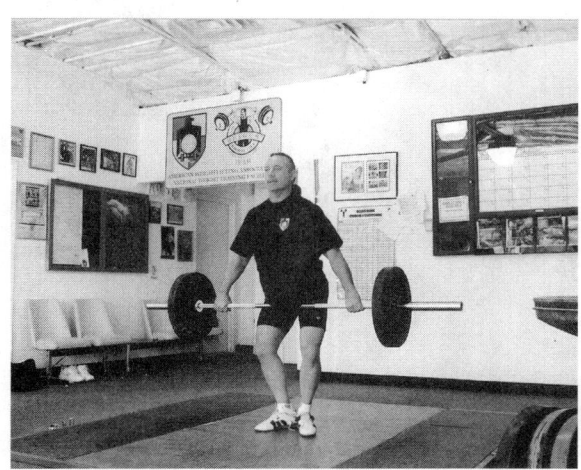
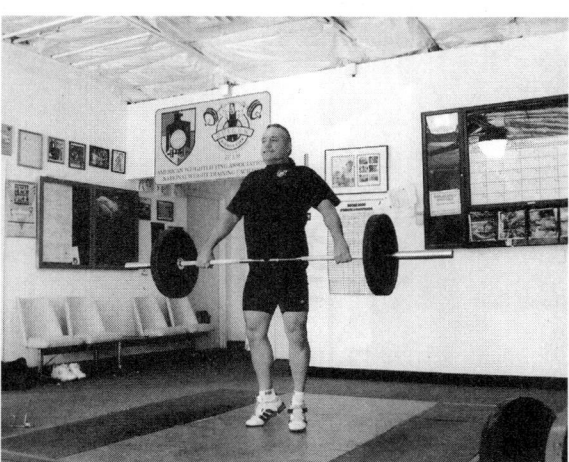

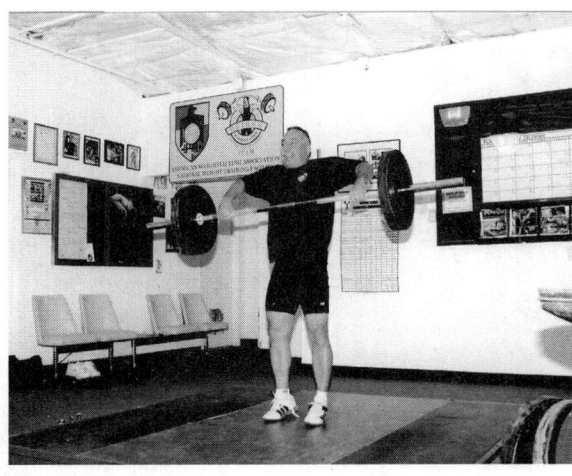
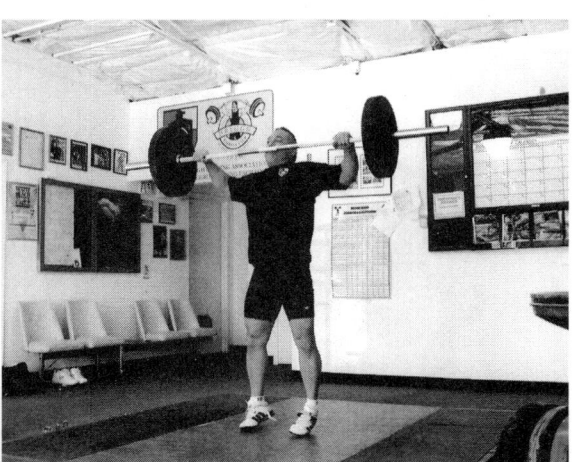

Clean Pulls

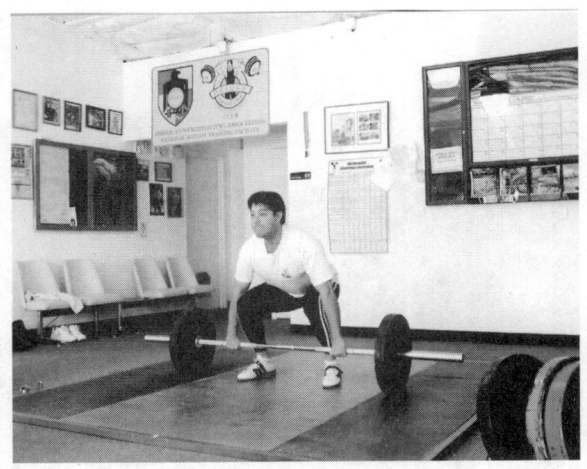 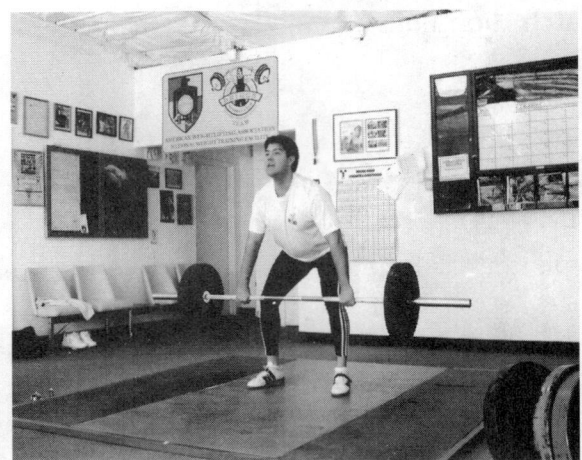

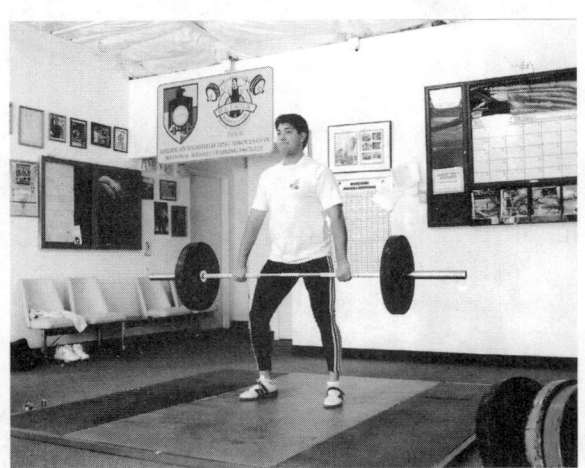 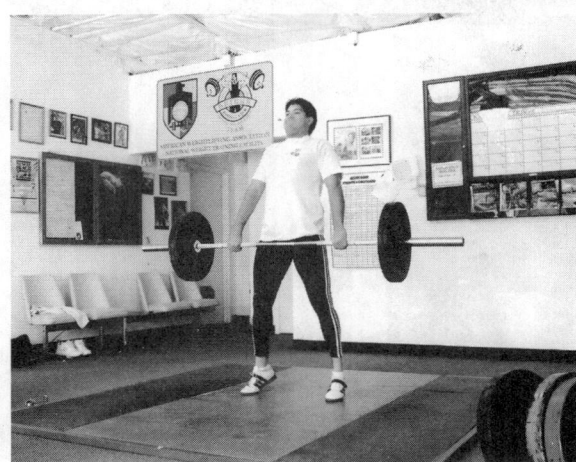

Front Squat

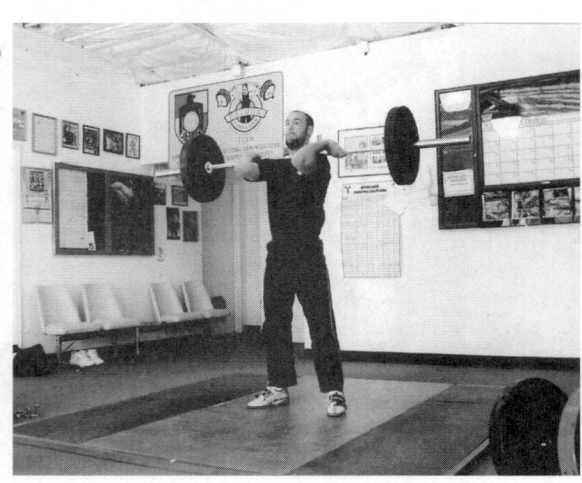 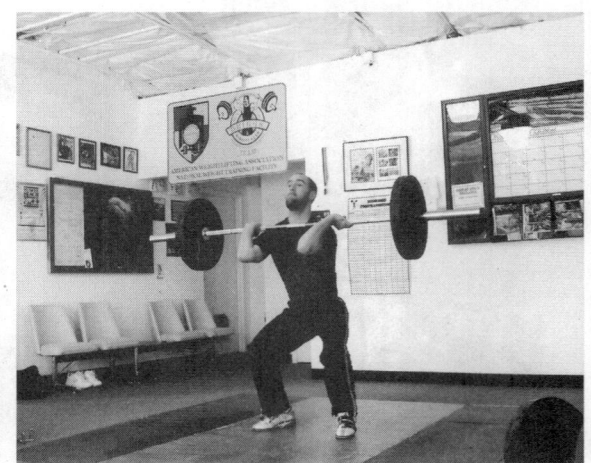

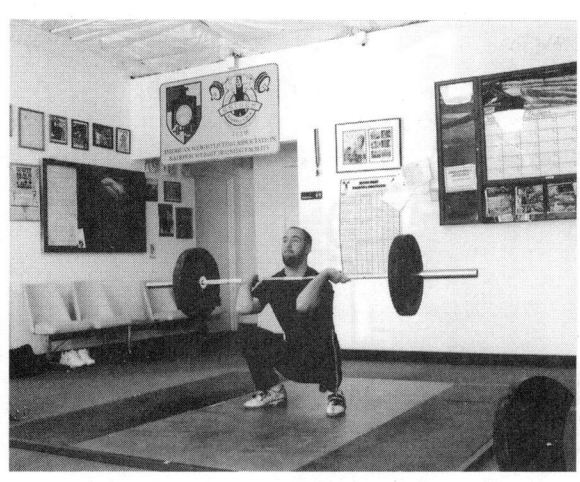
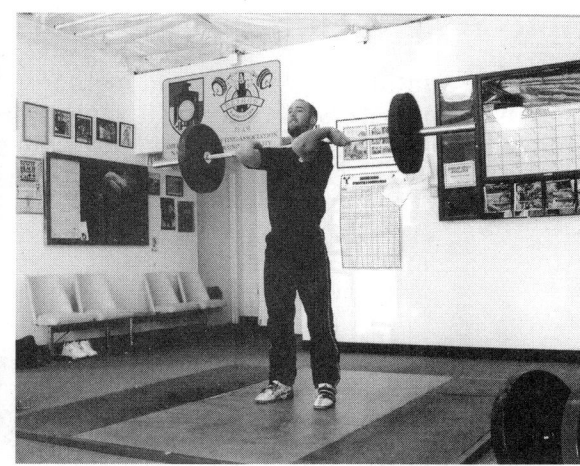

Overhead Squat

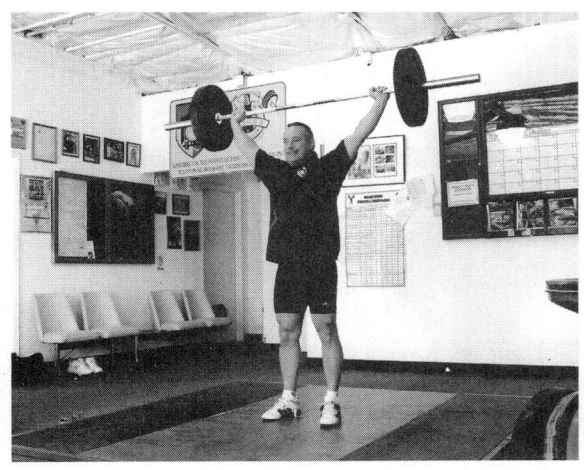
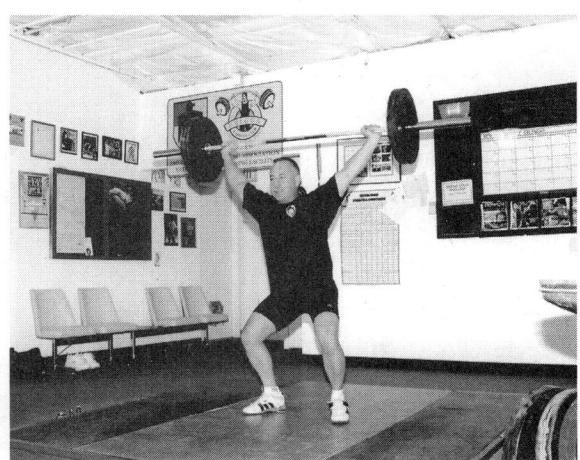

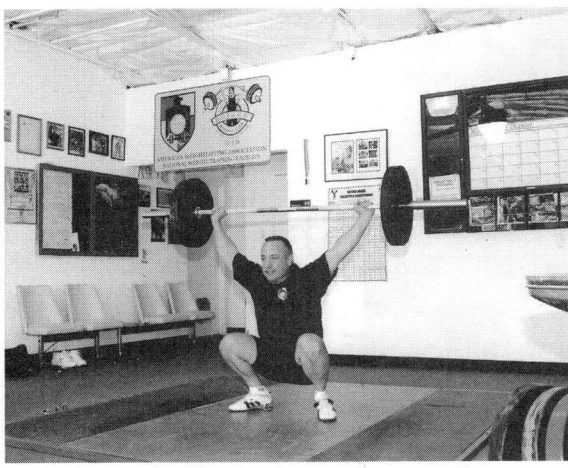
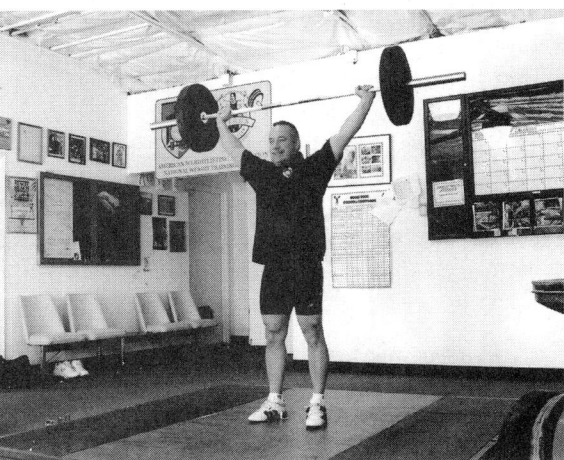

These are by no means the only assistance exercises for Olympic-style weightlifting, only a sample.

Olympic-Style Weightlifting Programs

Olympic-style weightlifting programs and methods of teaching them will be as diverse as the individuals who compete and coach in Olympic weightlifting. Find a good coach, work on the technique of the lifts, and gradually work into a program, advancing when your coach tells you that you are ready for the next level. Most importantly, have fun!

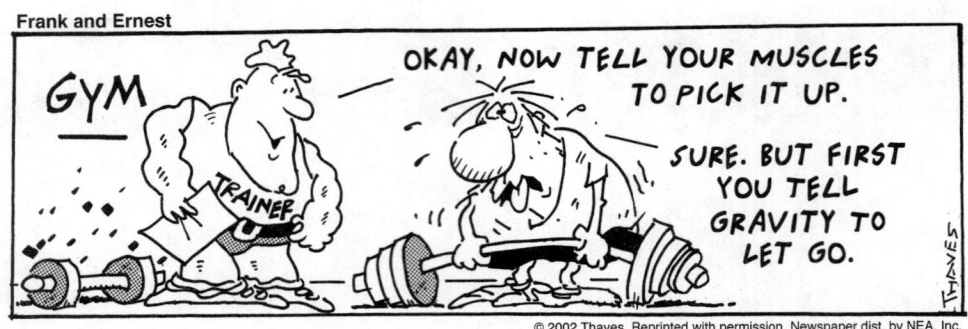

Frank and Ernest

© 2002 Thaves. Reprinted with permission. Newspaper dist. by NEA, Inc.

Weightlifting Organizations

The International Weightlifting Federation (IWF) is the governing body for world weightlifting and all the nations associated with it in the Olympics. Their address and phone number are:

International Weightlifting Federation
H-1374 Budapest, Pf. 614 Hungary
Phone: 36.1.353 0530
Website: www.iwf.net

The national governing body for weightlifting in the United States is USA Weightlifting. USAW conducts contests, seminars, and coaching clinics, as well as training at the Olympic Training Center (OTC) in Colorado Springs. Their address and phone number are:

USA Weightlifting
One Olympic Plaza
Colorado Springs, Colorado 80909
Phone: (719) 866-4508
Website: www.usaweightlifting.org

Another weightlifting association in the United States that conducts contests, seminars, clinics, and other events is the American Weightlifting Association, Inc. (AWA). The AWA is a grass roots organization founded in 1986 that believes in weightlifting for fun and sport. It is open to all ages. Their address and phone number are:

American Weightlifting Association, Inc.
721 Cheltenham Drive
El Paso, Texas 79912
(915) 845-2770
Website: www.americanweightlifting.bigstep.com

1. International Weightlifting Federation (2003). *Weightlifting History*. [On-line]. Available: www.iwf.net.

CHAPTER 8 SELF TEST

Please feel free to write on this page

True or False

1. _____ Olympic-style weightlifting is functional in that it works almost every muscle in the body.

2. _____ The arms are used to push the weights up in the snatch.

Multiple Choice

3. _____ In Olympic-style weightlifting, what 2 lifts are performed in competition?
   a. bench press / squat
   b. snatch / clean & jerk
   c. clean and jerk / bench press
   d. squat / clean and jerk

4. _____ Which muscles of the body do minimal work while performing Olympic-style lifts?
   a. pectoralis major and minor
   b. biceps brachii
   c. extensors of the forearms
   d. all of the above

5. _____ In competition, how many referees judge the lifts?
   a. 1
   b. 2
   c. 3
   d. 5

6. _____ At the end of the clean in the clean & jerk, where should the bar be resting on the body?
   a. above the head
   b. on the back of the shoulders
   c. on the clavicle and deltoids
   d. at the waist

7. _____ What year was the first world championship held?
   a. 1876
   b. 1891
   c. 1896
   d. 1996

8. _____ Where were the first modern Olympics held?
   a. London
   b. Rome
   c. Paris
   d. Athens

9. _____ How many weight classes are there for men?
   a. 3
   b. 5
   c. 7
   d. 8

10. _____ How many weight classes are there for women?
   a. 3
   b. 5
   c. 7
   d. 8

11. _____ At what Olympics did women first appear in the weightlifting competition?
   a. 2000 Sydney
   b. 1996 Atlanta
   c. 1992 Barcelona
   d. 1988 Korea

Please feel free to write on this page

Answers: 1. True   2. False   3. b   4. d   5. c   6. c   7. b   8. d   9. d   10. c   11. a

CHAPTER 9

Weight Training Programs

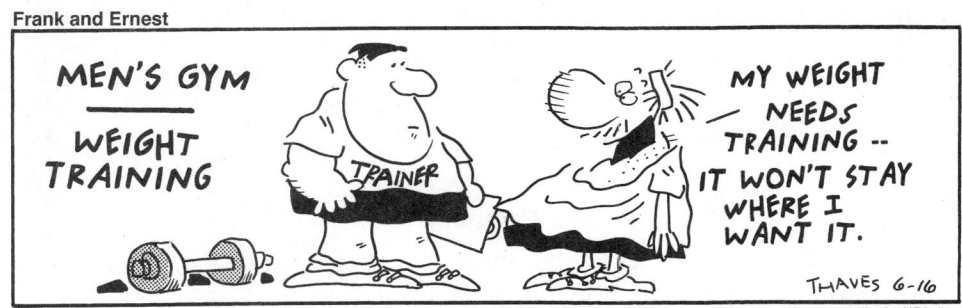

Frank and Ernest

© 1994 Thaves / Reprinted with permission. Newspaper dist. by NEA, Inc.

Training Is Specific

The #1 rule of weight training is that training is specific. What this means is that if you want to be a bodybuilder, you have to train like a bodybuilder, not a football player. Training is specific. You cannot train using a football program from high school or any other program for that matter, and become a bodybuilder. Your program must be a bodybuilding program, your diet must be a bodybuilding diet, and your lifestyle must be a bodybuilding lifestyle. This rule holds true for any other sport as well. An Olympic weightlifting program will not make you a powerlifter, and vice-versa, a program for heptathletes will not make you a decathlete, and a modern dance program will not make you a ballerina. You get the idea: training programs are different for every sport.

The one exception to this rule would be if you used a "cross-training" program. What this will do is make you a "well rounded" athlete and enhance your skills at a number of different sports, but an athlete that does not excel in any particular sport. In the case of triathletes, they are good at running, swimming, and biking, but if you took the same caliber athlete that trained in only one event such as running, that athlete would invariably beat the triathlete in running. The triathlete in a triathlon would beat the runner.

Decide what your goals are, and design a program to meet those goals. There is no such thing as a bad program, considering the choice between doing nothing as opposed to doing something, but there are some programs that are better than others. Always change your program every 4 to 6 weeks to keep the body and mind from becoming stagnant. Change means you would alter the sets, weight, or exercise order. Confuse the body and keep it guessing. That is how you will make progress. Do not expect miracles overnight. If you can work out for a year regularly, working out will become a lifestyle and you will miss working out if you take any time off. Another amazing benefit that will become apparent is that, as your diet improves, your cravings for "junk food" will decrease. No longer will you be running to the store for a donut, or Taco Bell, or Burger King; in fact, most junk foods will almost make you sick, because of the high sugar and/or fat content.

Cardio Before or After a Workout

The question of cardio before or after a workout comes up often, and the answer depends on what your goals are and what type of a training program you are using. Generally, if you are involved in a weight-training program, it is better to do the majority of your cardio workout *after* your weight-training workout. It is perfectly acceptable to do 5 to 10 minutes before a weight-training workout as a warm-up, but the majority of your cardio workout should come *after* your weightlifting routine. If you do too intense of a cardio workout before the normal weightlifting routine, you will find that you are unable to push as hard. You will have exhausted some of your energy stores, and this will affect your ability to push the weights with as much effort and enthusiasm.

Good ways to warm up are easy to find and can be done without too much effort. The goal is to elevate the heart rate, warm the body, and lubricate the joints. Some ideas:

1. Ride a bike between classes
2. Skateboard
3. Walk at a fast pace before your weight training session
4. Run in place
5. Run, jog, or walk the stairs in a building, stadium, or other facility
6. Use a stepper, treadmill, stationary bike, or other similar gym apparatus
7. Do a dynamic warm up, where you use your exercises as a part of your warm-up plan

To Stretch or Not to Stretch

Stretching is a personal preference, but not a good choice for weight training. The main thing here is that if you choose to stretch, always *warm up* first. *Warming up* is without a doubt the most important element before working out. Never stretch *cold,* as this will only lead to muscle injury at some time, generally in the form of muscle tearing. As you read in Chapter 1, current research does not support the myth of stretching before working out, and in fact may cause injury and a decrease in muscular power.

Program Basics

Rule #1: Decide what you want to accomplish with your weightlifting program. Do you want to lose weight? Do you want to get stronger? Do you want to get bigger? Do you want to become more powerful? Do you want to accomplish a little of all of the above?

Rule #2: Decide how much time you have to devote to working out. How many days per week can you work out? How many hours a day can you devote to working out?

Rule #3: How motivated are you to start and continue a workout program? Do you find yourself have a hard time getting started? If it is hard for you to get started, then you might consider working out with a friend who has similar goals, or hiring a personal trainer. Many times, when others are depending on you as a partner for their work out session, you will be more motivated to make the effort to show up and work out with them. This may be especially true for working out if you are paying a personal trainer.

Rule #4: Determine your current level of fitness. This can be accomplished through various strength tests, body fat measurements, and endurance tests. A personal trainer will generally perform all these tests during an initial visit. If you choose not to hire a personal trainer, then at the very least, take measurements and record them for the following areas:

1. Neck
2. Shoulders
3. Chest
4. Biceps, right and left

5. Forearms, right and left
6. Waist
7. Hips
8. Thighs, right and left
9. Calves, right and left

These measurements can be taken using a cloth tape available at any fabric store. Record your height, weight, and bodyfat percentage. Bodyfat can be determined using skinfold calipers, bio-impedance, hydrostatic weighing, or Body Mass Index (BMI). We will discuss the pros and cons of these methods in another chapter. Repeat the measurements no sooner than at one-month intervals. If you are trying to lose weight, do not worry about the weight per se, but the inches, and how your clothes fit, instead.

Rule #5: What type of equipment do you have to work out on? Is it home gym equipment or do you have a health club membership? Depending on the individual, results will come quicker to those with a health club membership or access to a weight room, because it is more motivating to work out among other people using a wide assortment of machines and free-weights. Not only will you be more motivated when you work out around others and see their progress, but boredom is less likely to become a problem, because of the variety of equipment available for your use.

Rule #6: Start out slowly. If you have not worked out in a while, take it easy. Start with a full body workout three times a week, and build on your program as your level of fitness increases. For your first workout, do one set of one exercise for all the major muscle groups of the body. Rest 48 hours and do another workout using two sets of one exercise for all the major muscle groups of the body. Rest 48 hours and do a complete three sets of one exercise for all the major muscle groups of the body. Do the three sets per major muscle group three times a week for at least four weeks before moving into a more advanced program. If you have not been working out for a while, your body will be deconditioned, and will need the time to adjust to the changes. Do not be discouraged, as this is normal.

Rule #7: When writing a workout program, always work the larger muscles before the smaller ones; do complex, multi-joint exercises (snatch, power clean, clean & jerk, etc.) first in the exercise order, and work toward simple, single-joint exercises last in the order. What this means is that a squat would come before leg curls, or bench presses would come before dumbbell flyes, or shoulder presses would come before dumbbell front lateral raises, and so on. It will take a little time to figure this out so don't be afraid to ask questions of others who are more experienced.

Basic Terminology

1. Reps—short for repetitions, the numerical count within a set. Each complete movement counts as 1 rep. An example: When doing dumbbell curls, the starting position would be standing with one dumbbell in each hand with your arms full extended and to your side. You would then curl the weight up, and at the top of the movement (approximately shoulder height) you would slowly lower the dumbbells to your side (the starting position). This would be one repetition.

2. Set—a group of repetitions. For instance, three set of 10 repetitions would mean that you do 10 repetitions a total of three times, with rest between each set. Do 10 repetitions, rest, do 10 repetitions, rest, do 10 repetitions, and you have completed three sets of 10 reps.

3. Routine—the total combined reps and sets for any single workout.

4. Program—the total combined routines for any given cycle. This could be four weeks, six weeks, 12 weeks, and so on.

5. Cycle—the total combined programs for any give predetermined period of time. In the example of periodization, cycles usually last about 12 weeks and have three distinct programs within a cycle.

6. 1 RM—The maximum amount of weight you can lift in an exercise for one repetition, thus the name 1 Rep Max.

7. DBs—short for dumbbells.

Training or Working Out

Athletes train; all others work out.

Sample Beginning Plan

TABLE 9.1   Week 1

Body Part	Exercise	Day 1	Day 2	Day 3
Warm-up	Bike, Treadmill, Stepper, etc.	10 minutes	10 minutes	10 minutes
Chest	Bench Presses	1 set of 10 reps	2 sets of 10 reps	3 sets of 10 reps
Back	Lat Pulldowns	1 set of 10 reps	2 sets of 10 reps	3 sets of 10 reps
Shoulders	Shoulder Presses	1 set of 10 reps	2 sets of 10 reps	3 sets of 10 reps
Biceps	Dumbbell Curls	1 set of 10 reps	2 sets of 10 reps	3 sets of 10 reps
Triceps	Dumbbell Kickbacks	1 set of 10 reps	2 sets of 10 reps	3 sets of 10 reps
Legs	Leg Presses	1 set of 10 reps	2 sets of 10 reps	3 sets of 10 reps
Abs	Machine Crunches	1 set of 10 reps	2 sets of 10 reps	3 sets of 10 reps
Cool Down	Bike, Treadmill, Stepper, etc.	5 minutes	5 minutes	5 minutes
Stretch	Personal preference			

This program incorporates all the major muscle groups for an overall body workout. It allows a build-up time so as to keep the body from becoming overly sore, and provides for an adequate recovery time between workouts. This would be a Week 1 type workout plan. For Week 2, do the same workout as Week 1, Day 3 for all three workouts. Continue for one month and change the entire workout to include more variety and more difficulty in exercises. This workout could be started on a Monday, in which case the workout would be on a Monday, Wednesday, Friday workout plan. Another possibility is starting it on a Tuesday, in which case it becomes a Tuesday, Thursday, Saturday workout plan.

A Slightly More Advanced Three-Day-a-Week Program

In this program, we will keep the same format of Monday-Wednesday-Friday or Tuesday-Thursday-Saturday. The point here is to allow 48 hours recovery time between workouts while increasing the intensity of the three-day-a-week routine.

TABLE 9.2

Body Part	Exercise	Day 1	Day 2	Day 3
Warm-up	Bike, Treadmill, Stepper, etc.	10 minutes	10 minutes	10 minutes
Chest		Incline Bench Presses	Flat Bench Presses	Decline Bench Presses
Back		Lat Pulldowns	1 Arm DB Rows	Machine Low Rows
Shoulders		DB Shoulder Presses	Military Presses	Machine Shoulder Presses
Biceps		Barbell Curls	Standing DB Curls	Cable Curls
Triceps		Bench Dips	Tricep Pressdowns	DB Kickbacks
Legs		Squats	Leg Presses	Lunges
Abs		Bent Knee Sit-ups	Machine Crunches	Wall Crunches
Cool Down	Bike, Treadmill, Stepper, etc.	5 minutes	5 minutes	5 minutes
Stretch	Personal preference			

The reps and sets for this program would remain at 3 sets of 10 reps; however, for more variety, the weight could be increased for the second set of 10 reps, and again for the third set of 10 reps.

A Different More Advanced Three-Day-a-Week Program

Using the same exercises and exercise order above, change the rep scheme. Whereas before you were doing three sets of 10 reps, we will now change to three sets using 10-8-6 repetitions. As the reps decrease, increase the weight. Thus, your first set might be with 50 lbs. for 10 reps.; the second set would be with 60 lbs. for 8 reps.; the final set might be with 70 lbs. for 6 reps. This introduces us to a key training principle called "progressive overload." Progressive overload is the foundation for making muscular gains in strength and size. In order to get stronger, more powerful, and have bigger muscles, we have to "overload" the muscle and make it work harder. By doing this, the muscle grows to accommodate the increased load. If you are a woman, do not worry. Your muscles will not become as big as those of a man, due to the factor of hormones. The main component in this difference is testosterone, which is produced in both men and women. However, men produce considerably more testosterone than women.

More Advanced Programs

There are an infinite number of possibilities when designing weight-training programs. There are upper/lower body programs, push/pull programs, light/heavy programs, high rep/low rep programs, or any combination imaginable in between. These programs are referred to as *split programs* because unlike the whole body programs, you are splitting the body into different muscle groups for training.

TABLE 9.3

Day	Upper/Lower	Push/Pull	Light/Heavy	High Rep/Low Rep
Monday	Upper	Push	Light	High Rep
Tuesday	Lower	Pull	Heavy	Low Rep
Wednesday	————	————	Rest_____	————
Thursday	Upper	Push	Light	High Rep
Friday	Lower	Pull	Heavy	Low Rep
Saturday	————	————	Rest_____	————
Sunday	————	————	Rest_____	————

TABLE 9.4   Another Possible Combination

Day	Upper/Lower	Push/Pull	Light/Heavy	High Rep/Low Rep
Monday	Upper	Push	Light	High Rep
Tuesday	————	————	Rest_____	————
Wednesday	Lower	Pull	Heavy	Low Rep
Thursday	————	————	Rest_____	————
Friday	Upper	Push	Light	High Rep
Saturday	————	————	Rest_____	————
Sunday	Lower	Pull	Heavy	Low Rep

This program allows for more recovery between workout days.

All of these programs would be referred to as *split programs* because you are dividing up the workouts by body part, muscle action (pushing or pulling), weight (light or heavy), or reps (high or low).

In the upper/lower program, you would work all upper body on one day and all lower body the next day or next workout session.

In the push/pull program, you would do all pushing exercises one day (bench presses, shoulder presses, etc.) and pulling exercises (low rows, barbell curls, etc.) the next day or workout session.

In the light/heavy program, you would do light exercises one day and heavy exercises in the next training session. In a program like this, Day 1 might be chest done lightly and Day 4 might be chest done heavy. Day 2 would be back done heavy and Day 3 would be back done lightly.

The high rep/low rep program combines one day doing high repetition routines and the next training session doing low repetition routines. Generally, when doing a high repetition routine, you would use a lighter weight, and when doing a low repetition routine, you would use heavier weights.

A *double split program* would be similar to a split program, in that you would work two body parts in the same day. Unlike the split program, in the double split program you would train the two body parts at different times in the day. You might work the chest muscles in the morning and the back muscles in the afternoon. Another possible combination might be the biceps in the morning and the triceps in the afternoon. However you choose to do it, you would work two body parts in one day at separate times. After the morning workout you might have lunch and a nap, and then do your afternoon workout.

A *priority split program* would be a program where you would work on body parts that are underdeveloped or not developing as rapidly as you would like. In this type of program, you might work the chest muscles three times a week and the back once a week, until you felt that they were balanced. This program selectively places more emphasis on a certain body part than on others.

More Terminology of Programs

There are many ways to describe programs, reps, and sets. A few are listed here:

1. Single set system—In this system a person does one set of exercises for every body part, and 8–12 reps per set. This is a good system for those that are deconditioned, new to weight training, or trying to maintain a specific level of fitness.

2. Multiple set systems   This would apply to almost all systems used in weight training where the person does a minimum of 3 sets after warming up.

3. Circuit training—A system of weight training that works the entire body in one session. Typically, in this type of system weight training is done 3 days per week, with at least 48 hours between workout sessions. There are two ways to go through a circuit: (1) All exercises for a particular body part are completed before moving on to the next body part; or (2) 1 set of exercises is done for each body part until 3 sets of exercises have been done. The reps are usually in the 10–20 range and rest is kept to 30 seconds between sets. Sometimes there will be a cardio station between muscle groups that must be performed, like running in place, squat thrusts, mini-trampoline, and so on. This is a good way to work the muscles and cardiovascular systems at the same time.

4. Pyramids—A pyramid is a system of training where the reps either decrease (ascending) or increase (descending) or do both. Generally, as the reps decrease the weight on the bar increases, and as the reps increase the weight on the bar decreases. An ascending pyramid would have a rep scheme of 10-8-6-4-2-1, whereas a descending pyramid would have a rep scheme of 1-2-4-6-8-10, and a complete pyramid would be something like 10-8-6-4-2-1-2-4-6-8-10. The complete pyramid will exhaust your muscles and give you a good "pump."

5. Supersets—Work both the agonist and the antagonist muscles by altering the muscle group being worked, as in one set for the chest and the next set for the back, or one set for the biceps and the next set for the triceps. Generally, in gyms you will hear people say they are supersetting when they are doing two different exercises for the same muscle group. In reality, a superset would be doing one set for an agonist and one set for an antagonist, otherwise, it would simply be a compound set. For the chest, they might do a set of bench presses and then immediately do a set of flyes.

6. Giant Sets—This is a superset using three exercises instead of two. It might be something like this: bench press, lat pulldowns, and barbell curls.

7. Negative Sets—These are sets in which you use more weight than you can normally handle. In the case of a bench press, you would load the bar with more weight than your maximum bench

press and then slowly lower the bar to your chest. At this point, your spotter would help you raise the bar back to the start position. A spotter is a necessity when doing this exercise.

8. Breakdown or Burnout Sets—In breakdown sets you start with a weight and do as many reps as possible, then you or someone else removes some weight and you do as many reps as possible, remove some more weight and do as many reps as possible, until you can't do anymore reps or go any lighter in weight. This also works well with selectorized machines, by dropping the weight one plate at a time

9. Forced Reps—In this system, you lift the weights until you can no longer lift them, and then your spotter helps you get a few additional reps, usually two to four reps.

10. Partial Rep Sets—In partial rep sets, the lifter, when unable to lift anymore weight, will go to partial movements. In this manner, the lifter may do a one-fourth rep, or a one-third rep, or a one-half rep. Many times this will be seen in curling, and can go by various names such as "21s." In 21s, the lifter raises the bar from the down position to the half-way point seven times, and then from the half-way point to the top of the lift seven times, and then for a full repetition seven times—thus the name "21s." This can be useful when trying to work past "sticking points."

11. One body part per day/per week or "Blitz programs"—One body part is worked one day and then another body part is worked the next day, until all the body parts have been worked once in a week. Not much scientific validity to this program.

There are an infinite number of types of programs in existence, such as pre-exhaustion, compound sets, and so on. Try out a few different ones and stick with the ones that have some scientific proof behind them.

Rep Schemes

Generally, different rep schemes produce different results. These are just guidelines and not etched in stone.

- 10–20+ reps produce muscular endurance. It can also produce hypertrophy by using adequate weight to properly tax the muscle.
- 8–10+ reps produce muscular hypertrophy.
- 6–10+ reps produce strength.
- 1–5 reps produce power.

TABLE 9.5 Goal Based Load, Repetitions, Sets, and Rest

Training Goal	Muscular Endurance	Muscular Hypertrophy	Strength	Power
Load as a % of 1 Repetition Max	Less than or equal to 67%	67–85%	Greater than or equal to 85%	Single effort, 80–90% Multiple effort, 75–85%
Repetitions	Greater than or equal to 12	6–12	Less than or equal to 6	Single effort, 1–2 Multiple effort, 3–5
Sets	2 to 3	3 to 6	2 to 6	3 to 5
Rest between sets	30 seconds or less	30 seconds to 1.5 minutes	2 to 5 minutes	2 to 5 minutes

Information extracted from Chapter 18, *Essentials of Strength Training and Conditioning*, Human Kinetics, (2000).

If 1 Repetition Max (1 RM) testing is not possible, the 1 RM may be calculated using tables providing data and predictions for a given weight lifted and the number of times the weight was lifted. This same chart should also be able to tell you how many times you can lift a weight based on a desired percentage of the 1 RM.

Training Variables

TABLE 9.6 Estimating 1 RM and Training Loads

Max reps (RM)	1	2	3	4	5	6	7	8	9	10	12	15
%1RM	100	95	93	90	87	85	83	80	77	75	67	65
Load (lb or kg)												
	10	10	9	9	9	9	8	8	8	8	7	7
	20	19	19	18	17	17	17	16	15	15	13	13
	30	29	28	27	26	26	25	24	23	23	20	20
	40	38	37	36	35	34	33	32	31	30	27	26
	50	48	47	45	44	43	42	40	39	38	34	33
	60	57	56	54	52	51	50	48	46	45	40	39
	70	67	65	63	61	60	58	56	54	53	47	46
	80	76	74	72	70	68	66	64	62	60	54	52
	90	86	84	81	78	77	75	72	69	68	60	59
	100	95	93	90	87	85	83	80	77	75	67	65
	110	105	102	99	96	94	91	88	85	83	74	72
	120	114	112	108	104	102	100	96	92	90	80	78
	130	124	121	117	113	111	108	104	100	98	87	85
	140	133	130	126	122	119	116	112	108	105	94	91
	150	143	140	135	131	128	125	120	116	113	101	98
	160	152	149	144	139	136	133	128	123	120	107	104
	170	162	158	153	148	145	141	136	131	12	114	111
	180	171	167	162	157	153	149	144	139	135	121	117
	190	181	177	171	165	162	158	152	146	143	128	124
	200	190	186	180	174	170	166	160	154	150	134	130
	210	200	195	189	183	179	174	168	162	158	141	137
	220	209	205	198	191	187	183	176	169	165	147	143
	230	219	214	207	200	196	191	184	177	173	154	150
	240	228	223	216	209	204	199	192	185	180	161	156
	250	238	233	225	218	213	208	200	193	188	168	163
	260	247	242	234	226	221	206	208	200	195	174	169
	270	257	251	243	235	230	224	216	208	203	181	176
	280	266	260	252	244	238	232	224	216	210	188	182
	290	276	270	261	252	247	241	232	223	218	194	189
	300	285	279	270	261	255	249	240	231	225	201	195
	310	295	288	279	270	264	257	248	239	233	208	202
	320	304	298	288	278	272	266	256	246	240	214	208
	330	314	307	297	287	281	274	264	254	248	221	215
	340	323	316	306	296	289	282	272	262	255	228	221
	350	333	326	315	305	298	291	280	270	263	235	228
	360	342	335	324	313	306	299	288	277	270	241	234
	370	352	344	333	322	315	307	296	285	278	248	241
	380	361	353	342	331	323	315	304	293	285	255	247

TABLE 9.6 Continued

Max reps (RM)	1	2	3	4	5	6	7	8	9	10	12	15
%1RM	100	95	93	90	87	85	83	80	77	75	67	65
Load (lb or kg)	390	371	363	351	339	332	324	312	300	293	261	254
	400	380	372	360	348	340	332	320	308	300	268	260
	410	390	381	369	357	349	340	328	316	308	274	267
	420	399	391	378	365	357	349	336	323	315	281	273
	430	409	400	387	374	366	357	344	331	323	288	280
	440	418	409	396	383	374	365	352	339	330	295	26
	450	428	419	405	392	383	374	360	347	338	302	293
	460	437	428	414	400	391	382	368	354	345	308	299
	470	447	437	423	409	400	390	376	362	353	315	306
	480	456	446	432	418	408	398	384	370	360	322	312
	490	466	456	441	426	417	407	392	377	368	328	319
	500	475	465	450	435	425	415	400	385	375	335	325
	510	485	474	459	444	434	423	408	393	383	342	332
	520	494	484	468	452	442	432	416	400	390	348	338
	530	504	493	477	461	451	440	424	408	398	355	345
	540	513	502	486	470	459	448	432	416	405	362	351
	550	523	512	495	479	468	457	440	424	413	369	358
	560	532	521	504	487	476	465	448	431	420	375	364
	570	542	530	513	496	485	473	456	439	428	382	371
	580	551	539	522	505	493	481	464	447	435	389	377
	590	561	549	531	513	502	490	472	454	443	395	384
	600	570	558	540	522	510	498	480	462	450	402	390

From *Essentials of Strength Training & Conditioning,* Human Kinetics, 2000.

Again, these are only general guidelines, and there are no "black & white" rules for rep schemes.

Periodization

The concept behind periodization is to reduce the instance of overtraining, by altering sets and reps through three or four training programs comprising a cycle. The complete cycle is referred to as a *macrocycle,* generally a period of time equivalent to one year; however, this period may last for several years. Within each macrocycle are mesocycles, usually three to four months in length; and within each mesocycle are microcycles of approximately one month.

There are generally four phases associated with mesocycles; the hypertrophy phase, the strength or power phase, the competition phase, and the transition phase. The hypertrophy phase is a conditioning phase using high-volume, low-intensity work. The strength or power phase uses less volume but more intensity. The competition phase uses low volume and high intensity. In the transition phase, the athlete will do many other sports or activities outside the area in which they normally compete. This phase could also be looked at as relaxation or recuperation. While training is not intense, it is nonetheless taking place.

When we speak of volume, we are speaking of the total amount of weight lifted in a workout session. This is calculated by multiplying the number of sets by the number of repetitions, and then multiplying this number by the weight lifted per repetition. Training intensity refers to the amount of weight lifted per repetition.

An Easy Way to Increase Your Workout Load

Many times, programs are written using even-numbered systems. An easy way to increase your workload is add one rep to each set. In the case of an ascending pyramid, instead of doing 10-8-6-4-2-1, your rep scheme would look like this, 11-9-7-5-3-1. This change would result in your performing an additional five reps, for an increase of 16.1% in reps.

Sample Workout Programs

Women's Intermediate Program

TABLE 9.7

Day 1	Body Part	Exercise	Repetitions
	Warm-up	Bike, Treadmill, Stepper, etc.	10 Minutes
	Chest	Bench Press w/bar or DBs	10-8-6-10
		Dumbbell Flyes	10-8-6-10
	Triceps	Tricep Pushdowns	15-12-10-15
		Dumbbell Kickbacks	15-12-10-15
	Back	Lat Pulldowns	10-8-6-10
		One Arm DB Rows	10-10-10
	Biceps	Barbell Curls	10-8-6-10
		Alternate Dumbbell Curls	10-10-10
Day 2			
	Legs	Squats or Leg Presses	10-8-6-10
		Lunges	10-10-10 (Repetitions Per Leg)
		Leg Curls	10-10-10
		Abductor/Adductor	15-15-15
		Calves—Standing	20-20-20
		Seated	20-20-20
	Shoulders	Machine Shoulder Press	10-8-6-10
		Dumbbell Side Laterals	10-10-10
	Abs	Crunches	20-20-20 (Holding a weight-plate)
	Cool Down	Bike, Treadmill, Stepper, etc.	5 minutes

Do the first workout on Monday and Thursday; do the second workout on Tuesday and Friday, or any combination of days that fit your schedule. Do cardio work on Wednesday and/or Saturday/Sunday.

Power Program

TABLE 9.8

Exercise		Week 1	
	Day 1		Day 3
Warm-up	Bike, Treadmill, Stepper, etc.	10 Minutes	
Bench Press	8-5-3-1-1-1-1-5		8-6-4-2-2-2-2-1
Incline Press	6-4-3-2-2-2-5		6-4-3-2-2-2-5
Parallel Squats	8-5-4-3-2-1-1-1-5		8-6-4-2-2-2-2
		Week 2	
Bench Press	8-6-4-3-3-3-3-5		8-5-5-5-5
Incline Press	5-4-3-2-1-1-1		5-4-3-2-1-1-1
Parallel Squats	8-6-4-3-3-3-3-5	8-5-5-5-5	
	Day 1 and Day 3		
Upright Rows	8-6-5-5		
Lat Pulldowns	10-8-6		
Tricep Extensions	8-6-5-5		
Standing Barbell Curls	10-8-6-6		
Sit-ups	40-40 with weight plate		
Side Bends	50 each side using a stick		
Leg Raises	40-40		
Twists	50 each side using a stick		

		Week 1	Week 2
		Day 2	Day 2
Power Cleans and Overhead Press		8-5-3-2-1-1-1-5	6-4-3-3-3-3
Bent Legged Deadlifts		8-5-3-2-1-1-1-5	6-4-3-3-3-3
Leg Curls		10-8-6-6-6-6	12-9-7-5-5
DB Side Lateral Raises		10-8-6	10-8-6
Standing DB Curls		8-8-8-8	8-8-8-8
Standing Tricep Pressdowns		8-6-5-5	8-6-5-5
Sit-ups		40-40 with weight plate	40-40 no plate
Side Bends		50 each side using a stick	50 each side using a stick
Cool Down	Bike, treadmill, stepper, etc.	5 minutes	

This is a three-day-a-week program, with different rep schemes on different days. Allow one day in between training sessions. The program repeats itself starting with Week 3.

Hardcore Workout Program

TABLE 9.9

Day 1

Warm-up	Bike, Treadmill, Stepper, etc.	10 Minutes
Chest	Bench Press	10-8-(3 × 3)-(3 × 2)-(3 × 1)-10
	Incline DB Press	10-8-6-10
	Flat DB Flyes	10-10-10-10
Back	Lat Pulldowns	10-10-10-10
	1 Arm DB Rows	10-8-6-10

Day 2

Biceps	Barbell Curls	10-8-(3 × 3)-(3 × 2)-(3 × 1)-10
	Seated DB Curls	10-10-10-10
	Hammer Curls	10-10-10-10
Triceps	Tricep Extensions	15-12-10-8
	Bench Dips	15-12-10-8
	DB Kickbacks	15-12-10-8

Day 3

Legs	Power Cleans	6-6-6-6
	Front Squats	10-8-6-10
	Leg Curls	10-8-6-10
	Standing Calf Raises	20-20-20
Shoulders	Military Presses	10-8-6-10
	Upright Rows	10-8-6-10
	DB Side Laterals	10-10-10-10

Day 4

Chest	Bench Press	10-10-10-10
	Incline Bench Press	10-10-10-10
	Incline DB Flyes	10-10-10-10
Back	Lat Pulldowns	10-8-6-10
	Low Rows	10-8-6-10

Day 5

Biceps	Barbell Curls	10-10-10-10
	Standing DB Curls	10-10-10-10
Triceps	Lying EZ Curls	15-12-10-8
	Rope Extensions	15-12-10-8
	Bench Dips	20-15-12-10

Day 6

Legs	Cleans	6-5-4-3-2
	Back Squats	10-8-6-4-10
	Leg Curls	10-8-6-10
	Lunges	10-10-10 (Repetitions per leg)
	Seated Calf Raises	20-20-20
Shoulders	Seated Behind the Neck Press	10-8-6-4-10
	DB Side Laterals	10-10-10
Cool Down	Bike, Treadmill, Stepper, etc.	5 minutes
Abs	Sit-ups, Crunches, etc.	50-50 on Calf Days

At the number of reps decrease, increase the weight. Where the reps remain the same, use a weight that is the maximum weight you can use and still complete the repetitions. Train your abs and forearms on calf days. For forearms, do flexion/extension exercises using a weighted barbell, handle with rope, grippers, and so on.

Research Review of Selected Programs/Systems of Resistance Training

The following table is compiled by Fleck, and Kramer[1]; the table does an excellent job of comparing and evaluating different training methods.

Research Review: Selected Programs/Systems of Resistance Training

Program	Description	Research Notes	Pros	Cons
Pyramids/Triangles: Light to Heavy	3-5 reps with relatively light weight; next set adds 5 lbs for another 3-5 reps. continued until only 1 rep is completed.	DeLorme (1952) system produces significant increases in static strength over short training periods.	• appears to be one of the more effective systems for increasing static strength in the legs, back and elbow flexors	• research suggests that the heavy to light method may be superior in increasing back and leg strength
Pyramids/Triangles: Heavy to Light	After a brief warm-up, heaviest set is performed first; resistance lowered each set thereafter. Oxford technique is 3 sets of 10 reps at 100% to 66% to 50% for a 10RM.	Oxford system (1951 1954 1967) exhibited significant strength gains in various studies. Results equivocal to light-to-heavy system.	• greater energy potential to perform heavier sets first	• higher intensity initial loads without a warm-up
Super Set (Also called agonist-antagonist or push-pull system)	Several sets of two exercises for agonist and antagonist muscles of one body part (leg curls & leg extensions). Generally consists of 8-10 reps with little or no rest between sets and exercises.	Kramer et al. (1987) concluded an increase in muscular endurance and bodybuilders demonstrated the ability to maintain a higher percentage of 1RM strength.	• muscular endurance and hypertrophy • localizes blood flow to tissue to enhance muscle fatigue	• muscular endurance and hypertrophy
Compound Set (Tri-set)	Alternating exercises for the same muscle group with little or no rest in between sets until the desired number of sets are completed. Active rest is implemented between sets.	Hatfield (1981) Bodybuilders implement this system to increase hypertrophy.	• time efficient and develops hypertrophy and muscular endurance	• may not be advantageous for muscular power and strength development
Pre-exhaustion	An initial set performed with a muscle in isolation with the intention to fatigue that muscle prior to a multi-structural movement in which that same fatigued muscle will not be able to contribute to the performance of that movement. Therefore the other muscles in the movement will be recruited at a greater rate to compensate for the fatigued muscle. (leg extensions to fatigue quads followed by a squat)	•Stowers et al (1983) one set to exhaustion of 10 repetitions causes significant gains in squat ability, but three sets of 10 reps, cause significantly greater increases in squat ability.	• more motor units recruited from non-fatigued and smaller supporting muscles	• groups trained with periodization had significantly greater increases in the squat and vertical jump ability
Circuit Training	Series of resistance exercises performed one after the other with minimal rest (15-30 sec.) between exercises. 10-20 reps of each set at 40-60% of 1RM.	Gettman and Pollock (1981) 8-20 wk program may increase VO2 max by 4-8% in both men and women.	• time efficient and some improvement of CV fitness	• rate of CV improvement substantially less than the 15-20% seen in traditional aerobic training over the same duration

Reproduced from Fleck, S. J., and Kramer, W. J. (1997) *Designing Resistance Training Programs.* Champaign, IL: Human Kinetics.

How Do I Know if I'm Overtraining?

Overtraining can become a problem for anyone obsessed with training for any physical activity. If the workout program does not allow for enough rest, and continues for a long enough period of time, chances are you will be overtrained. Many times this will happen when an exercise program is started because a person is very enthusiastic about the fact that they are exercising, or they want to see changes quickly, or they really like the sport that they are involved in. The problem starts when the fun of participating declines and the effort becomes more like "work." Some classic symptoms of overtraining are:

1. a decrease in performance
2. mood swings
3. changes in appetite or no appetite at all
4. lingering illnesses and upper respiratory infections
5. sleeplessness for more than a couple of nights
6. muscle fatigue and lack of strength
7. elevated heart rates and blood pressure
8. weight gain or loss, sometimes large, sometimes small

Fortunately, the solution may be as simple as rest. Depending on the degree of overtraining, rest may be only a couple of days or as long as a year or more. What will be learned after dealing with a bout of overtraining is that "more training" is not always "better training." The key here is to train intelligently, allowing the body ample time to recuperate.

How Long Should My Workouts Be?

Workouts with weights should never be longer than 1 to 1½ hours at a time. If you are spending more time than this in the gym, then you are wasting too much time talking and goofing off. I never spend more time than this with my athletes, with my personal training clients, or in my own training.

Training Information

The best publication I have found for issues and items relating to weight training, diets, nutrition, and other items of interest is *Pure Power Magazine*. This magazine presents information based on *FACT* and not fiction. Contact information:

Dan Wagman, Ph.D., CSCS
Pure Power Magazine
P.O. Box 77066
Colorado Springs, Colorado 80970
Phone: (719) 597-3525
Website: www.purepowermag.com

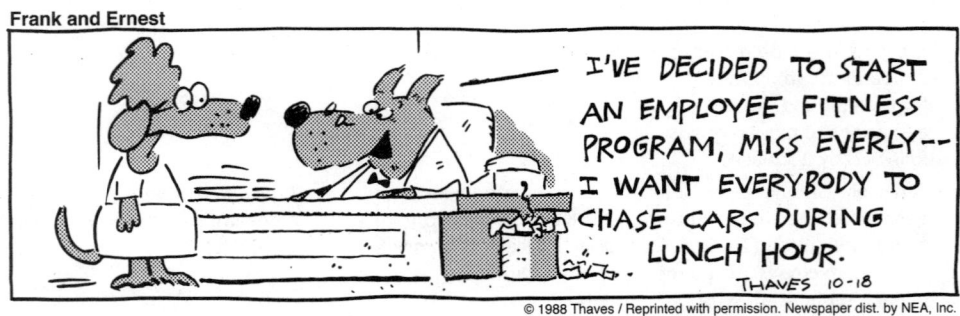

Frank and Ernest

I'VE DECIDED TO START AN EMPLOYEE FITNESS PROGRAM, MISS EVERLY-- I WANT EVERYBODY TO CHASE CARS DURING LUNCH HOUR.

THAVES 10-18

1. Fleck, S. J., and Kramer, W. J. (1997). *Designing Resistance Training Programs*. Champaign, IL: Human Kinetics.

Please feel free to write on this page

True or False

1. _____ To compete as a bodybuilder, you must train like a football player.

2. _____ Training programs are the same for every sport.

3. _____ A well rounded athlete excels in only one particular sport.

4. _____ There is no such thing as a bad program, but there are some programs that are better than others.

5. _____ Always warm up before stretching.

Multiple Choice

6. _____ What is the one exception to the #1 rule of weight training, that training is specific?
   a. cross-training
   b. warming-up
   c. stretching
   d. bodybuilding

7. _____ According to rule #6 of program basics, what should you do if you have not worked out in a while?
   a. go all out
   b. start with single-joint exercises
   c. enter a competition
   d. start out slowly

8. _____ What are the total combined programs for any given predetermined period of time called?
   a. set
   b. cycle
   c. routine
   d. repetitions

9. _____ What is a program where you would work on body parts that are underdeveloped or not developing as rapidly as you would like?
   a. double split program
   b. priority split program
   c. split program
   d. development program

10. _____ Lifting weights until you can no longer lift them, and then having your spotter help you get a few additional reps is called what?
    a. supersets
    b. burnout sets
    c. forced reps
    d. breakdown sets

Fill in the Blank

11. The #1 rule of weight training is that training is _____ .

12. Cross-training will make you a _____ _____ athlete.

13. Cravings for _____ _____ will decrease as your diet improves.

14. A _____ is a system of training where the reps increase, decrease, or do both.

15. The concept behind _____ is to reduce the instance of overtraining by altering sets and reps through three or four training programs comprising a cycle.

16. The _____ phase is a conditioning phase using high-volume, low-intensity work.

17. _____ can become a problem for anyone obsessed with training for any physical activity.

18. In the _____ / _____ program, you would do light exercises one day and heavy exercises the next training session.

19. _____ can be determined using skinfold calipers, bio-impedance, hydrostatic weighing, or Body Mass Index (BMI).

20. _____ is a personal preference, but not a good choice for weight training.

NOTES

Please feel free to write on this page

Answers: 1. False 2. False 3. False 4. True 5. True 6. a 7. d 8. b 9. b 10. c 11. specific 12. well rounded 13. junk food 14. pyramid 15. periodization 16. hypertrophy 17. overtraining 18. light/heavy 19. bodyfat 20. stretching

CHAPTER 10

Weight Training and Women

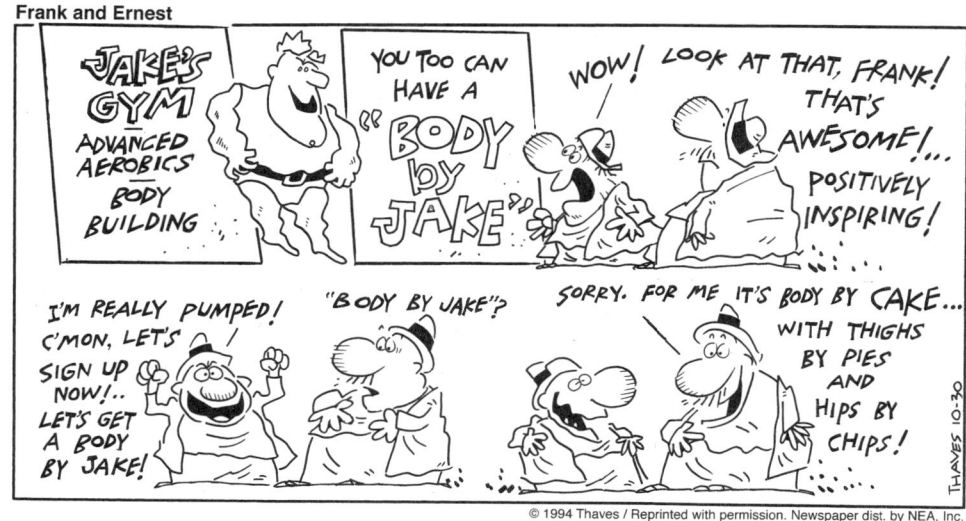

Frank and Ernest

© 1994 Thaves / Reprinted with permission. Newspaper dist. by NEA, Inc.

Is There a Difference between Men and Women?

Generally, there is no difference between men and women when we speak of muscles or fiber types. Women are beginning to realize that not only does weight training make them stronger, but it can also help them to lose body fat more quickly than by dieting or aerobics alone. In fact, aerobics does not preserve fast twitch muscle fiber, which is greatly needed to burn fat.[1] For women, weight training is the primary way to preserve or add muscle. The more muscle you have, the more calories you will burn, even when your body is at rest. Muscle is denser and occupies less space than a similar amount of fat. A pound of fat will occupy approximately 18 percent more space than a pound of muscle, and fat does not burn any calories. This is why women should be concerned with the inches they lose in their hips, waist, and so on, and not about the pounds lost. Many times when women initially start weight training, they will notice a slight increase in bodyweight and their clothes may fit a little tighter. This is because, as the muscle grows, it becomes larger and denser, and stores more glycogen. The trade-off here is that the muscle might be slightly larger and clothes slightly tighter, but the body will be burning more calories, which, will result in weight loss through a reduction in fat. In a study done by Westcott in 1996, research indicated that using an 8-week standard program resulted in lean weight gain of 2.4 pounds and a decrease in fat weight of 4.6 pounds.[2] As the body loses fat, the muscles will become noticeably more toned and visible.

In a study done by Bryner et al. in 1999, women who did resistance training for 12 weeks while on an 800 calorie per day diet were able to maintain their fat-free mass (FFM), i.e., bones, muscles, fluids, organs, and so forth and increase their resting metabolic rate (RMR). Women in the same study who consumed 800 calories per day and did aerobics, lost significant amounts of fat-free mass, and also experienced a decrease in RMR. However, 800 calories per day is a very low amount for women, and should not be tried on your own.

The gain in muscle sometimes scares women, because they don't want to get big like men. For the vast majority of women, this will never be a problem, thanks to hormonal influences. Before puberty, boys and girls exhibit similar levels of strength and fitness. Once puberty begins, boys produce increased amounts of the hormone testosterone, which will allow them to become larger and stronger than their female counterparts. Men and women both produce testosterone in their bodies, but the amounts produced by women are so small that it will never allow them to get "big," something in the neighborhood of 15 to 20 times less concentration of testosterone than men. Because of the lower levels of testosterone, women will not build the muscle mass of men, but will instead have a well defined muscle that is referred to as "toned;" however, they are capable of strength that is proportionate to that of a man. Becoming "toned" is a combination of increased muscle size and decreased body fat.

Muscle is good. For every pound of muscle you have, you will burn 35 to 50 calories per day. That is why FFM is so good. If you lose even 1/2 lb. of FFM, you could theoretically have a weight gain of almost 3 lbs. of fat in one year. In 10 years this would equate to about 30 lbs. of weight! Loss of FFM is one of the reasons that men and women gain fat as we age. A simple addition of only 25 extra calories per day could cause a 2.6 lbs. weight gain in 1 year![1] Remember that the next time some fast food server asks you, "Supersize that order?" Technically, food servers in major restaurants should be called "commissioned salespeople," according to Guy Andrews, M.S. of Exercise Etc. Inc. Their job is to sell you things you don't want in order to increase the price of your ticket, and thus increase the price of their tip and the profit of the restaurant. Many restaurant chains monitor the sales of their staffs to give the best sellers the best shifts. There will be more on the subject of restaurants in Chapter 12.

When women begin weight training, they should concentrate on developing muscular strength and endurance. Most women are significantly weaker in the chest and shoulders than comparably sized men, in part due to the width of their shoulders and the resulting loss of leverage, which in turn leads to a decrease in muscle size. There are any number of factors that can affect this difference, from genetics to childhood activities and societal influence. Areas of weakness should be addressed and prioritized to bring the body into balance. In this way, a woman may help prevent injury and provide for a lifetime of sports enjoyment.

In general, women should concentrate on doing sets that do not exceed 12 repetitions for overall fitness, and stay at or below 5 repetitions for strength and power development. Because women have higher concentrations of growth hormone (GH), the number of reps will become a factor in determining size gains. The GH production will be significantly higher during the menstrual cycle.[3] When training with weights, if women train at five reps and below for multiple sets, and take a three minute rest between sets, there will be no increase in growth hormone release. If, however, women train using 10 reps and multiple sets with a one minute rest between sets, there will be an increase in growth hormone release. Refer to Chapter 9 for more specific guidelines.

My advice to women: Throw away your scale and do not ever look at another one. Be concerned about the inches and not the pounds; exercise and insure that the number of calories you take in equals the number that go out everyday. Fat occupies more space, so it is possible to gain weight and not inches; in fact, most often you will lose inches. Concentrate on lowering your body fat percentage and not losing any fat-free mass.

Women, Boyfriends (or Husbands), and Weight Training

The best weight-training classes I have had the opportunity to teach have always been the women's weight-training classes. Why? Because women work hard, listen to directions, try what is presented to them, and do not come into the class with preconceived notions. Women are open to trying new things and are more in tune with their bodies than men. Men, on the other hand, seem to think they are born with the knowledge of how to weight train. Nothing could be further from the truth! The men are the worst to work with because they know everything there is to know about weight training, and if you don't believe them, ask their high school football coach who definitely, without a doubt, knows everything there is to know about weight training. Side note here: That is probably why the high school football coaches all look so good in their coaches shorts with their potbellies hanging out!

The same thing is generally true of husbands and boyfriends. Most of them think they know what exercises work what muscles, and how to train everybody and everything, from friends, family, men, women, and children to family pets.

Women, however, are the biggest cheats in the gym when it comes to counting reps or doing the full number of sets that are prescribed. I have never seen so many ways to miscount reps and sets, short of all of the accounting scandals currently taking place in the business world. It goes to show that creative accounting isn't just for the accountants! Enough said on this topic; listen, learn, and ask questions.

Women and Body Fat

Men and women vary in the body fat percentages they carry. See Chapter 14 for more information on body fat and body-fat testing. It is generally considered optimal for men to carry approximately 10 to 20 percent body fat, while for women, body fat is considered optimal at 15 to 25 percent. An athletic range of body fat for women is 14 to 18 percent. For females, essential fat is considered to be 10 to 12 percent, and a female should never drop below this percentage. When dropping below this percentage, women will often find that amenorrhea begins to appear. Amenorrhea is the cessation of menstruation. While there are many theories as to why this happens, it appears to be related to the drop below the essential fat range that is the trigger.

TABLE 10.1

Classification	Women (% Fat)	Men (% Fat)
Optimal	15-25%	10-20%
Athletic	14-18%	10-14%
Essential	10-12%	3%

Body fat in women is distributed in nine regions.[2] The nine regions are:

1. Buttocks
2. Low back
3. Trochanter or side of the leg, between the front of the thigh and the buttocks
4. Between the thighs
5. Navel
6. Pubis
7. Knee
8. Back of the upper arm
9. Breasts

Body-fat storage can be categorized in three different ways: subcutaneous (under the skin), intra-muscular (within the muscle, kind of like marbling in a steak), and intra-abdominal or visceral.[1] While fat distributions are similar in men and women, women of childbearing age carry more body fat as energy stores, in case of a pregnancy. During pregnancy, women will add additional fat, to aid in the nourishment and development of the fetus and as a protective mechanism, should it be needed. Body fat is a great cushion when it comes to protecting against injuries from impact, such as falls and other accidents. It also provides a blanket to help regulate the body temperature and protect the unborn.

On the average a female has approximately 27 billion fat cells, and many obese women may have as many as 75 billion fat cells.[1] Fat cells cannot be destroyed once they have been created. They will shrink in size, but they will not go away. Liposuction is probably the only method to remove fat cells. Typically, the fat cells in the body can store 50 to 60,000 kilocalories of energy. Fat is not deposited or removed from the body quickly, and when someone brags about losing 15 lbs. in one week, rest assured that it is not fat but most likely water weight.

Frederic Delavier, in *Women's Strength Training Anatomy,* makes an interesting observation concerning women and body fat. I have seen similar descriptions and I think they are worth repeating here. He observes that women in hot climates will carry body fat differently from women in cold climates. Specifically, women in hot climates will carry body fat primarily in one of three places: (1) buttocks—black Africans; (2) hips—Mediterraneans; and (3) navel—Asians. The logic is this: Since fat is an insulating mechanism, for women of hot countries it is carried in one primary area, but for women of colder countries, it is spread uniformly around the body for warmth—kind of like wearing a pair of long-johns.

At birth, infants are typically 12 percent body fat.[5] This changes rapidly increasing to 25 percent at six months and then rises to 30 percent by one year of age. After one year of age, body fat will typically decline until the age of five or six, and then it is again approximately 12 percent. After the age of five or six, body fat will rise slowly until the beginning of puberty. At puberty, the rise will continue in girls, but fall slightly in males.

The American Council on Exercise (ACE)[5] gives a little different breakdown of body fat. Their recommendations are as follows:

TABLE 10.2

Classification	Women (% Fat)	Men (% Fat)
Essential Fat	10-12%	2-4%
Athletes	14-20%	6-13%
Fitness	21-24%	14-17%
Acceptable	25-31%	18-25%
Obese	32% and up	25% and up

The goal here is to maintain a "natural weight;" that is, the goal is a weight you can comfortably stay at by eating for hunger (physiological need rather than psychological) and while exercising on a regular basis.[1] If you eat when you are hungry, that is physiological. If you eat because you are depressed, having a bad day, see food that you just have to have, because of peers, or any of a hundred other reasons, that is psychological and should be addressed. Losing weight and body fat is more than just a diet or working out; it is a change in lifestyle, and unless you address all the components, you will be doomed to repeated failures. If you are fat, you did not get that way overnight, and no diet in the world or wonder drug is going to get you thin again without a commitment to a change in diet and a good exercise routine.

A distinction needs to be made here concerning weight and fat. It is possible to be overweight but not overfat. A person who is overweight could very easily have a low body- fat percentage due to muscle mass, and still be healthy. Typically, charts for weight measures were developed using height and weight, with some adjustment being given for frame size. A 5'10" male weighing 220 lbs. with 13% body fat would be overweight but not overfat. A 5'10" male weighing 220 lbs. with 30% body fat would be overfat. Conversely, a 5'2" female weighing 95 lbs. with 20% body fat may not be overweight, but a 5'2" female weighing 95 lbs. with 30% body fat is overfat.

Women who are sedentary and untrained (not working out) burn approximately 50 percent carbohydrate and 50 percent fat while at rest and they take approximately 20 to 30 minutes to mobilize fat from fat stores during physical activity. Women who are active and trained will burn approximately 70 percent fat at rest, thus sparing the glycogen stores for other activities. This is important, because trained women will burn a higher percentage of fat than untrained women, and the trained women will be able to tap into the fat deposits faster.[1]

Women and Cellulite

Men and women can get cellulite. Cellulite is more predominant in women, and is sometimes called "cottage cheese" or "orange peels." It accumulates on the thighs and buttocks. Anytime the body consumes more calories than it expends, the excess calories are deposited somewhere on the body as "fat." Since the fibrous tissues in these areas are inelastic, the fat deposits itself subcutaneously in pockets that are similar to a "honeycomb" pattern, or like that of a net or quilt. Hormones, particularly estrogen, can cause water retention, which can also add to this phenomenon. As the water and fat retention increase, this can cause a compression of lymphatic and blood vessels, thus slowing down circulation and making it harder for the body to utilize these energy stores of fat. After all the other fat the on a woman's body is reduced, it is still possible to retain the fat in these areas and leave her with "cottage cheese thighs."[3]

One final point: spot reducing is a myth. The closest you may come to spot reducing would be liposuction, and even then the fat will return if you don't alter your eating and exercising habits.

Women, Aerobics, and Protein Consumption

The myth that aerobics are better than weight training has been reported and believed for entirely too long. I have had many aerobics instructors working for me who, in a period of five to six years, never increased muscle mass or tone. A gym member of average fitness can burn approximately 5 to 7 kilocalories per minute doing aerobic exercise and 5 to 8 kilocalories per minute doing strength training.[1] Why is this better? Because strength training will maintain or increase lean muscle mass, and this in turn increases the metabolic rate, which will increase the amount of fat burned even when you are at rest.

Most of the women I have had as students and clients did not get enough protein. Why? I don't really know, but I have an idea that it is because they typically consume diets very high in carbohydrates. Women who are doing aerobics and weight training should consume at least 1 gram of protein per pound of body weight per day.

Osteoporosis

Weight training helps females prevent osteoporosis, which is degeneration of bone tissue. Many studies have shown that weight-bearing exercises develop more bone density. Lack of bone density is a major problem for many women in the United States. While there are many factors in the onset of osteoporosis, and the exact mechanism is unknown, it is somehow related to menopause and the body's utilization of calcium.

Weight Training Programs

Weight-training programs do not need to be any different for women or men. The goal of the individual is the determining factor in the type of weight training program that is utilized. This goes back to the "training is specific" principle discussed in the previous chapter. Decide what the desired goal is—muscle gain, weight loss, or physical endurance or even a combination—and design the program based on the need of the individual. Incorporate the time element into it, keep it new, and success will come naturally. Most of all, make it fun!

A Word of Caution

Women need to be careful if they are trying to lose size in the thighs, particularly the upper thighs. Common exercises I see women doing endlessly are the adduction/abduction exercises. These exercises, if not done correctly, can actually *add* size to the thighs, because the muscles will grow. This will make your pants fit very tight and give you the impression that you are not losing size or weight. This is particularly true of the tensor fascia latae, since it crosses over the hip joint. I would limit these exercises to no more than five repetitions and three sets, if you do them. Personally, I prefer walking lunges.

Women and High Heels

While walking, working, and dancing in high heels may be sexy and appealing, the downside is that it can cause shorter calf muscles, shorter Achilles tendons, and more stress on the knees. In a study done in Boston,[6] researchers using special cameras and sensors found that high heels—those at least two inches high and higher—increased the torque (twisting force) at the knee, and that this force placed additional strain behind the kneecaps and inner knee joint. For women consistently working in high heels, this force could cause a permanent degenerative change by wearing down and destroying the cartilage that cushions the knee. This wear and tear could ultimately lead to osteoarthritis. Also, 87 percent of foot surgery is performed on women, and two times as many women as men suffer from osteoarthritis.

While high heels have a slimming effect on the legs by elevating the heel and causing the woman to walk in plantar flexion, the price you pay later in life may not be worth the attention you receive when you are younger. If you wear high heels, stretch your calves regularly, even daily; on days you work out, stretch them before and after working out. Another good idea would to be to wear low heels or tennis shoes as often as possible when working or after work.

Women and Make-up

Ladies, let's get real here. You are in the gym to work out, not participate in a Victoria's Secret fashion show. Between the overdone make-up that leaves a mark on every piece of equipment you use and the absolutely totally inappropriate dress, I often wonder if I'm in a gym or a nightclub. Save the pore-clogging, sweat-inhibiting make-up for your night out. Oops, my mistake. Doesn't the old saying go something like *"Ladies glisten, men perspire, and horses sweat"* or is that *"horses sweat, men perspire, and ladies glisten"*? Either way, carry that towel and sweat away; sweating is good for you.

Women and Perfume in the Gym

Many people are allergic to perfume, and it can be especially annoying in a confined space where people are inhaling and exhaling deeply. Perfume is not much better than B.O. (body odor) when it comes to working out. Neither is desirable. While I personally like perfume on women and find it makes them very appealing, in the gym it is nothing short of environmental pollution. Work out without the perfume!

Women and Rep Ranges

Use the following guidelines when deciding what you want to accomplish with your training program:

TABLE 10.3 Goal Based Load, Repetitions, Sets, and Rest

Training Goal	Muscular Endurance	Muscular Hypertrophy	Strength	Power
Load as a % of 1 Repetition Max	Less than or equal to 67%	67–85%	Greater than or equal to 85%	Single effort, 80–90% Multiple effort, 75–85%
Repetitions	Greater than or equal to 12	6–12	Less than or equal to 6	Single effort, 1–2 Multiple effort, 3–5
Sets	2 to 3	3 to 6	2 to 6	3 to 5
Rest between sets	30 seconds or less	30 seconds to 1.5 minutes	2 to 5 minutes	2 to 5 minutes

Information extracted from Chapter 18, *Essentials of Strength Training and Conditioning*, Human Kinetics, (2000).

If 1 Repetition Max (1 RM) testing is not possible, the 1 RM may be calculated using tables providing data and predictions for a given weight lifted and the number of times the weight was lifted. This same chart should also be able to tell you how many times you can lift a weight based on a desired percentage of the 1 RM. 1 RM chart is available in Chapter 9.

Women and Squatting Exercises

Can women squat using bars and weights? The answer is an unequivocal YES! In fact, it is one of the better exercises for hip, thigh, and leg development. The only difference between men and women has to do with hip width and pelvic structure. Typically, women have wider hips to allow for childbirth. Wider hips change the convergence angle of the femur in relation to the knee, and thus create more stress on the knee joint.

Another very important point to remember here is that, due to the convergence angle, the patella (knee cap) in women is forcefully being pulled toward the outside of the knee. The vastus medialis is attached to the patella and pulls it toward the inside of the thigh and leg to overcome this tendency. An easy way to strengthen the vastus medialis is to use the leg extension machine and externally rotate the foot. This will further emphasize the development of the vastus medialis and correct this tendency; in other words, this exercise will aid in properly aligning the patella in its groove.

When squatting, women should start out slowly, gradually building up strength in the lower limbs, and paying particular attention to keeping the knees from knocking (moving toward one another). It is a good idea to point the toes outward slightly, which will place more emphasis on the adductors.

It is very important to drive through the heels when squatting, rather than through the balls of the feet. The feet should stay firmly planted on the floor throughout the exercise. If necessary, lift your toes up in your shoes to help you learn to drive through your heels. Do not use a board under your heels. This is analogous to squatting in heels, low or high, depending on the height of the board. If you can do a squat with no weight and keep your heels firmly on the floor, then you can do a regular squat with a bar and weights.

Many times I have seen women squat using a Smith Machine. I do not recommend this practice for men or women. In the squat, the weight and the bar do not travel in a straight line, as does the weight on the Smith Machine. What is required is flexibility. This machine will do nothing but teach you improper form in the squats. Squats, when done in the Smith Machine, can also lead to a difference in muscle balance, because the hamstrings are not worked as effectively as in a regular squat. The trunk muscles will be similarly affected, since there is not the same need for stabilization as in a regular squat. Refer to Chapter 6 and how to squat in order to develop picture perfect form.

Again, do not use a board under your heels when squatting. Using a board will be similar to squatting in high heels. If you have to use a board, start working on lengthening the Achilles tendon and calf muscle, by stretching the calf muscle until you no longer need a board under your heels. Refer to the section on "High Heels" on page 141 for more information about this condition and its causes. Another suggestion would be to point your toes up in your shoes when you squat, and drive through your heels. You will be amazed at what happens!

Women and Strength Training

In a position paper titled, *"Strength Training for Female Athletes,"* the National Strength and Conditioning Association (NSCA)[8] published its findings concerning the use of resistance exercise by female athletes. Of particular interest are some of the committee's recommendations for designing training programs:

1. Female athletes should be exposed to weight training in junior high and high school.

2. Strength and conditioning personnel need to be sensitive to the individual needs of the female athlete.

3. It has been found through interviews with strength coaches that strength levels of female athletes diminish more quickly than male athletes. Therefore, female athletes should train at a higher percent of their max weights for strength maintenance.

4. Strength and conditioning professionals should explain the concept of "specificity of training," and encourage the female athlete to approach training with a high degree of enthusiasm and arousal.

5. More multi-joint exercises (power cleans, snatches, etc.) should be introduced to the female athlete sooner in her exposure to weight training.

6. Female athletes are capable of handling a high volume and high intensity, and performance standards need to be set and records kept.

7. Females should be encouraged to strengthen the entire body, but particular attention should be given to the upper body in general, and the triceps and low back in particular.

Using these guidelines, it will be possible to improve the athletic performance and physiological function of not only the female athlete, but the average woman as well. Since women have physiological responses similar to men there is no reason to train women any differently.

The most important thing in training women is the assessment of needs, and appropriate training to meet those needs.

Why is the list of recommendations on page 143 included in this book, you ask? Because if you take out the terminology of strength and conditioning professional (strength coach) and insert the words "Personal Trainers," you will have a guideline for how a Personal Trainer should be training you; or if you are self-trained, this is how you should design a program that best suits you.

A Recommendation for Further Study

I would highly recommend the book *Women's Strength Training Anatomy*, by Frederic Delavier, for any ladies serious about weight training and their bodies. This book will give you a very clear understanding of the female body, and exercises that are unique to it. Who knows? Maybe then you will be able to counteract all that bad advice received from your boyfriend, husband, or self-proclaimed fitness expert!

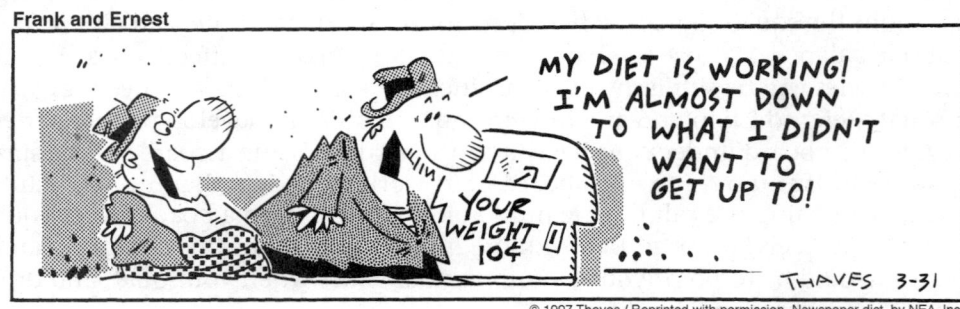

© 1997 Thaves / Reprinted with permission. Newspaper dist. by NEA, Inc.

1. Lecture 2/23, Exercise Etc., Inc. Seminar, Houston, Texas (2003).

2. Lecture 2/23, Exercise Etc., Inc. Seminar, Houston, Texas (2003). Based on research by Wayne Westcott, 1996.

3. Bryner, et al. (1999). Effects of resistance vs. aerobic training combined with an 800 calorie liquid diet on lean body mass and resting metabolic rate. *Journal of American College of Nutrition.* 18:115-121.

4. Burger, M. & Burger, T. (2002). Neuromuscular and hormonal adaptations to resistance training: Implication for strength development in female athletes. 24(3), 51-59. *National Strength and Conditioning Journal.*

5. Delavier, F. (2003). *Women's Strength Training Anatomy.* Champaign: Human Kinetics, p. 8-10.

6. Growth And Physical Development. (February 12, 2003). *The Merck Manual.* [On-line]. Available: www.merck.com/pubs/mmanual/section19/chapter256/256d.htm.

7. Understanding Your Body Fat Percentage. (February 12, 2003). *HealthCheck Systems.* [On-line]. Available: www.healthchecksystems.com/bodyfat.htm.

8. High Heels Means High Stress on Knees. (January 20, 2003). *Valley General Hospital Consumer Guide.* [On-line]. Available: www.valleygeneral.com/TipsHighHeelsMeansHighStressonKnees.htm.

9. Delavier, F. (2003). *Women's Strength Training Anatomy.* Champaign: Human Kinetics, p. 45, 63.

10. Position Paper: *Strength Training for Female Athletes.* (1990). Colorado Springs: National Strength and Conditioning Association.

Please feel free to write on this page

True or False

1. _____ Women should be more concerned about the inches they lose rather than the pounds.

2. _____ A desired goal must be determined before developing a training program.

3. _____ Female athletes should not train at a higher percentage of their maximum weight for strength maintenance.

4. _____ The most important thing in training for women is the assessment of needs and the appropriate training to meet those needs.

5. _____ Sweating is not good for you while working out.

6. _____ Perfume is better than B.O. (body odor) when it comes to working out.

7. _____ If you wear high heels you should stretch your calves regularly before and after working out.

8. _____ Women don't produce testosterone.

9. _____ For women it is a good idea to point the toes outward slightly in squatting, that way it will place more emphasis on the adductors.

10. _____ Two times as many women as men suffer from osteoarthritis.

Multiple Choice

11. _____ When should more multi-joint exercises be introduced to the female athlete in weight training?
    a. Later
    b. Sooner
    c. Never
    d. All of the above

12. _____ Weight training helps women prevent what?
    a. Osteoporosis
    b. Arthritis
    c. Tendinitis

13. _____ Women in hot climates will carry body fat primarily in one of three places; what are these places?
    a. Buttocks
    b. Hips
    c. Navel
    d. All of the above

14. _____ Since women have physiological responses similar to males, how are they supposed to be trained?

    a. The Same

    b. Differently

    c. None of the above

15. _____ What can cellulite be called that is more predominant in women?

    a. Cottage cheese

    b. Orange peels

    c. Both of the above

16. _____ What is the optimal body fat percentage for women?

    a. 10 to 20 percent

    b. 25 to 30 percent

    c. 15 to 25 percent

17. _____ What percentage of body fat will women have in the fitness category according to age?

    a. 10 to 12 percent

    b. 14 to 20 percent

    c. 21 to 24 percent

18. _____ Women squatting, using bars and weights, is one of the better exercises that will help what?

    a. Hip

    b. Thigh

    c. Leg

    d. All of the above

19. _____ For women, working, walking, and dancing in high heels can use what?

    a. Shorter calve muscles

    b. Shorter Achilles tendons

    c. More stress on the knees

    d. All of the above

20. _____ Female athletes are capable of handling what?

    a. High volume

    b. High intensity

    c. Performance standards

    d. All of the above

NOTES

Please feel free to write on this page

CHAPTER 11

Muscles, Tendons, and Ligaments

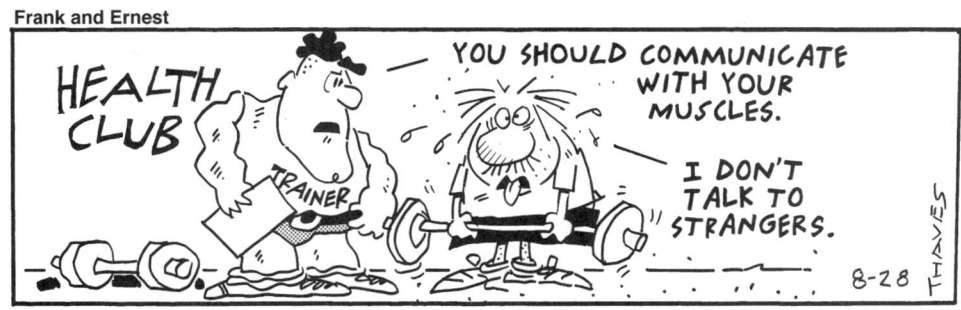

Frank and Ernest

HEALTH CLUB

TRAINER

YOU SHOULD COMMUNICATE WITH YOUR MUSCLES.

I DON'T TALK TO STRANGERS.

8-28 THAVES

© 1998 Thaves / Reprinted with permission. Newspaper dist. by NEA, Inc.

Did You Ever Wonder?

Did you ever wonder why so many bodybuilders walk so funny? Their shoulders are rounded forward, their arms have a fixed bend at the elbow, and they walk with their toes pointed out and kind of hunched over. If you were to take the time to analyze how they train, it wouldn't take to long to realize that many of them do an excessive amount of chest, biceps, ab, and leg exercises. What happens is that, by overworking the chest and neglecting the back, the chest muscles become unbalanced with the back muscles and pull the shoulders forward. The same thing happens with the biceps when they neglect the triceps. The biceps become too strong in relation to the triceps, causing a bend at the elbows as a result of a shortening of the biceps. Do too much ab work and not enough lower back work, and you'll walk hunched over. Fortunately, there is a solution. Work the neglected part, using a priority split system, until you get the muscle groups back in balance with each other. So much for walking like a Neanderthal. Now if we could only do something about that ridge above the eyebrows!

Muscles

There are four normal functions associated with skeletal muscle: (1) movement; (2) posture; (3) joint stabilization; and (4) heat production through contractions to keep the body at 98.6 degrees Fahrenheit.[1]

Muscle have four distinct properties: (1) They contract; (2) They extend; (3) They are elastic; and (4) They are irritable (respond to electrical stimulus).

The main purpose of the over 600 skeletal muscles is contraction. Of these 600 muscles, approximately 430 are voluntary muscles, meaning we consciously control their movement. Muscles contract to produce voluntary movement by converting chemical energy into mechanical energy. The muscles are attached to the bones by tendons. Your total body weight is roughly 50 percent muscle. Ligaments attach bones to other bones at the joints.

When muscles contract, they force movement of the bones by pulling on the tendons. This action is the result of the myofilaments—actin and myosin—sliding across one another. The myofilaments make up muscle units called myofibrils, which in turn make up muscle fibers. The smallest contractile unit of the myofilament is the sarcomere, as shown in Diagram 1.

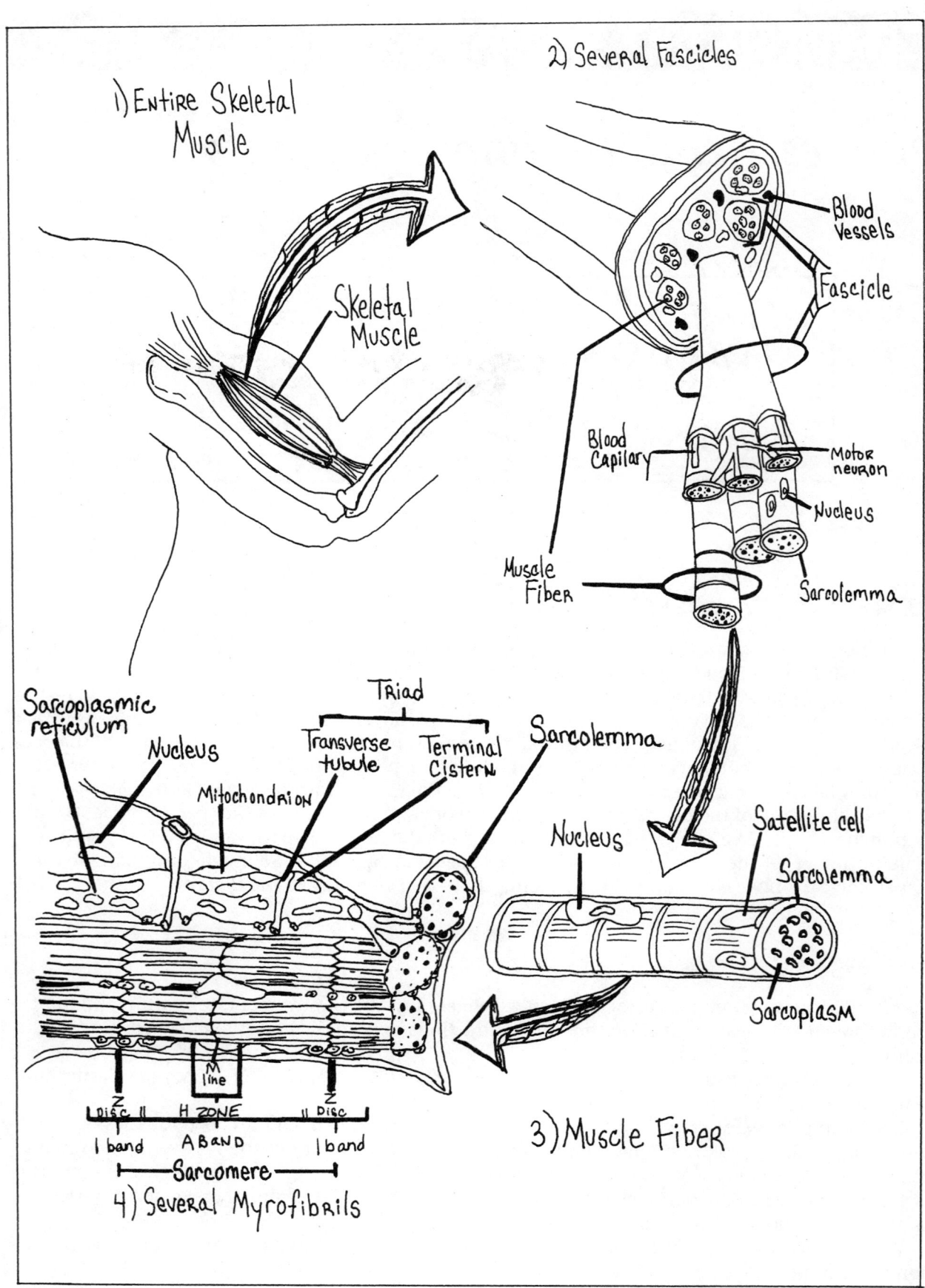

1) Entire Skeletal Muscle

Skeletal Muscle

2) Several Fascicles

Blood Vessels

Fascicle

Blood Capilary

Motor neuron

Nucleus

Muscle Fiber

Sarcolemma

3) Muscle Fiber

Nucleus

Satellite cell

Sarcolemma

Sarcoplasm

Sarcoplasmic reticulum

Nucleus

Mitochondrion

Triad

Transverse tubule

Terminal Cistern

Sarcolemma

Z Disc II

M line

H ZONE

Z II Disc

I band

A BAND

I band

Sarcomere

4) Several Myrofibrils

Drawing by Monica Rabel.

The sarcomere is composed of actin and myosin. When the sarcomere is stimulated by the nervous system, it contracts. All of the sarcomeres in a muscle contract when stimulated by the nervous system. This is where the principle of "all or none" originates, and this is why you cannot "target" a specific portion of the muscle. Either all of the muscle cells contract, or none of the muscle cells contract. As the myosin filaments pull on the actin filaments, the muscle shortens, causing the movement of the bone. This is known as the "sliding filament theory of muscle contraction," and is shown in Diagram 2.

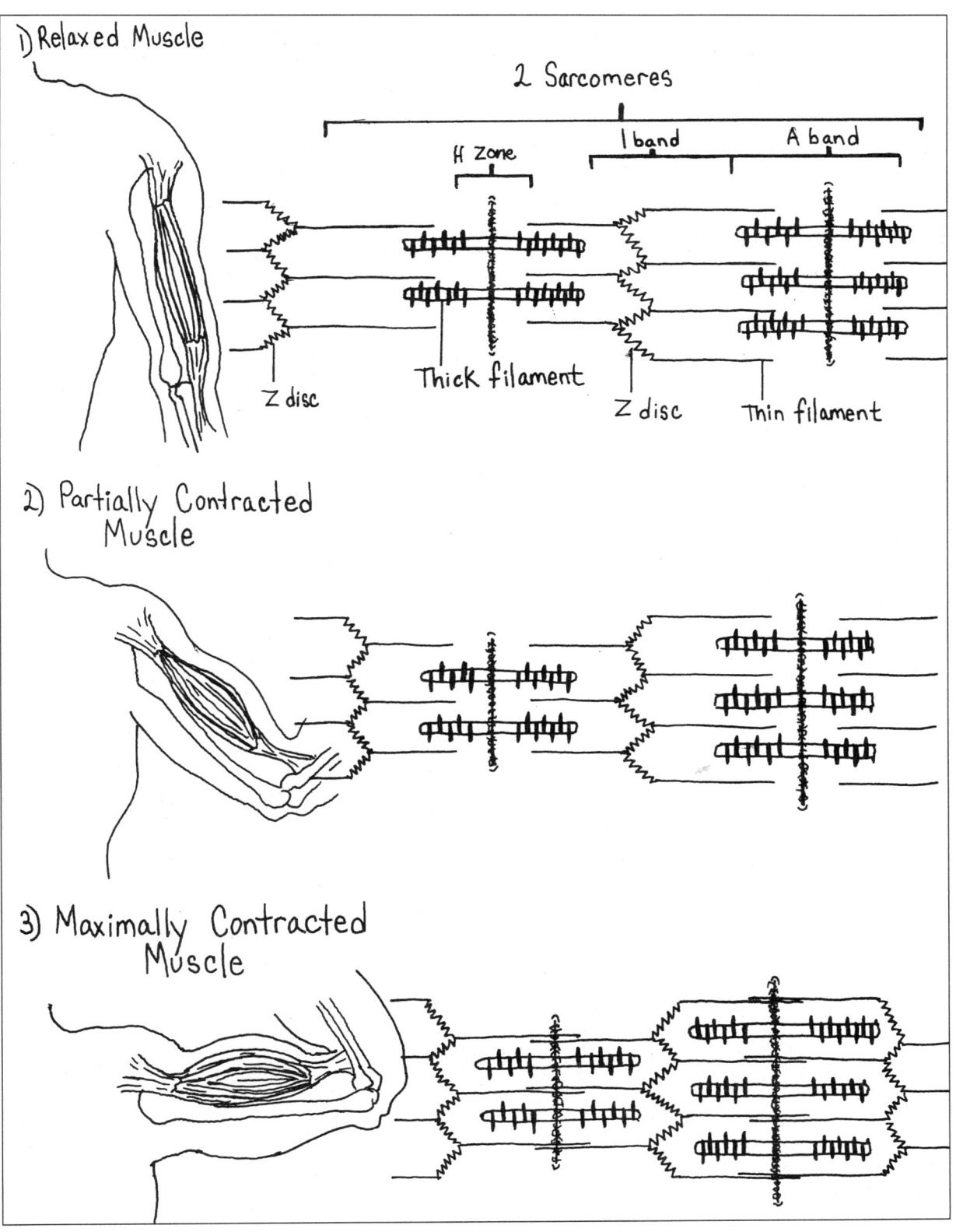

Drawing by Monica Rabel.

The movement that muscles produce is generally the result of muscles working as a group, rather than individually. Skeletal muscles are usually arranged in opposition to one another at the joints. In such groupings, one muscle is the "prime mover" or agonist, and the other muscle is the antagonist. The agonist contracts and causes movement, while the antagonist lengthens or stretches in response to the effort of the agonist. The agonist and antagonist are on opposite sides of a bone, that is, the biceps and the triceps. In curling a weight with the biceps, the agonist would be the biceps. The triceps would be the antagonist; however, when lowering the weight to the starting position in a controlled manner, the muscles would reverse roles, with the triceps becoming the agonist and the biceps becoming the antagonist. If both muscles contracted at the same time, there would be no movement.

The lifting movement utilizing the biceps is called a concentric movement, whereas lowering the weight to the starting position would be called the eccentric movement.

Strength will be determined by four factors: (1) limb length, (2) muscle length, (3) tendon insertion, and (4) muscle fiber type. Shorter people will have a mechanical advantage over taller people. This is why, in the Olympics, you will see the shortest weightlifters lifting the most weight proportionately to their body weight. Many times the weight lifted in the clean & jerk in the lightest weight classes will be 3x their bodyweight, while the weightlifters in the heaviest weight classes will be lucky to get 2x their bodyweight. The same is true of muscle fiber types. If a world-class marathoner is compared to a sprinter, the marathoner will have about 90 percent slow twitch fiber (endurance) versus the sprinter, who will have about 75 percent fast twitch fiber (power). In the normal population, a person's muscle fiber type will be approximately 55 percent slow twitch and 45 percent fast twitch. Muscle fiber type is genetically predetermined.

The study of muscles is known as "myology."

Types of Muscles

There are three types of muscles:

1. Skeletal muscles, so named because their function is to move the bones of the skeleton.
2. Cardiac muscles, which are only found in the heart.
3. Smooth muscles, which are in the blood vessels, organs, and airways.

Skeletal muscles are voluntarily controlled in a conscious manner, whereas the autonomic system and hormones involuntarily control cardiac and smooth muscles.

Slow Twitch Muscle Fibers

Slow twitch muscle fibers are known as Type I red fibers, and are the smallest fibers in diameter. They are dark red in color, because of the many capillaries and large amounts of myoglobin contained within them. Myoglobin is a protein contained in the sarcoplasm that is iron-rich and oxygen-abundant. The sarcoplasm itself contains a considerable amount of glycogen that can be split, resulting in glucose, used for muscular energy. This fiber type is used for long-duration, low-intensity types of exercise. A bodybuilder would recruit more of this type of muscle fiber because of high rep sets and the relatively low weights used. This would be the same for a person doing aerobics. Slow twitch muscle fibers show great endurance during the performance of low-intensity exercise. These muscle fibers are ideally suited for long-distance running and maintaining body position.

Fast Twitch Muscle Fibers

Fast twitch muscle fibers are known as Type II white fibers, and are the largest fibers in diameter. They are white in color, because they have few capillaries and small amounts of myoglobin. Fast twitch fibers are used for short-duration, high-intensity types of exercise. An example would be that of an Olympic weightlifter in the performance of the snatch. Fast twitch fibers fatigue quickly.

Intermediate Muscle Fibers

Intermediate muscle fibers have a diameter somewhere between a slow twitch and fast twitch muscle fiber. They are dark red in color, because they have many capillaries and large amounts of myoglobin. These muscles contract very fast, and they have great endurance, but not as great as slow twitch muscle fibers. Muscle fibers of this type are well suited for walking.

Atrophy

Atrophy is a decrease in muscle size due to the lack of training or injury. The decrease in muscle size is the result of a decrease in the size of the muscle cells. There is no decrease in the number of muscle fibers.

Hypertrophy

Muscle hypertrophy is the increase in the size of a muscle due to an increase in the size of the muscle cells. This is done without cell division, which is known as hyperplasia. For bodybuilders, this would mean that the size of the slow twitch fibers would increase. For powerlifters or Olympic weightlifters, this would mean that the fast twitch muscle fiber size would increase. To bring about the maximum gain, the theory of "progressive overload" would need to be applied.

Hyperplasia

Hyperplasia is an increase in the number of muscle cells due to an increase in the frequency of cell division. Another name for this would be "muscle splitting."

Components of Muscular Strength, Endurance, and Power[2]

Muscular Strength: The ability of a muscle or group of muscles to produce and exert maximum force, classified as either dynamic or static strength. Dynamic strength is the force exerted by a muscle group as a body part moves through a range of motion, whereas static strength is the force exerted against an immovable object. In this instance, no movement occurs. Muscular strength is often measured by doing one-repetition maximum resistance tests in exercises like the bench press, squat, deadlift, curls, or many other exercises. An example of this type of athlete would be a powerlifter.

Muscular Endurance: The ability of a muscle or group of muscles to resist fatigue and make repeated contractions. If the force is sub-maximal, it will be dynamic endurance. Static endurance is the ability to maintain force over a period of time.

In weight training, a high-resistance (high-weight) program with low repetitions (5 and under) will produce muscular strength, while a program with low resistance (low weight) and high repetitions (10 repetitions and up) will produce muscular endurance. I have trained with bodybuilders like Serge Nubret who would routinely do sets that started with 20 reps and increased by two reps each set until 30 reps were attained, and then do a final set with 40 reps! We did this in bench press and it went like this: 20, 22, 24, 26, 28, 30, and a final set of 40 in case you missed what I was saying two sentences ago (and the weight wasn't light either, typically—185-225 lbs. in the bench press!). In the squat and deadlift, we would start at 20 reps and decrease by 2 reps each set while adding 10 lbs. to the bar. Typically, we would do a 20, 18, 16, 14, 12, 10, and a final set at 20 for reps!

Muscular Power: The ability of a muscle or muscle group to generate maximum force in the fastest possible time in an explosive manner. An example of this type of athlete would be an Olympic weightlifter. The formula for calculating power is:

$$\text{Power} = \frac{\text{Force} \times \text{Distance}}{\text{Time}}$$

In this instance, force would be equal to the weight being lifted, multiplied by the distance, and then divided by the time it takes to complete the lift. Power, simply put, is the ability to produce and exert force very rapidly. Often, power is associated with powerlifters; however, Olympic weightlifters are more "powerful" by definition, while powerlifters are actually "stronger." The name "powerlifter" is really a misnomer; it should be "strengthlifter" or some other word implying strength. Work is usually expressed in terms of ft-lbs. or kcal, and power is expressed in terms of ft-lbs./sec, kcal/sec, or watts.

In fact, in work done by Dr. John Garhammer entitled "A Review of Power Output Studies of Olympic and Powerlifting: Methodology, Performance, Prediction and Evaluation Test",[3-4] some compared power outputs of elite Olympic weightlifters and powerlifters are as follows, when looking at the watts generated per kilo of body weight (w/kg):

During the entire snatch or clean pull movements in Olympic weightlifting:

34.3 watts/kg for men

21.8 watts/kg for women

In the second pulls:

52.6 watts/kg for men

39.2 watts/kg for women

In the squat and deadlift:

12 watts/kg for men

Thus, a 100-kilo male Olympic weightlifter would produce:

3420 watts in the clean

5260 watts in the second pull

and a similar 100-kilo male powerlifter would produce:

1200 watts in the deadlift

This is a considerable difference in power outputs. The output of power in the cleans is 2.85 times greater than a deadlift, and second pulls are 4.38 times higher than deadlifts. If we put this into horsepower, there are 746 watts per one horsepower; thus a deadlift would generate 1.6 horsepower, whereas a clean would generate 4.6 horsepower.

While this information may not apply to the type of weight training you do, it is nonetheless very interesting and it helps differentiate between the concepts of muscular power and muscular strength!

Strength and Muscle Balance[5]

Muscle balance testing compares the strength of opposing muscle groups. This testing is important in injury prevention and to maximize speed of muscle contraction. The following ratios are generally accepted, and will help to assess which areas to devote more training time and effort to:

1. The leg press-to-bodyweight ratio is important in determining how fast the body can get to and maintain high speeds. This is important in making speed improvements in short-distance running. Good ratios would be 2.5:1 or higher. This would mean that the leg press exercise would be 2½ times bodyweight.

2. The leg strength test is a functional test used in predicting sprinting and jumping ability. A one-repetition maximum score of 2 times bodyweight for men and 1.5 times bodyweight for women, when doing a squat, would be a good score.

3. Hamstrings-to-Quadriceps strength ratios can be determined by doing a 1-repetition maximum for both legs, using the leg curl and leg extension exercises. Divide the leg extension weight by the leg curl weight to find the ratio for each leg. The leg curl percentage should be 80 percent of the leg extension weight. Any score less than 75 percent would be cause for concern, and could lead to injury in the hamstrings. Target this area to get the scores closer to the 80 percent range.

4. The bench press will check for upper body strength. For males, a score of 1.25 times bodyweight and, for women, 0.8 times bodyweight would be good. Any score above these numbers would be excellent.

Lactic Acid Burn

When exercising with weights or doing any repetitive movement, you may feel a "burn" in the muscle. This sensation is due to the accumulation of lactic acid, which will cause muscular fatigue. To get rid of the burning sensation, stop doing the exercise causing it. Sometimes if you do light exercises after a rest period, the lactic acid burn will go away.

Muscle Soreness

For many years, there was a myth floating around that said the culprit for muscle soreness was lactic acid. This myth is still around. True muscular soreness is the result of an amino acid called hydroxyproline. After an intense training session, muscle cells are damaged, and some have breaks in the cell wall. The break allows hydroxyproline to be released, which acts as a nerve agitator. The cell dies and must be sluffed off into the bloodstream for disposal. This intense type of soreness actually sets the weightlifter or exerciser back from their goals for a period of time, as new muscle cells must be created. The best way to avoid this condition is to gradually increase exercise intensity and duration. Usually, pain associated with overuse of the muscle will appear within 12 to 24 hours and disappear within 48 to 96 hours. Small muscles such as biceps will recover faster than the large muscles of the legs.

Another possible explanation is called delayed onset of muscle soreness (DOMS). This condition can be identified by stiffness, soreness, tenderness, and sometimes swelling. The belief is that it is caused by microscopic muscle tears resulting from excessive mechanical force on the muscle.

To relieve this condition after it appears, do one set of 10 reps for the muscle group that is sore. Use a light weight, and flush the muscle of the by-products from the previous workout. A massage, Jacuzzi, and/or a session in the sauna may be all it takes to relieve this condition and allow you to return to working out.

When Working Muscles

Work your muscles in the direction of its line of pull (direction of muscle fibers) for maximum results. An example would be a person trying to work the obliques. Since the direction of muscle fibers in this muscle is oblique or diagonal, it will not be properly engaged when doing a twist with a stick while sitting on a bench. However, if you flex the rectus abdomens (abs) and then twist as normal, you will engage the obliques, since you are working in the direction of the muscle fiber. The same is true of every muscle in the body.

Frank and Ernest

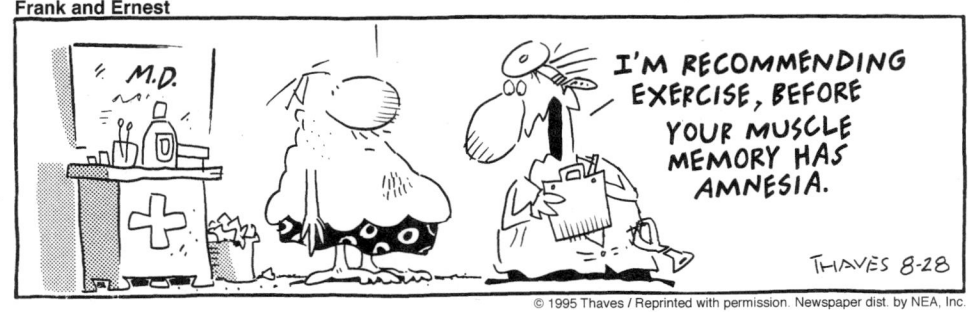

1. Marieb, E. N., Mallat, J. (2003). *Human Anatomy* (3rd Edition). San Francisco: Pearson Education, Inc., p. 244.

2. Miller, D. (2002). *Measurement by the Physical Educator* (4th ed.). New York: McGraw-Hill. p. 141.

3. Croxdale, K. (2/10/03). The "No Deadlift" Deadlift Program. *STRENGTHCATS* [On-line]. 2. Available: www.strengthcats.com/nodeadlift.htm

4. Garhammer, J. (1993). A Review of Power Output Studies of Olympic and Powerlifting: Methodology, Performance Prediction, and Evaluation Tests. *Journal of Strength and Conditioning Research, 7.* pp. 76-89.

5. http://www.brianmac.demon.co.uk/sambc.htm *Sports Coach—Strength & Muscle Balance Checks.*

Please feel free to write on this page

True or False

1. _____ Ligaments attach bones to other bones at the joints.

2. _____ Antagonist means "prime mover."

3. _____ The study of muscles is known as myology.

4. _____ Muscle hypertrophy is the increase in size of a muscle.

5. _____ Skeletal muscles are usually arranged in opposition to one another at the joints.

Multiple Choice

6. _____ Which of the following is a recommended way of getting rid of the muscle burning sensation when you are exercising with weights or doing any repetitive movement?
   a. Stop doing the exercise causing it.
   b. Increase tempo and rhythm of movement.
   c. Do light exercises after a rest period.
   d. Both A and C.
   e. B and C.

7. _____ Which of the following is NOT a recommended way of relieving delayed onset of muscle soreness (DOMS), which can be identified as stiffness, soreness, tenderness, and sometimes swelling?
   a. A massage
   b. A cold bath or shower
   c. A Jacuzzi
   d. A session in the sauna

8. _____ Which of the following is NOT one of the four normal functions associated with skeletal muscles?
   a. Movement
   b. Posture
   c. Joint stabilization
   d. Heat production
   e. Stimulation of nervous system

9. _____ The ability of a muscle or group of muscles to produce and exert maximum force is known as
   a. Muscular strength
   b. Muscular endurance
   c. Muscular power
   d. None of the above

10. _____ Which of the following muscles will most likely recover faster than the others from muscle fatigue and soreness?
    a. Pectoralis major
    b. Quadriceps
    c. Trapezius
    d. Biceps

11. _____ Intermediate muscle fibers contract very fast and have great endurance. This type of muscle fiber is well suited for
    a. Running
    b. Walking
    c. Driving
    d. None of the above

12. _____ The ability of a muscle or muscle group to generate maximum force in the fastest possible time in an explosive manner is
    a. Muscular endurance
    b. Muscular strength
    c. Muscular power
    d. Olympic weightlifting

13. _____ The decrease in muscle size is
    a. Hyperplasia
    b. Hypertrophy
    c. Atrophy
    d. None of the above

14. _____ Muscle-balance testing is important in which of the following?
    a. To prevent injury
    b. To improve endurance
    c. To maximize speed of muscle contraction
    d. Both A and C

15. _____ Muscle soreness is caused by which of the following?
    a. Damaged enzymes
    b. Lactic acid
    c. Amino acid called hydroxyproline
    d. All of the above
    e. None of the above

16. _____ The increase in the size of a muscle due to an increase in the size of muscle cells is known as
    a. Hyperplasia
    b. Hypertrophy
    c. Atrophy
    d. Intermediate muscle fibers

17. _____ The ability of a muscle or a group of muscles to resist fatigue is
   a. Muscular strength
   b. Muscular endurance
   c. Muscular power
   d. None of the above

18. _____ Slow twitch muscle fibers are known as Type I red fibers, and are the
   a. Largest fibers in diameter
   b. Smallest fibers in diameter
   c. Depends on the muscle
   d. None of the above

19. _____ Which of the following examples of muscle-balancing testing is NOT a test used for muscle-balance testing?
   a. The leg press-to-bodyweight ratio test
   b. The leg extension and reverse leg curl
   c. The hamstring-to-quadriceps strength ratio test
   d. The bench press test

20. _____ Fast twitch muscle fibers are known as
   a. Type II red fibers
   b. Type II blue fibers
   c. Type II white fibers
   d. Type III red fibers

NOTES

Please feel free to write on this page

Answers: 1. True 2. False 3. True 4. True 5. True 6. d 7. b 8. e 9. a 10. d 11. b 12. c
13. c 14. d 15. c 16. b 17. b 18. b 19. b 20. c

CHAPTER 12

Diet, Nutrition, and the Use of Supplements

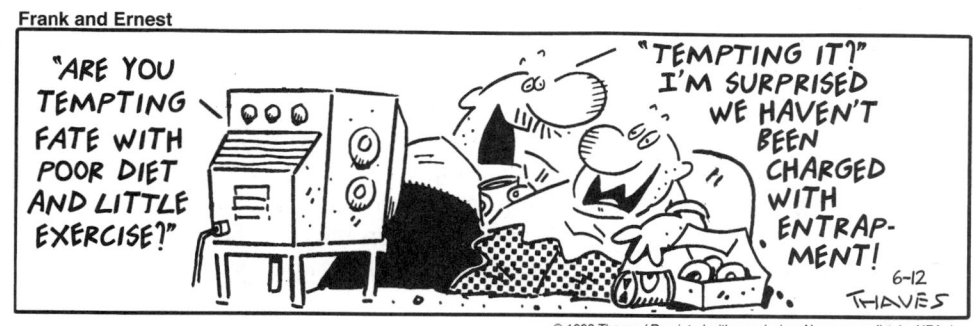

Frank and Ernest

© 1998 Thaves / Reprinted with permission. Newspaper dist. by NEA, Inc.

"Would ya get your dog up in the morning and give him a cup of coffee, a cigarette and a doughnut?"—Jack LaLanne[1]

Even Our Family Pets Are "Eating Themselves to Death"

David Crary, in an article for the Associated Press, states, "Family pets are eating themselves to death."[2] The article states that veterinarians consider obesity in America's dogs and cats to be the leading health problem of an estimated 30 percent of the animals. Pet-food manufacturers are meeting the problem head-on by offering diet products similar to those of humans. There are even weight-loss clinics for our pets. Julie Churchill operates one at the University of Minnesota's College of Veterinary Medicine. Ms. Churchill states, "The average American dog these days is a couch potato." Sounds familiar, like many of the people I know, and the advice is the same: reduce the quantity and richness of the food. Moreover, don't forget to exercise! Have you ever heard that saying about pets and how they resemble their owners? Fact is indeed stranger than fiction.

Not Only Our Pets, but Our Children as Well

In a report to the president on youth activity and sports, it is noted that the percentage of children who are overweight has doubled since 1980 to about 25 percent. The National Health and Nutrition Examination Survey, completed in 2000, sets the overall prevalence of overweight children to be 15%, which is a doubling of the rate in children 6-11 years old, and a tripling of the rate in children 12-19.[3] At the same time, enrollment in high school physical education classes has dropped from 42 percent to 29 percent in 1999. Overall participation in each of the most popular sports in America has dropped between 1990 and 1999, with the only two exceptions being basketball and soccer, and both of these have also shown weaknesses. Is it any wonder that we are becoming fatter as a society when we no longer value and recognize the importance of physical education in establishing habits that allow us to live not only longer, but with a better quality of life? In fact, the World Health Organization (WHO) has labeled obesity and inactivity the number one threat to health in the western world!

Diet

When speaking of diet, most people immediately assume the worst—weight loss! However, the first definition of diet, as defined by "Webster's New World Compact School and Office Dictionary,"[4] "is what a person or animal usually eats or drinks." The usual food and drink are composed of everything we eat, whether it is for weight loss, weight gain, or weight maintenance. Everything we eat can be further broken down into six categories of nutrients essential to our health: protein, carbohydrates, fats, vitamins, minerals, and water. The seventh category, which has nothing to due with nutrition but affects calorie intake, is alcohol.

Nutrients

Protein: Hippocrates, the Father of Nutrition, wrote 2500 years ago that protein was the most important nutrient. Proteins are composed of complex organic compounds made up of amino acids. In the human body, there are 9 essential and 11 nonessential amino acids. Essential amino acids cannot be synthesized, but must be obtained from plant or animal proteins ingested in the diet. Nonessential amino acids can be synthesized from other amino acids and other substances such as carbohydrates. The amine portion of the molecule needs to come from a nitrogen source that is not a carbohydrate. Proteins are responsible for muscle tissue growth and repair. Protein can be used as a fuel source when carbohydrates and fats are not available. Protein contains 4 calories per gram of weight.

Carbohydrates (carbs): There are two forms of carbohydrates: simple and complex. Carbohydrates provide the body with energy. Simple carbohydrates are commonly known as sugars, and have little nutritive value. Complex carbohydrates are found in grains, cereals, whole-grain breads, vegetables, and fruits. Carbohydrates contain 4 calories per gram of weight.

Fats: Fats are also an energy source for the body in a concentrated form, and are essential for the proper absorption of certain fat-soluble vitamins (A, D, E, and K). Fats also transport the hormones of the body. Fat provides the feeling of fullness after a meal and delays the onset of hunger pangs. Fats, as known by their correct name, are called lipids, and are made up of fatty acids. These fatty acids can be called either saturated or unsaturated. Saturated fat usually comes from animal products, coconut oils, and palm oils. Saturated fats are usually solid at room temperature. Unsaturated fat are usually liquid at room temperature and can be called monounsaturated or polyunsaturated. Fats contain 9 calories per gram of weight.

Vitamins: Many essential biological functions within the body are dependent on vitamins and minerals. Vitamins are organic substances that perform a specific metabolic function.

Minerals: Minerals are essential in regulating many body functions, such as muscle contraction, protein synthesis, and heart function.

Water: A full 60 percent of the total bodyweight of a human is water. Water contains no calories or vitamins. The body's need for water is second only to the need for oxygen; while a person may live for up to 50 days without food, the same person will generally die within a week without water. Muscle is 72 percent water, while fat is 20 to 35 percent water.

Alcohol: Alcohol has no nutritive value, but figures prominently in many diets. Alcohol contains 7 calories per gram of weight and the calories are often referred to as "empty calories," meaning they have no nutritive value. When figuring daily calorie requirements for weight loss, weight gain, or weight maintenance, it is essential to include these calories.

Popular Diets

At a seminar that I recently attended, offered by Exercise ETC., Inc., Jeannie Patton, M.S., presented some interesting facts concerning the current fad diets, facts that support my belief in "calories in must equal calories out." When the fad diets are all compared, no matter what is recommended concerning the products to be consumed and in what quantities, the one common factor is a reduction in calories consumed. This was the one common thread among all of the diets. It had nothing to do with high protein, high carbs, low fat, or any other combination. It had to due with a reduction in CALORIES! Couple this with exercise, and bingo! A new you! These are the guidelines as offered by Exercise ETC., Inc. when deciding on a diet:[5]

1. Author's or Promoter's Credentials—look for ties to reputable academic/research institutions and expertise in diet, nutrition, or weight loss.

2. Premise of the Diet—how do the claims being made fit in with the current research on the subject of weight loss?

3. Calories, Foods Allowed, and Use of Supplements—do the recommendations allow for sufficient calorie intake on a daily basis (for women, approximately 1,400 to 2,000 calories per day, and for men, approximately 1,600-2,000 calories per day)? Are you required to eliminate certain foods or food groups, and are they labeled as "good" or "bad"? Are supplements recommended?

4. Sustainability—will you be able to stay on this diet for a long period of time? Does it allow for proper nutrient intake, and will the diet fit into your lifestyle? Are there options in food choices and flexibility?

5. Weight loss—is there proof of weight loss on the particular diet, and at what rate? What weight is being lost? Is it fat, or water weight or, worse yet, is it muscle?

6. Scientific Basis/Research—are there any studies to support the claims, and are they published in peer-reviewed journals? Is the diet based on sound nutrition principles?

According to Dr. Wanda Eastman, the key phrase is "not too much and not too little" of a nutrient.

Please see the ten accompanying charts at the end of this chapter for a comparison of the popular diets. My belief still holds true: balance and moderation are the key! Fiber is a non-digestible form of carbohydrate.

A very important element in weight loss and health is fiber intake. Americans do not get enough fiber! Adult men need to get a minimum of 30 to 38 grams of fiber per day, and women should get 20 to 25 grams a day. On the average we get somewhere between 12 to 15 grams of fiber a day. Fiber is found in plants, and is what makes up the structure of the plant, similar to the framing on a house. Fiber consists of leaves, stems, roots, and other related materials, including the skins of fruit and the seeds that plants bear. This is why whole-grain foods are preferable over refined foods. Whole-grain foods have more fiber, vitamins, and minerals than refined or processed foods. Does it make any sense to take everything out of grain and then enrich it when it is made into bread? When we eat fiber, it aids in digestion by a scraping action on the intestinal walls. It also binds, dilutes, and inhibits the absorption of harmful chemicals, and shortens the amount of time that food remains in the body, which may reduce the incidence of intestinal problems and cancer, since food passes more quickly through the body. Fiber slows the absorption of carbohydrates by slowing the rate of absorption. Fiber should be acquired from food and not supplements. On the other side of the equation, too much fiber can slow the absorption of minerals.

How to Reduce or Stop Muscle Gains

In a review of literature about low-carbohydrate diets, there is convincing evidence that a low-carbohydrate diet will reduce performance in endurance events; however; resistance exercise is more affected by low dietary energy intake than carbohydrate intake.[6] Dietary energy intake is the calories derived from an intake of protein, carbohydrates, and fat. While it could be all of one source, say protein, hopefully it would be from a combination of protein, carbohydrates, and fat. The important point here is that calorie consumption is very important in gaining lean muscle mass. Eat!

Calories In = Calories Out

In order to maintain the same body weight, the calories consumed must equal the calories expended. If you consume more calories than your body needs, the excess calories will be deposited as fat. Calories are used for the production of energy—energy for walking, running, lifting weights—as well as energy for normal bodily functions such as respiration, circulation, body temperature maintenance, and so on. Basal Metabolic Rate (BMR) is the minimum amount of energy the body needs to conduct the vital processes. It is measured while the body is at rest.

A kilocalorie is the measure of the energy value of food expressed in terms of heat. This is the amount of heat required to raise the temperature of one kilogram of water one degree Centigrade. Calorie is the term most often used to describe a kilocalorie, and is the term most of us are familiar with using. The energy value is measured using a sample of food, which is placed in a "bomb calorimeter." The sample is burned under conditions allowing for complete combustion and termed "heat of combustion." The heat of combustion is the energy produced by the combustion of the material being tested.

By combining BMR and daily activity level, we arrive at the total caloric expenditure for a day. This is dependent on a number of factors, including normal daily activities, bodyweight (lean muscle mass vs. fat), metabolism, exercise time per day, exertion level during exercise, sex, body condition, hormones, and age, to name a few.

Another way to estimate daily caloric needs is offered by the United States Department of Agriculture (USDA). They recommend a person take their bodyweight in pounds and multiply it by a factor correlated to activity level as shown below.

TABLE 12.1   Estimated Daily Caloric Needs

Activity Level*	Less than 1 hour daily	1 hour daily	More than 1 hour daily
Men	16	21	26
Women	14	18	22

* Amount of exercise per day.

For a male weighing 200 lbs., exercising one hour a day, the equation would look like this:

$$200 \times 21 = 4200 \text{ calories per day.}$$

For a female of the same weight, exercising one hour a day:

$$200 \times 18 = 3600 \text{ calories per day.}$$

These estimations appear to be high, and do not take into consideration age, physical condition, height, and so on.

I have found that a more accurate representation in the athletes I have trained would be:

TABLE 12.2   Estimated Daily Caloric Needs for Athletes

Activity Level*	Less than 1 hour daily	1 hour daily	More than 1 hour daily
Men	14	19	24
Women	12	16	20

* Amount of exercise per day.

Thus, a 200-lb. male training 1 hour per day would need approximately 3800 calories, and a 100-lb. female training 1 hour per day would need 1600 calories.

When the caloric intake is equal to the caloric expenditure, there will be no change in bodyweight. The bodyweight will change when this balance is not maintained. One pound of bodyweight has the caloric equivalent of 3500 calories. To gain 1 pound and individual would need to consume an extra 3500 calories and to lose 1 pound an individual would need to expend 3500 calories. The calorie count is cumulative. What this means is that if you consume 100 extra calories per day for 35 days, you will gain one pound. Conversely, if you subtract 100 calories a day from your diet, over 35 days you will lose one pound of bodyweight. Granted, these numbers would work like this in a perfect world, but since very few of us have the means to determine our exact caloric intake per day, it is merely a guideline.

When altering the diet for weight loss or weight gain, most individuals will use 500 calories per day as a marker. By adding 500 calories per day, an individual will gain approximately 1 pound per week, whereas by subtracting 500 calories per day, an individual will lose 1 pound per week. These estimates are just examples, and there are many other factors that would need to be considered.

It is generally considered safe for women to lose 1 pound per week and for men to lose 2 pounds per week. By "safe" I mean reasonable, and I mean weight that will stay off. With a gradual reduction, the body will have a tendency to keep the weight off; the gradual reduction, also allows the body to reset itself in terms of what the body considers "normal" weight.

In all the years of training I have done with people, I have recognized that however long it took a person to gain weight is approximately how long it will take them to lose the weight. The weight did not appear overnight by surprise, and it won't disappear overnight by surprise either. How many of you can honestly tell me that you didn't notice when you gained weight? I have often wondered how people can kid themselves about gaining weight when they are buying larger dresses, larger pants, and larger belts. We are only kidding ourselves! All of our family, friends, and acquaintances are seeing the weight gain.

Weight Loss Example Using Calories

A male with a bodyweight of 200 lbs. would like to lose 10 lbs. of weight. He works out approximately 1 hour per day. What is his starting caloric demand, and what will be his adjusted caloric demand to lose 2 lbs. per week to reach his goal weight of 190 lbs.?

Current weight: 200 lbs.

Activity level: 17

Goal weight: 190 lbs.

Using the formula of bodyweight × activity level = daily calories, we would have:

200 (lbs. of bodyweight) × 17 (activity level, 1 hour per day) = 3400 calories.

To maintain this weight he would have to consume 3400 calories per day.

500 calories per day × 7 days per week = 3500 calories or 1 lb. of weight loss per week.

1000 calories per day × 7 days per week = 7000 calories or 2 lbs. of weight loss per week.

To lose 2 lbs. of weight per week, he would have to deduct 1000 calories per day from his diet. Since he is consuming 3400 calories per day, his new total calories per day would be 2400. At this rate, it would take him 5 weeks to lose the 10 lbs.

The same formula to gain 10 lbs. at 2 lbs. per week would be used for weight gain; only we would add 1000 calories per day instead of subtracting it.

This is a simplistic approach to weight loss and weight gain, and will not work for those who have underlying medical conditions. In order for this formula to work, the individual would have to keep a log detailing quantities and types of food consumed. The individual would then have to convert calories to see how many they are consuming per day, and adjust accordingly.

Number of Meals per Day

A number of factors are associated with the number of meals consumed per day. It is fairly well established that smaller meals, spread out through the day, will have an influence on the depositing of fat. The more meals consumed, the less likely an individual is to deposit them as fat, provided the daily required calories are not exceeded. This does not mean six large meals, but six smaller ones instead. The daily required calorie figure is divided by six meals to arrive at the calories per meal. There is some room for variation, here as an individual could eat two or three larger meal and then divide the remaining calories into a couple of snacks during the day. In our example above, for the weight loss of 2 lbs. per week, we would take 2400 calories per day and divide it by six meals. This will give us six meals at 400 calories per meal. By adding more meals that are smaller in size, it has been shown that the body will deposit less fat and burn more calories, due to the speeding up of the metabolism to digest the six meals. We will also have better utilization of the nutrients in these meals.

Daily Protein Requirements

For sedentary individuals, the USDA Recommended Daily Allowance (RDA) is probably adequate; however, for active individuals the protein requirements fall short. The RDA for adults is thought to be about 0.8 grams per kilogram of bodyweight. One kilo is roughly 2.2 lbs. Again, this figure is for the sedentary individual. Numerous studies on protein confirm that active individuals need more protein than sedentary individuals, particularly athletes. A minimum amount of protein for an athlete would be 0.75 to 1 gram per POUND of bodyweight. This amount will help improve strength and muscular development in athletes. While many nutritionists do not agree, strength coaches and others who deal with athletes and can see the difference protein makes will attest to the fact that athletes need more protein. I do not know of *any* strength athletes or bodybuilders who do not consume large quantities of protein. They include protein in their diets from a variety of sources, including red meat, chicken, fish, turkey, cheese, milk, eggs, and protein supplements. Very few of these same athletes consume large quantities of vegetable-based proteins such as soy. Protein is *very* important for individuals engaged in weight training.

Athletes, particularly those engaged in weight training (and women in general) do not get enough protein. A simple rule of thumb for daily protein intake that will work for men and women is this: Take in 1 gram of protein for every pound of bodyweight, every day.

Nitrogen Balance

Nitrogen balance is the sum of all nitrogen content of all food intake compared to the amount of nitrogen that is excreted from the human body and is a way to measure protein status. If the nitrogen balance intake is equal to the nitrogen excretion, the body is said to be in nitrogen equilibrium. This is indicative of the protein intake being sufficient to repair existing body tissue, but no new growth is occurring. A positive nitrogen balance happens when nitrogen intake exceeds excretion, thus allowing for muscular growth to occur. This means that muscles are being built faster than they are being destroyed. In negative nitrogen balance, excretion is exceeding intake, and muscles are breaking down at a rate faster than they are being repaired. With a positive nitrogen balance, the body is said to be in an anabolic state, whereas with a negative nitrogen balance, the body is said to be in a catabolic state. The body will gain protein in the positive state, but lose protein in the negative state.

Testing for nitrogen balance can be done using nitrogen sticks, available from a pharmacist.

Vegetarians and Weight Training

I know of very few vegetarians involved in weight training or other strength sports at the competitive level. Personally, I do not believe in vegetarian diets and believe that humans are omnivores, as evidenced by our teeth. If we were supposed to be vegetarians, we wouldn't have teeth designed for ripping and tearing meat. However, I recognize that being a vegetarian is a personal choice and may be for reasons such as religion, ethical, or ecological.

I'm going to make a generalization here about strict vegetarians, not the lacto-ovo variety or others, but the hard-core vegetarians whom I have trained. They are generally a pale white color; lack muscle tone and strength, and they look "stringy." The female vegetarians I have trained have disproportionately large hips in relation to their shoulders. This is possibly due to the lack of muscle in the upper body.

In a paper titled "Effect of Vegetarian Diets on Performance in Strength Sports,"[7] Chris Forbe-Ewan explored a debate on the *Sportscience* mailing list about vegetarians and strength sports. Three categories were included:

1. Non-vegetarians or omnivore's. This group eats foods of plant and animal origin, including meat, fowl, fish, eggs, milk, and other dairy products.

2. Lacto-ovo vegetarians. This group eats predominantly foods of plant origin, with milk, dairy products, and eggs being the only foods of animal origin.

3. Vegans: This group eats foods only of plant origin.

Since the Vegan diet is less common than the lacto-ovo diet, the discussion was limited to the lacto-ovo vegetarians and the non-vegetarians.

Hebbelinck et al. (1999) conducted a study of vegetarian children, adolescents, and young adults in the Netherlands. The researchers conducted anthropometric analyses (stature, weight, skinfold thicknesses), puberty ratings (where appropriate), and physical-fitness testing (handgrip strength, standing long jump, sit-ups in 30 seconds, and heart-rate recovery following a step test). When the results were compared to reference values:

1. Vegetarian adolescents were of significantly lower stature, weight, and body mass index. There were no differences in stature or weight for the other age groups.

2. Vegetarian children were equally fit, but the vegetarian adolescents scored lower on the standing long jump and 30 second sit-up tests.

3. The heart rate of vegetarian adolescents and young adults recovered substantially faster after the step-test.

The conclusion of Hebbelinck et al. is that vegetarian adolescents and young adults performed better at the cardiorespiratory test, but vegetarian adolescents scored lower on the strength and explosive tests that were administered.

Observationally, I would agree with this assessment.

The following conclusions were derived from the discussion:

1. Different kinds of vegetarianism could have different effects on strength.

2. It appears that there is a preponderance of meat-eaters among strength athletes at the elite level. Whether this is because of meat consumption, placebo effect, supplement consumption, or other effects is unclear.

3. Diets of gorillas, chimpanzees, and Paleolithic humans cannot be relied on to indicate the optimal diet for health and fitness or strength athletes.

4. Vegetarian diets that are well planned, especially those including milk and/or eggs, can provide all essential nutrients for good health and a high level of sports performance.

5. Vegetarian diets associated with improved health outcomes do not mean that vegetarian diets are superior for performance in strength sports or strength-dependent activities.

6. One recent study of resistance training in older males showed that omnivores had a bigger gain in muscle mass than vegetarians.

7. If strength is enhanced by meat consumption, the mechanism could be increased testosterone or increased storage of creatine phosphate in the muscle.

8. More research is required.

If you are still not convinced that it is permissible to eat meat, chicken, fish, and fowl, then eat a balanced diet by combining complementary foods to insure that you get a balanced amino acid profile. Depending on your degree of vegetarianism, it could be difficult to get enough high-quality protein in your diet. The addition of milk and egg products will greatly enhance your protein intake, as will the use of protein powders such as whey, milk, and egg. As a vegetarian, you will need to work closely with your trainer and nutritionist.

Recommended Percentages of Protein, Carbohydrates, and Fat

It is often stated that the typical diet should consist of between 50 to 60 percent carbohydrates, 25 to 30 percent fat, and 10 to 15 percent protein. Currently, the average American diet is 49% carbohydrates, 34-35% fat, and 16% protein according to the National Health and Nutrition Exam.[3]

For weight training, I would recommend an intake of approximately 30 percent protein, 40 percent carbohydrates, and 30 percent fat. Some would say that this is too much protein and fat. Dr. Kevin Vigilante of Brown University School of Medicine has stated that diets containing less than 25 percent fat may raise heart attack risk, because these diets reduce the levels of good cholesterol (HDL) as well as that of bad cholesterol (LDL). Consumed in moderation, fat actually promotes weight loss.

As a nation, we have heard for two to three decades that a high-carbohydrate, low-fat diet is the way to go. However, we have become more obese on these diets. We have also cut our fat intake at the same time, yet we continue to get fatter. Currently, roughly 60 percent of Americans are overweight, and

30 percent are obese. Something is not right with our diets. Maybe it is because we consume too many "simple" carbohydrates as compared to "complex" carbohydrates. Maybe it is the fault of the food service industry with their "all you can eat buffets" and their "super-sized portions" or maybe it is our fault because we are just "pigs" when it comes to eating. Foods high in sugar and fat taste good, and an extra hundred calories here or there is not noticeable at the time of consumption. Whatever the reason, I can't help but believe that the main reason we are fat is because we consciously choose to be fat. It is impossible not to notice the increasing size of our clothes on the way to "fatdom." We may deny it or be in denial about it, but the bottom line is that we know we are fat. I know from personal experience that the easiest way to lose weight is to eliminate the "simple" carbohydrates. While this may not work for everybody, it has certainly worked for me when I have needed to cut weight. The problem of obesity is more complex than carbs, fats, and proteins; the #1 reason is lack of physical activity. Calories consumed have to equal calories burned (calories in = calories out), otherwise weight gain or weight loss will occur!

How to Read a Food Label

Food labels, required by the Food and Drug Administration (FDA), are very important in determining product ingredients. The labels will include information about calories, fat, cholesterol, sodium, carbohydrates, protein, and other vitamins and minerals. The labels also show the "Percentage of Daily Value" or % DV, which is based on a diet containing 2000 calories, the reference point of the average daily energy requirement for most people. This percentage is designed to show how much of certain nutrients are being supplied by the food being consumed. Larger, more muscular individuals would require more nutrients, while smaller and leaner individuals might require less. Most food labels also provide the fat, cholesterol, sodium, carbohydrate, and fiber counts for a 2500-calorie diet as well as the 2000-calorie diet.

The amount of each nutrient per serving is divided by the total recommended daily amount. This division gives us a percentage on which to base how much of the daily value of that particular nutrient we are eating per serving. If the daily value of fat is 65 grams and we consume a serving that contains 6.5 grams of fat, we have consumed 10 percent of the recommended daily value.

If you are an athlete or dieter, or are pregnant or nursing, your daily value will probably differ from the 2000-calorie-a-day reference point. A dietitian or nutritionist will help you develop a program that will meet your needs, whether it be weight gain, weight loss, or just a change in eating habits to shed fat and add muscle. A great website for finding a registered dietitian is www.eatright.org.

Ingredients

Ingredients are listed in descending order on a label. The ingredient that makes up most of the product will be listed first, followed by the second most plentiful ingredient, and so on. The ingredient that is the least of the product will be listed last. All ingredients are listed on the label.

The label will state the serving size and the servings per container. The serving size and servings per container will vary by product. Many products are designed to have one serving per container, while other products may have many servings per container. The calories listed on the label will be per serving.

As an example, we will use a 6 oz. can of Star Kist Tuna (solid white albacore in spring water). The label claims the following:

TABLE 12.3   Star Kist Tuna

White Albacore in Spring Water

Nutrition Facts	Saturated Fat 0 g
Serving Size: 2 oz. drained	Cholesterol 25 mg
Servings Per Container: About 2.5	Sodium 250 mg
Amount Per Serving	Total Carbohydrates 0
Calories 70 Fat Calories 10	Protein 15 g
Total Fat 1 g	

Ingredients: White Tuna, Spring Water, Vegetable Broth, Salt, Pyrophosphate

Taking the servings per can and multiplying by 15 grams of protein per serving, we see that the total protein content of this can is approximately 37.5 grams.

Taking the servings per can and multiplying by 1 gram of fat per serving, we see that the total fat content of this can is 2.5 grams.

Taking the servings per can and multiplying by 70 calories per serving, we see that the total calories for this can are 175.

Eating the contents of this can of Star Kist Tuna will provide us with 62.5 mg of cholesterol and 625 mg of sodium.

By reading the ingredients on the label, we see that white tuna is the #1 ingredient, followed by spring water, vegetable broth, salt, and finally the last ingredient in the smallest amount, pyrophosphate.

Sodium

Sodium chloride is a mineral required for good health, however, we consume too much of it because it is hidden in almost everything that we eat. We require only about 2000 milligrams a day, but we consume as much as six times this amount! Table salt, as it is called, is in everything from potato chips to canned vegetables and lunchmeats; even the tuna used in the example on how to figure calories contains salt.

Too much sodium in a diet can lead to an increase in blood pressure, which is known to be a risk factor in heart disease and kidney disease. Sodium causes water retention as well, and this is not a desirable side effect for most athletes. Never salt food until you taste it and then only salt it to taste. Most foods are prepared using salt, and by salting it you are missing out on the true flavor of what you eat.

Caffeine

Caffeine is a stimulant found in many things such as coffee and tea. It is also found in chocolate, soft drinks, various spiked waters, over-the-counter (OTC) medications, beer, and too many other sources to mention. Caffeine is addictive.

Caffeine stimulates the brain and body, and in small amounts is not harmful. However, in large amounts it can lead to insomnia, anxiety, heart rhythm irregularities, higher blood pressure, nervousness, and upset stomach. Too much caffeine can also lead to fatigue and irritability.

The amount of caffeine in a product varies widely. The average 12 oz. cup of coffee probably has between 100 and125 mg of caffeine, whereas the average shot of espresso has only about 25 to 30 mg of caffeine. Compare this to a No-Doz or Vivarin tablet that has 100 to 200 mg of caffeine per tablet.

Coffee served at coffee houses usually will have more caffeine if it is a light roast, and less caffeine if it is a dark roast.

For most people it is probably not a good idea to have caffeine after the noon hour, as those sensitive to caffeine will have a restless night of sleep and be more tired the next day. It is a vicious cycle. Withdrawal from caffeine can cause excruciating headaches, drowsiness, and nausea that will last for several days to a week. It is recommended that pregnant women and those that are nursing not use caffeine. Caffeine may cause birth defects.

It makes one wonder, how can anything that causes withdrawal symptoms and birth defects be good for us?

Caffeine Decontamination Regime

In order to cleanse your body of caffeine, simply follow the program below.

Week 1   Cut caffeine consumption by 1/2

Week 2   Cut caffeine consumption by 1/2 again

Week 3   Cut caffeine consumption by 1/2 again

Week 4   No caffeine.

If you are drinking four cups of coffee a day at the start of Week 1, cut it down to two cups a day. Beginning Week 2, cut it down to one cup a day. Beginning Week 3, cut it down to 1/2 a cup a day. Beginning Week 4, you are caffeine-free, without all of the negative side effects with getting caffeine out of your system. I have used this program successfully with my athletes, and they have had no ill effects from the withdrawal.

Body Pollutants

"Remember, the food you eat today is walking and talking tomorrow!"—Jack LaLanne[1]

Nothing could be truer than the above quotation. In a news conference held on January 31, 2003, David Fleming, MD, of the Centers for Disease Control (CDC)[8] spoke about an extensive assessment of exposure the U.S. population is getting to environmental chemicals. In the two years since the CDC first released a report focusing on 27 chemicals, the list has expanded to include 116 chemicals. The chemicals invading our bodies are factually known, not guesswork. The data of actual blood and urine measurements of thousands of Americans has been collected and analyzed. The 116 chemicals include secondhand tobacco smoke, pesticides, metals, dioxins, PCBs and other chemicals known to cause cancer and/or other health problems in animals.

While not every chemical was found in everyone tested, and the findings don't necessarily mean they will suffer disease, all chemicals were found in at least some people. While the body can handle many kinds of exposure to a degree, the real question will be to what degree before a disease begins.

The most troubling find for Richard Jackson, MD, MPH, was the fact that more than half of our kids still have environmental smoke exposure and one-third of all cancers are from tobacco. Environmental smoke has been linked to sudden infant death syndrome (SIDS) and respiratory infections.

Jim Pirkle, MD, PHD, says, "From a public health point of view, it is a giant step forward for us (the CDC). It will make big differences in our ability to identify and prevent disease."

Bottom Line

The bottom line is this: Steer clear of anything refined, enriched, processed, or white. By white, I mean sugar, white flour, white pasta, and so on. Get your carbohydrates from fresh fruit and vegetable sources that have not been processed or concentrated.

When purchasing your food, try to buy natural, organic, pesticide-free, chemical-free, fungicide-free, and herbicide-free. Also, stay away from anything using genetically modified organisms (GMO's), or containing hormones (growth or otherwise) or antibodies such as might be found in meat and milk.

Beginning on October 21, 2002, the USDA is implementing a national standards and food-labeling program designed to replace state and private certification standards as to what is "organic." Under the new guidelines, in order to be considered organic, the product must be 95 to 100 percent organic in order to carry the USDA Organic seal. Other products can be labeled as "Made with Organic" if they contain 70 to 94 percent organic ingredients.

Organic and natural products can be found in a wide variety of stores, including Wild Oats, Sun Harvest, Albertson's, Coop's, and many more. Surprisingly enough, they are not that much more expensive than regular products, and in many cases are as cheap or cheaper.

While modern medicine is a wonderful thing and life expectancies have increased, what we are talking about here is not how many years you live, but instead the "quality" of those years. What good is it to live to be 100 if you are bedridden and incapable of going outside to play with a child or a dog? There is only one reason we cannot live to be 100 and active, and that reason is our individual lifestyle!

Supplements

It has been my experience from 25 years of weight training, competitive weightlifting, teaching, owning a gym, and working for a supplement company, that 90 to 95 percent of the supplements on the market as advertised in health & fitness magazines, bodybuilding magazines, and so on, are a complete waste of money, and the only thing you get out of them is expensive urine and feces!

With that said, let's look at some supplements that could have some potential. Dr. Med. B. Dorr at the 72nd Men's and 15th Women's World Weightlifting Championships Annual Congress held in Warsaw, Poland, November 18, 2002, did a presentation on nutritional supplements.[9] Some of the facts presented:

1. It is necessary to use nutritional supplements in sport sometimes.

2. 94 of 634, or 15% of the substances in samples acquired from 13 countries were contaminated; and an Austrian study showed a contamination rate of 22% (12 of 54 samples). By contamination it is meant that we are talking about substances that would yield a positive drug test for banned substances as governed by the International Olympic Committee (IOC). Olympic athletes are responsible for whatever substances are found in their bodies.

3. Three questions were posed:

   a. Are the supplements useful?

   b. Are the supplements dangerous?

   c. How can safety of the supplements be guaranteed?

4. Do scientific studies exist proving the supplements work and, if so, for what kinds of supplements?

The answers to the three questions are: Maybe, maybe, and yes if the company producing the supplements does not produce hormones or prohormones, and no contact with these two groups of compounds has occurred. It is also necessary that there is a quality-control component for anabolic substances.

So what works, you ask?

1. Glutamine, because of its anticatabolic effect due to increased intracellular volume.

2. BCAAs (Valine, Leucine, and Isoleucine) may work because protein decreases during exercise and they may help against symptoms of overuse.

3. Creatine has shown to allow for increased training intensity, and hypertrophic effects have been observed in weightlifting.

4. HMB (Beta-Hydroxy-Beta-Methylbutyrate) shows positive effects for *untrained* persons and possible effects for endurance athletes, but no confirmed effects for trained athletes.

Additional Supplements

I would recommend the following supplements in addition to eating a balanced diet:

1. Protein in various forms, i.e., soy, whey, milk, egg, etc. An excellent source for information about protein and custom blending can be found at: www.proteinfactory.com. The Protein Factory has been very consistent in providing me with quality products. Not only can you custom-blend your protein through this company, but they also offer ready-to-purchase powders at a reasonable cost.

2. Daily vitamin and mineral supplement, ideally one that would be taken in the morning and again in the evening. I prefer the vitamins and minerals to be either capsules or soft gels since there won't be any fillers, binders, etc. in the product. Many times tablets will pass through the body unabsorbed due to the tremendous pressure required to form and make the ingredients into tablets.

Don't Even Think about These

Do not consider any supplement or liquid that contains ephedra, ephedrine, or ma huang. There are more studies than I care to cite detailing ephedra-based products and the potential health risks associated with these products, however, one is worth mentioning. In a study to be posted on the *Annals of Internal Medicine's*[10] website, February 4, 2003, it is reported that there were 1,178 adverse reactions reported to U.S. poison-control center's in 2001. The report states that ephedra is unsafe at any dose, even the recommended dose. Ephedra is typically found in weight-loss products and bodybuilding supplements, and as an over-the-counter (OTC) medication in many stores, gas stations, truck stops, and so on. It is used primarily as a stimulant. In May 2003, the state of Illinois banned the sale of ephedra products. This move is long overdue and should become a nationwide ban on these products. According to the U.S. Food and Drug Administration, 117 deaths and 18,000 reports of other medical problems have been linked to ephedra.

Isn't It Amazing?

I find it absolutely amazing that people will put anything in their bodies when trying to lose weight. If you think about it, what do these supplements for weight loss do? Generally, they speed up the metabolism, increase heat in the body, and cause water loss. Isn't that the exact same thing that exercise does? If you exercise, your metabolism speeds up, the heat in the body increases, and your body sweats! Sounds like the same thing to me, only there is *one* big difference: exercise is good for you, weight loss products or other drugs aren't. Which would you rather do? On the one hand we have exercise, which is healthy; on the other hand we have drugs, potions, and gimmicks that could potentially kill you. But then again, some people also believe in "live fast, die young, and leave a good-looking corpse!"

Drug or Supplement Questions?

If you ever have a question about a particular drug or supplement and its legality in competition, call the United States Anti-Doping Agency (USADA) at 1-800-233-0393 (www.usantidoping.org). The USADA is an independent anti-doping agency for Olympic sports in the United States, and they are determined to eliminate the doping in sports while maintaining the integrity of the sports and the competitive spirit of clean participants in the U.S. I have discovered that if a drug or supplement isn't banned by the USADA, chances are it doesn't work, with a few notable exceptions like creatine. If a drug is banned, that could mean many things, not the least of which is that the drug could be dangerous to your health. Just because it is banned does not mean that you should take it, and it also does not mean that it will enhance your performance!

Why Do Most Supplements Work?

The perception that most supplements work can be attributed to a phenomenon known as the "placebo effect." In other words, if you think it will work, it will, but the question is, for how long? If the supplement has not been studied and published in a journal that is peer-reviewed, don't waste your money! An excellent source of information on supplements is: www.consumerlab.com. Their goal is to identify the best health and nutrition products on the market through independent testing. Consumer Lab (CL) will tell you if the product contains what the label claims, and if it contains things the label doesn't claim. CL is not affiliated with any manufacturer.

Another way to tell if a product is a quality product is to look for the "USP" designation. The USP stands for United States Pharmacopeia. The USP provides standards for over 3,800 medicines, dietary supplements, and other health care products. The USP ensures that consumers receive quality medicines and dietary supplements by establishing standards that manufactures must meet for strength, purity, quality, packaging, and labeling. Their website is: www.usp.org.

Check the next dietary product you buy, chances are about 1 in 100 that it will have either the CL or USP stamp of approval. Does this tell you anything?

Smoking Makes You Ugly

While smoking and tobacco products are not supplements, they will detract from optimal athletic performance. In a study done by scientists from St. John's Institute of Dermatology in London and published in *The Lancet* medical journal[11] it is suggested that smoking turns on a gene that is involved in destroying the collagen in the skin, which is a structural protein that gives skin its elasticity. The gene is also implicated in wrinkles due to sunbathing, and it was found that the same gene was very active in smokers, but not in nonsmokers. The indication is that something in smoking is injurious to skin in a fashion similar to sunbathing, or at least using the same pathways, according to Dr. James Leyden, a professor of dermatology at the University of Pennsylvania Medical School. Dr. Leyden was not connected to the research. Dr. Leyden also states that contributing factors to premature aging in smoking can be attributed to screwing up the face and pursing the lips when one drags on a cigarette.

For more information on aging skin, go to:

www.skincarephysicians.com/agingskinnet/index.html.

It has been known for years that there is a link between smoking and wrinkles, and if this doesn't prove it, then go ahead and make yourself ugly!

One Final Note

My mom has said many times that when you are young, you live to eat, and when you are old, you eat to live. Thinking back, I think she must be right, for I remember being eighteen and always thinking about my next meal. I never gained weight, no matter how much I ate. Now, my level of enthusiasm to eat has diminished and I eat when I need to according to my training schedule, but never with the anticipation I had when I was eighteen. If I go on a bout of eating and no exercise, I gain weight. After considering this statement, I have concluded that it means when we are young, our bodies are calorie-burning machines and we need to feed them constantly to keep the machine going; however, as we age, the machine slows down and does not burn the calories it once did. In later years, as studies have shown, a person must eat to survive, because the first step to death for many elderly is when they quit eating and their bodies waste away from lack of nourishment. This is all the more reason to put premium foods in our bodies, rather than the junk foods. A long life is not about the age, but more about the quality of life.

The Center for Science in the Public Interest (CSPI)

The CSPI is a nonprofit education and advocacy organization with a focus on improving safety and nutritional quality. They offer many good self-tests and information on their website, www.cspinet.org, that focus on nutrition, food safety, food additives, and alcohol. The site also has many special reports on items from eating raw shellfish, to eating liquid candy, to the obesity epidemic. This is a must-see website.

3 Fat Chicks

One of my favorite websites for great information on commercial diets, fast food restaurants, diet supplements, food reviews, and many other interesting items related to nutrition is www.3fatchicks.com. If you click on "Fast Food Nutrition" you will find the nutritional breakdowns for many popular chain food restaurants and the items they serve. This site also has low-carb and low-fat recipes, a forum, weight loss articles, and a whole host of other fun things relating to food. I highly recommend that you access this website; in fact, it has been named "Best of Web" by *Forbes Magazine* for a third time!

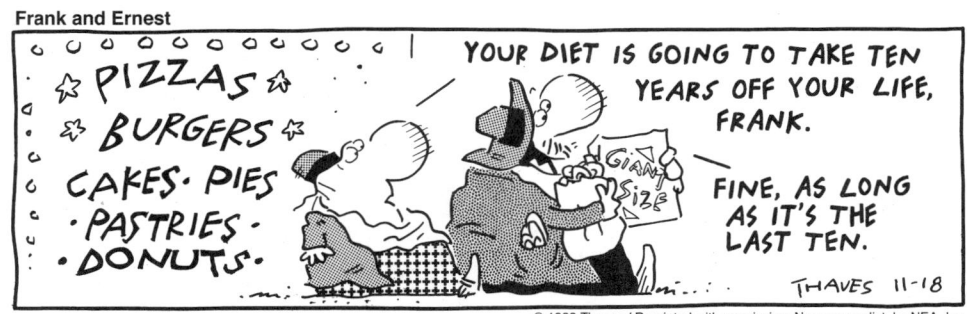

Frank and Ernest

© 1993 Thaves / Reprinted with permission. Newspaper dist. by NEA, Inc.

Foods You Eat on this Diet

Red meat, chicken and turkey, seafood, eggs, high fat dairy foods like cheese, butter, and cream, oil, nuts, some vegetables that do not contain a lot of starch, artificial sweeteners.

General Facts: There are three phases of this diet: induction, weight loss, and maintenance

Can you keep it off on this type of diet? No long term studies have been provided to date. High fat diets are not associated with health weight maintenance.

Positives: Some people may enjoy the fatty foods and meat on this diet and the rapid weight loss at first.

Drawbacks: This is a high fat diet, high in animal foods, and limited in carbohydrate, so it teaches people to choose calorie dense foods that are likely to lead to weight gain and heart disease once the diet is over.

Safety and Health Issues

This diet limits many healthy vegetables and nutrient rich carbohydrates. Eating a diet high in saturated fat raises blood cholesterol levels and increases risk of heart disease.

- Associated with heart disease. High in saturated fat, the number one nutrient associated with this disease
- Low in fruits, whole grains, and other sources of carbohydrate
- Low in phytochemicals - cancer fighting substances founds in fruits and vegetables
- Lack of fiber may cause constipation
- Rapid loss of water weight at first may provide a false sense of diet success

Diet Surf's Recommendation: Not Recommended

Dietitians Comments about the Atkins Diet: Many people may enjoy eating the fatty foods allowed on this diet but may find it monotonous and restrictive over time. Any diet that restricts calories will cause weight loss, a reduction in blood pressure, reduced blood sugar (if it was abnormally high), and reduced blood cholesterol and triglycerides in the typical overweight person. There is no magic in restricting carbohydrates. Eventually, carbohydrates need to be added to this diet. Adding back carbohydrates on top of foods high in saturated fat brings people back to square one, the typical American diet, associated with obesity, heart disease, cancer, and high blood pressure.

If this diet was a true cure for obesity and heart disease, it would have worked the first time it was introduced over 30 years ago.

The preceding table has been reprinted with permission from the webmaster of DietSurf.com as it originally appeared.

THE ZONE DIET   Type of Diet: Low Carbohydrate, High Protein, Moderate Fat

Foods You Eat on this Diet

Low fat protein foods such as skinless chicken breast, fish, low fat cottage cheese, some fruits and vegetables, and small amounts of olive or canola oil.

Comments: Emphasis is on eating a specific balance of foods at every meal so that you stay in "the zone" for peak efficiency and energy. Focus is on eating on low-glycemic index foods.

Can you keep it off on this type of diet? This diet is quite low in calories (800-1200 Calories), designed for short term, quick weight loss, not long term.

Positives: Good amounts of fruits and low starch vegetables, and low in saturated fat. Restricts refined carbohydrates that are low in nutrition.

Drawbacks: Meals must be calculated with exact balance of fat, protein and carbohydrate for proper "zone". Diet is very restricted in calories, so it is difficult to stay on long enough to lose weight, especially if you exercise.

Safety and Health Issues

Basically safe on the higher calorie level (1200) but too low in essential nutrients.

- Low in whole grains and calcium
- Low in carbohydrate - eliminates many highly nutritious foods without proven scientific rationale

Diet Surf Recommendations: Not recommended

Dietitians Comments: The challenge of combining certain foods may be too complex and a hassle for many people to follow for an extended period of time. Amounts of carbohydrate containing foods (even the good ones like whole grains and beans) are restricted so that it may be difficult to stay on this diet long enough for long term results. Overemphasis is placed upon the notion that carbohydrates promote fat storage due to increased insulin levels, and that reducing carbohydrates is the solution to obesity. Restricting total **calories** and amounts of food causes weight loss and improves insulin sensitivity, not just restriction of carbohydrates. Any diet that restricts calories (of any source - fat, carbohydrate, and protein) will cause weight loss. There is no magic in restricting carbohydrates and it is unnecessary to limit the "good" carbohydrates like starchy vegetables, whole grains, and beans.

The preceding table has been reprinted with permission from the webmaster of DietSurf.com as it originally appeared.

Foods You Eat on this Diet

Whole grains, fruits, vegetables with low a glycemic index, avoids grains, fruits, and vegetables with high a glycemic index and avoids refined sugar.

Comments: Emphasizes that sugar is "toxic" to the body and is based on the glycemic index of foods instead of nutrient composition or calories.

Can you keep it off on this type of diet? Emphasis on avoiding highly processed foods helps keep many low nutrition foods (like most desserts) out of the diet, and this can help with calorie control, which is important for long term weight maintenance.

Positives: Eliminates a lot of "junk" foods

Drawbacks: Overemphasis on glycemic index to determine food choices, therefore eliminates many healthful, beneficial foods unnecessarily.

Safety and Health Issues

Generally safe, although athletes and hard core exercisers need high glycemic carbohydrates for fuel and should avoid this diet.

- Eliminates many healthy carbohydrates
- Focus is on a single dietary issue

Diet Surf Recommendations: Recommended with reservations - diet is basically safe but goes overboard on the sugar toxicity issue and overemphasizes one aspect of food metabolism, the glycemic index.

Dietitians Comments about the Sugar Busters Diet: Although Sugar Busters helps people to reduce their intake of "empty" calories from refined carbohydrates like sugar, it overemphasizes the importance of the glycemic index, which is a measure of a food's effect on raising blood sugar levels. The glycemic index of a single food changes when that food is eaten with something else. So, since most people eat meals and snacks that are mixed (fat, protein, and carbohydrate) the glycemic index doesn't have the impact that this diet asserts. Sugar is nutritionally useless, but it is not toxic. Insulin resistance comes from obesity, and eating too many calories, not just a single carbohydrate source.

The preceding table has been reprinted with permission from the webmaster of DietSurf.com as it originally appeared.

Foods You Eat on this Diet

Your blood type determines what foods you are allowed ranging from modified vegetarian to large amounts of animal foods. The premise is that if you eat right for your blood type your digestion will improve, avoid viruses and infections, and prevent disease as well as lose weight.

Comments: This is not necessarily a weight loss diet and has a long list of specific food restrictions for each blood type.

Can you keep it off on this type of diet? Unknown, this diet is not really a weight loss plan.

Positives: Gives structure telling you what you can and can't eat.

Drawbacks: Very complicated to follow, many nutritious foods are eliminated. No scientific evidence supports the premise that people should eat certain foods based upon their blood type.

Safety and Health Issues

Basically safe because it lists specific foods that must be avoided but all others can be eaten. However:

- Eliminates nutritious foods without reason
- Practicality is difficult—especially for family members with different blood types
- Lacks scientific proof

Diet Surf Recommendations: Waste of time and effort

Dietitians comments: Many healthy foods are eliminated for different blood types, which encourages odd food practices and micro-managing your diet. Eating healthfully is much easier than this! Weight loss will result from restricting your food intake, just like any other diet.

The preceding table has been reprinted with permission from the webmaster of DietSurf.com as it originally appeared.

Foods You Eat on this Diet

Mostly fruits and vegetables. Recommends eating foods in specific combinations and at certain times of the day.

Comments: Specific foods are eaten in combination throughout the day at specific times. Their claim is that this results in improved energy and a natural weight reduction.

Can you keep it off on this type of diet? There is no scientific basis for combining foods to cause weight loss or to assist in weight maintenance. Because the diet has many severe limitations on nutritious foods, it cannot be followed safely for healthy weight maintenance.

Positives: Not based on counting calories or grams of fat. You can eat as much of the specific foods as you desire.

Drawbacks: Lean protein foods such as lean meats and low fat dairy foods are restricted. Food combining rules are complex and difficult to follow, plus they are without scientific merit.

Safety and Health Issues

Combining foods and eating them at specific times is not a proven way to lose weight or improve health.

- Severe food restrictions makes this an unhealthy diet to follow over time.
- Severe limitations on foods allowed, not enough variety to provide good nutrition
- Requires serious changes in your diet habits. Food combining can be complex without any real benefit except to limit food choices so that calories are reduced.

Diet Surf Recommendations Not recommended

Dietitians Comments about the Fit for Life Diet: Food combination diets are just a fancy way to restrict calories. Since they aren't based upon valid or proven nutritional principles, they can make eating well and losing weight much more complex and tedious than it needs to be. Diets that severely restrict healthy foods and insist upon having people combine foods at certain times of the day make them difficult to follow if you have something else to do besides eat. There are much easier ways to lose weight that make much more sense.

The preceding table has been reprinted with permission from the webmaster of DietSurf.com as it originally appeared.

MEDITERRANEAN DIET   Type of Diet: Balanced, Heart Healthy

Foods You Eat on this Diet

Variety of whole foods, similar to the diet of people who live in the Mediterranean - mostly Greece, Crete, Southern Italy. Foods include whole grains, fruits, vegetables, seafood small amounts of poultry, and limited red meat and dairy products. The fat source is mostly olive oil or monounsaturated fat.

General Facts: This diet is based on research that showed that a Mediterranean style of eating lowers cholesterol and reduce risk of heart disease and that Mediterranean people have reduced risk of heart disease.

Can you keep it off on this type of diet? If this diet is followed along with proper portion control and exercise, it should lead to healthy weight control.

Positives: A good variety of healthy foods associated with reduced risk of heart disease. Does not require special diet foods or supplements, and foods and recipes are easy to find.

Drawbacks: Diet is just one aspect of the Mediterranean lifestyle and may not be the sole cause of reduced heart risk. Still, this is a very healthy way to eat.

Safety and Health Issues

This is a well balanced, safe diet to follow and people have thrived on it for centuries.

Diet Surf Recommendations: Highly recommended.

Dietitians Comments about the Mediterranean Diet: Translating the Mediterranean diet for Americans can be a little tricky. Food portions need to be controlled, and even good fats like olive oil are high in calories. Mediterranean restaurants still serve portions that are too large for anyone on a weight loss diet. Get some professional help (preferably a dietitian's) and some lower fat, lower calorie Mediterranean cookbooks if you want to eat a Mediterranean diet and want to lose weight at the same time!

The preceding table has been reprinted with permission from the webmaster of DietSurf.com as it originally appeared.

Foods You Eat on this Diet

Grapefruit-meat- and high fat foods like fried foods. No complex carbohydrates are included in this diet.

Comments: Although it is called the "Mayo Clinic" diet, this diet is not endorsed by the Mayo Clinic. This diet claims that grapefruit has special properties that allow you to burn fat, and that eating large amounts of fat will cause weight loss.

Can you keep it off on this type of diet? Depending upon grapefruit to burn fat and eating until you are stuffed is not a short term or a long term weight loss solution.

Positives: People who love to eat grapefruit, meat and fatty foods might enjoy unlimited amounts of these foods.

Drawbacks: This diet is too limited in carbohydrates and may cause low energy, and is based upon the unfounded notion that eating grapefruit burns fat.

Safety and Health Issues

This diet is unbalanced nutritionally and encourages unhealthy food choices and overeating.

- Fried foods and other fatty foods associated with heart disease and cancer are encouraged
- Complex carbohydrates (the body's chief source of energy) are eliminated on this diet.
- Eating large portions of food is not a good health practice

Diet Surf Recommendations: Not Endorsed by the Mayo Clinic and not recommended by Diet Surf

Dietitians Comments about the Mayo Clinic Diet: The Mayo Clinic Diet is typical of fad diets that use scientific sounding names or famous people and places to promote a diet program. It is unfortunate that these ploys fool so many people looking for help.

The preceding table has been reprinted with permission from the webmaster of DietSurf.com as it originally appeared.

Foods You Eat on this Diet

Combines different foods on the premise that they should be eaten together for particular health effects. Fruits and vegetables are encouraged.

General Information: This diet promotes food combining without scientific evidence to support its claims of benefits.

Can you keep it off on this type of diet? This diet reduces calories and eliminates many junk foods which can be helpful in maintaining healthy body weight. Food combining, however is not required to accomplish this.

Positives: Reduces "junk" foods, encourages fruits and vegetables. Encourages frequent small meals.

Drawbacks: Unnecessarily complex meal planning required to combine different foods without a real benefit.

Safety and Health Issues

- Unsupported by scientific evidence
- Promotes invalid nutrition practices
- Eliminates healthful foods without valid reasons

Diet Surf Recommendations: Not Recommended

Dietitians Comments about the Sommersizing Diet: Since food combinations plans like this have no science to support their diet claims, it promotes invalid beliefs about how to maintain a healthy diet. These diets complicate the process of choosing and eating healthful foods which may turn a lot of people off before they get long lasting benefits from reducing unhealthy foods. The human body is designed to be smart enough to digest all types of foods at once, and separating them doesn't make a bit of difference in losing weight. Reducing calories, increasing the amount of lower fat, nutrient rich foods, and reducing the number of times that low nutrient foods are eaten are the keys to losing weight.

The preceding table has been reprinted with permission from the webmaster of DietSurf.com as it originally appeared.

SCARSDALE DIET Type of Diet: Low Carbohydrate, High Protein

Foods You Eat on this Diet

lean animal foods, fruit, vegetables, herbal appetite suppressants

Comments: Rigid meal plan without snacks. Extreme carbohydrate restriction induces rapid water weight loss. Goal is rapid weight loss.

Can you keep it off on this type of diet? This is a diet designed for one to two weeks only, not long term weight control.

Positives: Rapid weight loss for those who thrive on quick results.

Drawbacks: Weight regained after going off the diet and returning to former eating habits.

Safety and Health Issues

Extreme restriction of carbohydrate makes this diet unhealthy. Herbal appetite suppressants can be dangerous for many people.

Diet Surf Recommendations: Not recommended for anyone.

Dietitians Comments about the Scarsdale Diet: This diet has been around for many years. If it was the magic cure for obesity, it would have worked a long time ago. Rapid weight loss and extreme diets can produce quick results but are typically very disappointing to the dieter when weight loss returns just as quickly.

The preceding table has been reprinted with permission from the webmaster of DietSurf.com as it originally appeared.

PRITIKIN DIET Type of Diet: Low Fat, Low Caloric Density

Foods You Eat on this Diet

unprocessed fruits and vegetables, lean animal foods, non fat dairy foods, low fat carbohydrate foods

General Facts: Diet is based upon choosing foods that contain 400 Calories or less per pound.

Can you keep it off on this type of diet? This approach should help with keeping portions and calories in check, which should help with weight maintenance.

Positives: Lots of fruits and vegetables and low fat carbohydrate foods encourages healthier eating and controls calories.

Negatives: May be difficult to follow long term as diet is quite low in fat

Safety and Health Issues

This diet is nutritionally safe if you choose a variety of foods.

Diet Surf Recommendations: Recommended as a healthy diet, but may be too restrictive for most people to follow long term.

Dietitians Comments about the Pritikin Principle Diet: This diet is quite low in fat and may be too restrictive for people to follow long term. Otherwise it is a safe diet and may be especially beneficial for those with risk of heart disease.

The preceding table has been reprinted with permission from the webmaster of DietSurf.com as it originally appeared.

1. Dougherty, M. (2003, February). Jumping Jack. *Reader's Digest,* 133-136.

2. Crary, David. (Friday, February 18, 2000). Pets and nutrition. *Associated Press.*

3. Jama, Vol. 288, 1728–1732, 2003 and reported by the National Center for Health Statistics, 2002, www.cdc.gov/nchc.

4. Neufeldt, V. (EIC) & Sparks, A., (PE). (1995). (Updated). New York: Simon & Schuster.

5. Exercise ETC. Inc. (2003). *Analyzing Popular Diets.*

6. Huff, F. (2001). Roundtable discussion: Low carbohydrate diets and anaerobic athletes. *NSCA Strength and Conditioning Journal.* 23 (3), 42-61.

7. Forbes-Ewan C. (2003). Effect of vegetarian diets on performance in strength sports. *SPORTSCIENCE* {On-line.} Available: www.sportsci.org/jour/0201/cf-e.htm

8. DeNoon, D. (2003). CDC measures pollution in Americans. *WEBMD Medical News* {On-line}. Available: http://aolsvc.health.webmd.aol.com/content/article/60/66968.HTM?z=1728_00000_1000_LN_02

9. Dorr, Med. B. (2002, November). Nutritional Supplements. Paper presented at the 72nd Men's and 15th Women's World Weightlifting Championships Annual Congress, Warsaw, Poland.

10. INBRIEF: Researchers: Ephedra unsafe at any dosage. (2003, February 4). *The El Paso Times,* 3A.

11. (2001, March 23). NATION: Study: Smoking triggers gene in forming wrinkles. *The El Paso Times,* 5A.

CHAPTER 12 SELF TEST

Please feel free to write on this page

True or False

1. _____ When consumed in moderation, fat actually promotes weight loss.

2. _____ 90-95% of supplements on the market are good investments.

3. _____ Protein is not very important for individuals engaged in weight training.

4. _____ In order to maintain the same body weight, the calories consumed must equal the calories expended.

5. _____ By combining BMR and daily activity level, we arrive at the total caloric expenditure for a day.

6. _____ When the caloric intake is not equal to the caloric expenditure, there will be no change in body weight.

Multiple Choice

7. _____ How many calories does fat contain per gram of weight?
   a. 4
   b. 5
   c. 9
   d. 10

8. _____ Which statement(s) is/are true about protein?
   a. is responsible for muscle tissue growth and repair
   b. can be used as a fuel source
   c. contains 4 calories per gram
   d. all of the above

9. _____ What is the Recommended Daily Allowance of protein for adults in grams per kilograms of bodyweight?
   a. 0.8
   b. 0.5
   c. 1
   d. 0.7

10. _____ Most food labels provide information based on a _____ calorie diet.
    a. 1000
    b. 2000
    c. 3000
    d. 4000

11. _____ The average 12 oz cup of coffee probably has between _____ mg. of caffeine.
    a. 0-75
    b. 100-125

c. 150-225

d. 250-325

12. _____ According to the Centers for Disease Control, there are _____ chemicals invading our bodies.

    a. 50

    b. 78

    c. 116

    d. 127

13. _____ Which of the following is not a form of protein?

    a. potatoes

    b. milk

    c. eggs

    d. soy

14. _____ Daily vitamin and mineral supplements should be taken in _____ .

    a. morning

    b. afternoon

    c. evening

    d. both a and c

Fill in the Blank

15. _____ is a stimulant found in many things such as coffee and tea.

16. _____ Carbohydrates are found in grains, cereals, whole grain breads, vegetables and fruits.

17. _____ _____ _____ is the minimum amount of energy the body needs to conduct the vital processes.

18. It is often stated that the typical diet should consist of between 50 to 60% _____ , 25 to 30% _____ , and 10 to 15% _____ .

19. Numerous studies on protein confirm that _____ individuals need more protein than _____ individuals, particularly athletes.

20. In order to be considered organic, a product must be _____ in order to carry the USDA Organic seal.

Please feel free to write on this page

Answers: 1. True   2. False   3. False   4. True   5. True   6. False   7. c   8. d   9. a   10. b   11. b   12. c   13. a   14. d   15. Caffeine 16. Complex   17. Basal Metabolic Rate   18. carbohydrates, fats, protein   19. active, sedentary   20. 95-100% organic

CHAPTER 13

Weight Training Injuries

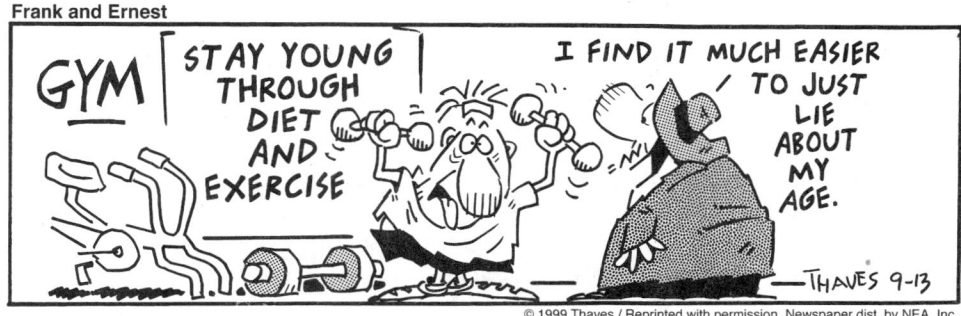

Weight Training Injuries

Injuries in weight training are rare and generally nothing more serious than muscle soreness, although callouses, strains, sprains, tendinitis, and bursitis sometimes occur. Research has shown that weight training is actually one of the safest sports.[1] Some of the more common injuries are:

1. Blisters, scrapes, cuts, and other minor injuries.
2. Muscle soreness: Can be caused by overexertion, overuse, or many other factors. Recovery is usually nothing more than resting the sore muscle. A warm shower, sauna, or Jacuzzi combined with a little aspirin, ibuprofen, or other pain reliever may be all it takes to get rid of the pain and get back to training.
3. Callouses: Usually develop over time because of contact with weightlifting bars and apparatus. Cut them off or sand them down with an abrasive stone. Not too many things hurt as bad as having a callous ripped off.
4. Strains: Are stretches or tears in the muscle or tendon, caused by rapidly applying force to a muscle causing the muscle to tighten and/or not warming up thoroughly.[2] Symptoms may include:
   a. a burning or popping when the injury occurs
   b. muscle pain
   c. lack of use of the injured muscle
   d. swelling or bruising
5. Sprains: Stretches or tears in the ligaments; may be classified as mild, moderate, or severe. A twisting or severe stretching of a joint causes sprains. Sprains are typically associated with accidents, and occur in the ankle.[2] Symptoms may include:
   a. swelling and pain in the joint
   b. loss of mobility in the joint
   c. the skin may be red and within a few days look bruised

6. Tendinitis: Usually caused by overuse of a particular muscle, and is indicated by soreness and sometimes swelling of the affected area. Rest is good for this injury.

7. Bursitis: Caused when the bursa sac becomes inflamed. Inflammation of the bursa may be caused by overuse or injury. The bursa sacs are located in or near joints. Rest is required and sometimes if the bursitis is bad enough, it will be treated with cortisol injected directly into the bursa sac.

Treatment of Weight Training Injuries

The front line of defense in treating injuries is R-I-C-E. Rest it, Ice it, Compress it, and Elevate it.[2]

Rest—avoid all activities that cause pain and keep the weight off the injury.

Ice—apply ice packs for 20 to 30 minutes every 3 to 4 hours for 2 to 3 days.

Compress—wrap an elastic bandage or tape if necessary around the injured part.

Elevate—keep the injured muscle above the heart when resting.

R-I-C-E is especially important in treating strains and sprains. By using this method, you will allow the muscle or joint to rest; apply ice to reduce the pain and swelling, apply an elastic bandage to compress and reduce swelling, and elevate the limb to also reduce swelling.

For any injury there should be a progressive decrease in symptoms over 7 to 10 days, if not, then medical attention should be sought from your physician.

Training When You Are Sick

Don't. Many people insist on training when they are sick. DO NOT TRAIN OR WORK OUT WHEN YOU ARE SICK! If you train or work out when you are sick, you will only extend the length of time that you are sick. The body views working out as a stress like any other stress. The body does not differentiate between the stress of work, family, or anything else. It is all stress, so why add to it? By placing the additional demands of working out on a sick body, you will only extend your recovery time, not to mention that it is rude to work out around other people when you are sick. No one wants your illness and it would be very inconsiderate for you to give it to him or her. Stay home, recover, and then go back to the gym.

Frank and Ernest

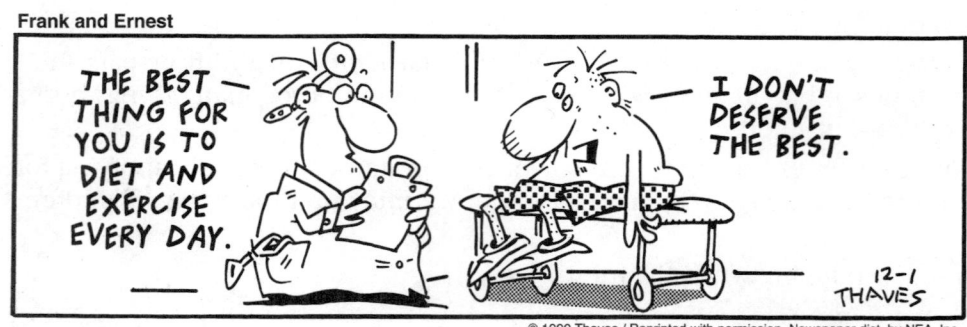

© 1999 Thaves / Reprinted with permission. Newspaper dist. by NEA, Inc.

1. Chandler, T. J., and Stone, M. H. (1991). The Squat Exercise in Athletic Conditioning a Review of the Literature. *National Strength and Conditioning Association Journal.* 13(5): 56.

2. Rouzier, P. (1999). *The Sports Medicine Patient Advisor.* Amherst: SportsMedPress.

Please feel free to write on this page

True or False

1. _____ Strains are stretches or tears in the muscle or tendon.

2. _____ Tendinitis is usually caused by overuse of a particular bone and is indicated by numbness and sometimes swelling of the affected area.

3. _____ A twisting or severe stretching of a joint causes sprains.

4. _____ It is good to workout when you're sick because you are able to combat the illness.

5. _____ For any injury there should be a progressive decrease in symptoms over 7 to 10 days.

Multiple Choice

6. _____ Which of the following is not recommended when muscle soreness occurs?
   a. Warm Shower
   b. Sauna
   c. Ice
   d. Jacuzzi

7. _____ Sprains are stretches or tears in the ligaments that may be classified as:
   a. Mild
   b. Moderate
   c. Severe
   d. All of the above

8. _____ The frontline of defense in treating injuries is R-I-C-E. What does I mean in the word, and what are the recommendations for it?
   a. Inertia, apply ice packs for 50-60 minutes every 5-6 hours for 7-8 days
   b. Ice, apply ice packs for 20-30 minutes every 3-4 hours for 2-3 days
   c. Ice, apply ice packs for 10-20 minutes every 1-2 hours for 2-3 days
   d. Impulse, apply ice packs for 40-50 minutes every 7-8 hours for 4-5 days

9. _____ Sprains are common in injuries. What are the symptoms that could come along with them?
   a. Swelling and pain in the joint
   b. Loss of mobility in the joint
   c. The skin may be red and within a few days look bruised
   d. All of the above
   e. None of the above

10. _____ When you are sick, what should you do?
    a. Do not train or work out
    b. Keep going outside to get fresh oxygen because the air will decrease sickness
    c. Keep on training because it is not a bid deal
    d. Slow down your training and do not go vigorously at it

NOTES

Please feel free to write on this page

CHAPTER 14

Evaluations and Fat Considerations

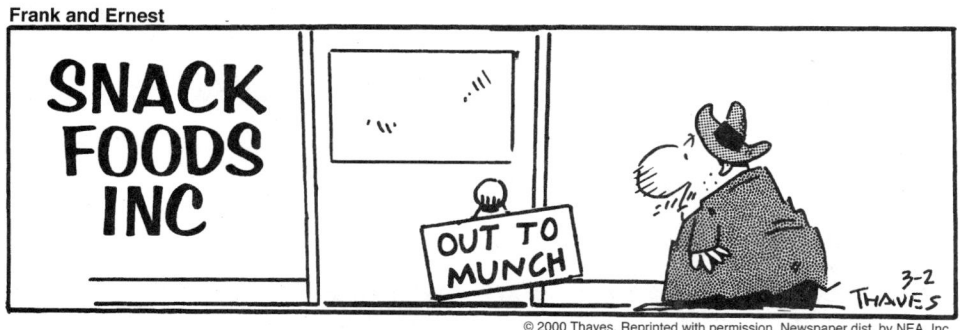

Frank and Ernest

SNACK FOODS INC

OUT TO MUNCH

THAVES 3-2

© 2000 Thaves. Reprinted with permission. Newspaper dist. by NEA, Inc.

Body Composition

Body composition is the relative proportion of body fat to lean mass. Lean mass is also known as Fat Free Mass (FFM). There are numerous ways to measure body fat, such as the Body Mass Index (BMI), skinfold thickness, hydrostatic (underwater) weighing, bioelectrical impedance, whole body potassium method, and dual energy x-ray absorptiometry (DEXA). Why is body fat so important? It is important because more and more we are associating diseases and health issues with being overweight. Today, approximately 60 to 65 percent of Americans are overweight, and 30+ percent are considered obese. Obesity for women would be when 32 percent or more of their bodyweight is fat, and for men the figure would be when 25 percent or more of their bodyweight is fat.

Body Typing[1,2]

Human bodies may be broken down into one of three types:

1. Ectomorphs: Those who are slender and small-boned, with long, slim arms and legs. They will also have what appears to be a long neck and little definition in their muscles, with a frail and delicate appearance and skeletal features that are readily visible. Ectomorphs will usually have high metabolisms and burn large quantities of calories. They will have a hard time gaining weight and must consume more protein than other body types. After a training session, they will recuperate faster than mesomorphs or endomorphs. Many ectomorphs are good endurance athletes. Ectomorphs will have a low percent of muscle mass, and upon doing body fat tests, may actually have high percentages of body fat.

2. Mesomorphs: Those who are athletic, with broad shoulders, narrow hips, big bones, and thick joints. They have visible muscle tissue and definition. These are the athletes in strength sports requiring large amounts of muscle per proportion of body weight and size. Most mesomorphs are not good at endurance events, but add muscle easily.

3. Endomorphs: Those who are pudgy and have thick arms and legs, which are short compared to the torso. The neck will be thick, and the chest and waist will be roughly the same size, with

many having "potbellies." Their metabolisms may be slower, requiring longer recuperation periods after a training session, and the body will require fewer calories to maintain their weight.

While no one is a perfect example of an ectomorph, mesomorph, or endomorph, we all exhibit some characteristics that will make us more of one type or the other. This is an important factor when deciding how to train. The three types will use completely different training and eating patterns from one another. The hardest thing about weight training is finding out what works for you and your body type. There is no one formula for all of us. It is imperative that you keep records of your weight, exercise programs, pounds lifted, sets, reps, and so on, in a training logbook in order to determine what works for you. Include in your logbook how you feel before, during, and after a work out. Don't forget the nutritional component. Note when you had a lot of energy and a great work out, and try to tie this to what you had to eat before a work out, maybe even the day before. Notice the rest required also. Did you get a good night's sleep? Do you recover faster working out two days in a row and taking one off, or do you do better working out one day and taking one off. This is the secret to making weight training work for you: figuring out what works with YOUR body! When it comes to working out, more is not always better!

Body Fat Measures and Variability

According to Ellen Coleman, MA, MPH, RD, desirable body fat for men should be around 15 percent and for women around 22 percent.[3] Essential fat for men is 3 percent; for women it is 12 percent. However, optimal body fat may vary by as much as 10 percent among athletes in the same sport, and similar variations may be seen between athletes in different sports.

Most importantly, body fat measurements done using skinfold measurements, circumference and bone diameter, or height to weight ratios, should be considered estimates, not absolute values!

Body Mass Index

The body mass index (BMI) is a measure of body composition based on the ratio of body weight in kilograms to height in meters squared, or BMI = weight (kg)/height (m^2). The resulting number is expressed in a percentile ranking or fixed values.

The problem with this index is that it does not take into account whether an individual is heavily muscled or has a lot of body fat. Never the less, it is probably one of the least reliable indicators of body composition.

Skinfold

The skinfold method is based on a measure of subcutaneous (under the skin) fat. The measurement is done using a skinfold caliper, which measures subcutaneous fat thickness by "pinching" the skin together at selected sites on the body. The pinching doesn't hurt and allows the person doing the measurement to get a reading in millimeters (mm) of subcutaneous fat. The skinfold method is one of the most valid and reliable methods for body fat assessment when done by a trained tester, yielding reliability measurements in the 99 percentile range.

Hydrostatic Weighing

Hydrostatic weighing (underwater weighing) uses the principle of displacement to determine body volume. The volume of water that is displaced can be measured, or the tester can determine the loss of body weight while the person is underwater. Hydrostatic weighing is the "standard" against which other body fat methods are compared. It is usually more accurate with athletes and individuals who undergo the test most often.

Bioelectrical Impedance

In bioelectrical impedance, a small electrical current is applied to the body and the resistance to that current is measured. The current is usually applied at the extremities, such as the right hand and right foot. This method of assessment is fast and convenient to use. It is fairly accurate in measuring body fat, and very accurate in showing percent of change in body fat. Factors that may influence this test are hydration and mineral content of the body.

Whole-Body Potassium Method

In the whole-body potassium method, emissions of potassium-40 are measured. This is a radioactive form of potassium that occurs naturally in the body in tiny amounts, mostly in muscles. The body fat is then calculated by subtracting lean mass from the bodyweight.[3]

Dual Energy X-Ray Absorptiometry

In the dual energy x-ray absorptiometry (DEXA) method, bone mass and other lean mass, connective tissue, organs, and water are measured. Lean mass would include muscle.[3]

Both the whole-body potassium method and DEXA are very sensitive, yielding accurate measurements. Neither is invasive, but don't expect to see them at your local health club any time soon!

What Is Considered FAT?

T. G. Lohman, in *The Physician and Sportsmedicine* (1982), offers the following percentages for consideration when determining health as related to fat:

TABLE 14.1

Fat Content as Related to Health	Males	Females
Optimal	10-20%	15-25%
Moderately High	20-25%	25-30%
High	25-31%	30-35%
Very High	>31%	>35%

I would like to add the following ranges to this chart to take into consideration athletes:

TABLE 14.2

Fat Content as Related to Health	Males	Females
Athletic	10-14%	14-18%

Obesity

There has been much written about the obesity problem facing the United States for both adults and children. But what is considered "obese"? According to D. C. Nieman in *Fitness and Your Health*, Palo Alto, CA., (1993), a body-fat percentage greater than 25 for men or a body fat percentage greater than 32 for women would be considered obese.

Essential Fat

Essential fat is the fat that is stored in bone marrow, heart, lungs, liver, spleen, kidney, intestines, muscles, and the central nervous system. This fat is called "essential" because normal physiological functioning requires this minimum amount of fat.

	Males	Females
Essential Fat	3%	10-12%

In females the essential fat also includes fat that is termed sex-specific essential fat, and is important in childbearing, menstruation, and other functions related to hormones.

When dropping below the essential fatty ranges, body functions change and can cause such things as hair loss, lethargy, cessation of menstruation, and ultimately death.

Physique Measurement

In Chapter 1, it was suggested that you take measurements in order to be able to detect changes in your physique. For the men, I have a physique chart to track their changes, and to record how proportional/symmetrical their bodies are. David P. Willoughby[3] devised the Symmetrometer in 1944, based on over 50 years of observation and study of well developed athletes and bodybuilders. It is as applicable now as it was then, and is one of my favorites for measuring proportionality. Unfortunately, I have not seen one for women. By plotting your measurements, you will be able to determine which of your body parts are out of symmetry, and adjust your training using the "priority split" system to bring them into symmetry.

Willoughby Symmetrometer

The Symmetrometer is simple to use, basically it is a detailed height and weight chart. Measurements are to be taken by another person to insure that the tape is not slanted, pulled too tight, or held too loose. Measurements are to be taken *before* exercise, since after exercise body parts will be larger.

To measure:

1. The neck—hold the head erect, eyes straight ahead, and neck muscles relaxed. The measurement is taken at the smallest girth, just above the Adam's apple.
2. Upper arm—raise the arm to the side and shoulder height with the lower arm straight and elbow locked. The palm should be down and the fist should be clenched. The measurement is made around the bicep at the largest point for both the left and right biceps.
3. Forearm—same as above in Number 2, only measure the forearm below the elbow at the point of greatest girth for both the left and right forearms.
4. Wrist—the palm is facing up, with the fingers extended in line with the forearm. Take the measurement at the base of the hand and the bony protuberance on the little-finger side of the hand for both the left and right wrists.
5. Chest normal—with the body and head erect, and eyes looking straight ahead, take the measurement around the chest at the largest part. The tape should be straight across the back and just above the nipples. Do not contract the latissimus dorsi and do not include the arms in the measurement.
6. Chest expanded—same as Number 5, but the person inhales deeply and the person doing the measurements notes the increase. Again, do not flex the latissimus dorsi muscles.
7. Waist—with the body erect and the abdominal muscles relaxed, measure at the smallest point, typically slightly above the navel.

8. Thigh—with the body erect, feet hip width apart, weight equally distributed on each foot and the thigh muscles relaxed, measure at the largest part, which is usually just below the buttocks, for both the left and right thighs.

9. Calf—with the body erect, heels on the floor, weight equally distributed on each foot, measure at the largest part of the calf for both the left and right calves.

10. Ankle—with the body erect, heels on the floor, weight equally distributed on each foot, measure the smallest part, which is usually about two inches above the ankle bones, for both the left and right ankles.

Take your weight in pounds and divide by your height in inches, and draw a straight line from the top to the bottom of the Symmetrometer corresponding to the number that is derived.

Once you have taken all measurements, plot them on the chart on the following page. Make heavy dots at the appropriate points on the chart. Plot the larger of the two arms as the right arm, regardless of whether it is the right or left, and vice-versa. Using a heavy line, connect the dots. A variation off of the straight line of +/− 2.5% is acceptable. To visualize the limits of 2.5%, draw a line parallel to the first line at 0.95% of the weight-to-height number and again at 1.05% of the weight-to-height number.

Good luck with this chart, and welcome to proportionality!

Willoughby Symmetrometer

Status of Ratio or Measurement →	Minimum	Small	Medium	Large	Maximum
Weight ÷ Height	1.6 1.7 1.8	1.9 2.0 2.1 2.2	2.3 2.4 2.5 2.6	2.7 2.8 2.9 3.0 3.1	3.2 3.3 3.4 3.5 3.6

Girths		Minimum	Small	Medium	Large	Maximum
	Neck	13.0	14.0	15.0 16.0	17.0	18.0 19.0
	Biceps, R.	12.1 13.0	14.0	15.0	16.0	17.0 18.0
	,, L.	12.0 13.0	14.0	15.0	16.0	17.0 18.0
	Forearm, R.	10.1 11.0	12.0	13.0	14.0	15.0
	,, L.	10.0 11.0	12.0	13.0	14.0	15.0
	Wrist, R.	6.0	6.5	7.0 7.5	8.0	8.5
	,, L.	6.0	6.5	7.0 7.5	8.0	8.5
	Chest (normal)	34.0 35.0 36.0 37.0 38.0	39.0 40.0 41.0 42.0 43.0	44.0 45.0 46.0 47.0	48.0 49.0 50.0 51.0	
	Waist	25.0 26.0 27.0	28.0 29.0 30.0 31.0	32.0 33.0 34.0	35.0 36.0 37.0 38.0	
	Hips	30.0 31.0 32.0 33.0 34.0	35.0 36.0 37.0 38.0 39.0	40.0 41.0 42.0 43.0	44.0 45.0 46.0	
	Thigh, R.	18.0 19.0 20.0	21.0 22.0 23.0	24.0 25.0 26.0	27.0	
	,, L.	18.0 19.0 20.0	21.0 22.0 23.0	24.0 25.0 26.0	27.0	
	Knee, R.	12.0 13.0	14.0 15.0	16.0	17.0 18.0	
	,, L.	12.0 13.0	14.0 15.0	16.0	17.0 18.0	
	Calf, R.	12.0 13.0	14.0 15.0	16.0	17.0 18.0	
	,, L.	12.0 13.0	14.0 15.0	16.0	17.0 18.0	
	Ankle, R.	7.0 7.5	8.0 8.5	9.0 9.5	10.0 10.5	
	,, L.	7.0 7.5	8.0 8.5	9.0 9.5	10.0 10.5	

Instructions: Make the required measurements according to the directions given earlier and plot the data on the appropriate scales by making heavy dots at the proper points. Plot the larger of the two arms as the right arm, regardless of whether it is actually the right or the left, and vice versa. Connect the dots by means of a heavy line. The more nearly this coincides with a line drawn perpendicularly from the Weight/Height point to the bottom of the chart, the more symmetrical are the proportions of the body. A variation of ±2.5 percent is acceptable. The help in visualizing these limits, parallel lines may be drawn at 1.05 and 0.95 percent of the Weight/Height figure. In obese individuals, body weight will take care of itself if the oversized areas, particularly the waist, are brought into line with the other girth measurements, particularly the wrists and ankles. Source: David P. Willoughby.

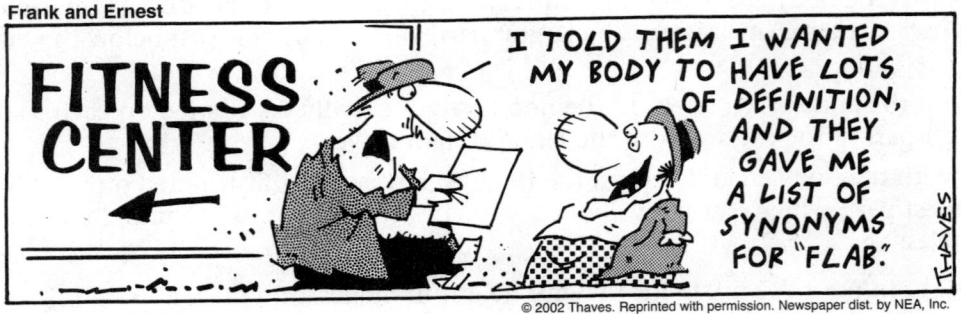

Frank and Ernest

FITNESS CENTER

I TOLD THEM I WANTED MY BODY TO HAVE LOTS OF DEFINITION, AND THEY GAVE ME A LIST OF SYNONYMS FOR "FLAB."

© 2002 Thaves. Reprinted with permission. Newspaper dist. by NEA, Inc.

1. Miller, D. (2002). *Measurement by the Physical Educator* (4th ed.). New York: McGraw-Hill, p. 141.

2. Delavier, F. (2002). *Exercises pour une belle ligne.* [Women's Strength Training Anatomy]. Paris: Editions Vigot.

3. Be Realistic: Optimal Body Fat Percentages May Vary Up to 10 Percent Among Athletes. (March 1, 2001). *Georgia Institute of Technology: Press Release.* [On-line]. Available: www.gatech.edu/news-room/archive/news_releases/bodyfat.html.

4. McBride, J. (June, 1996). America's Kids—Scanning for Growth Trends. *Agricultural Research.* [On-line]. Available: www.ars.usda.gov/is/AR/archive/jun96/growth.pdf.

5. Rasch, P. J., (1990). Willoughby Symmetrometer. *Weight Training* (5th ed.). Dubuque: Wm. C. Brown Publishers, pp. 76-78, 82-83.

Please feel free to write on this page

True or False

1. _____ When performing the symmetrometer test, measurements are to be taken by another person.

2. _____ Body-fat testing is important because more and more fitness professionals are associating diseases and health issues with being overweight.

3. _____ Body mass index is the most valid and reliable method for body fat assessment and measurement.

4. _____ Only top-notch, peak-performing, athletic people use the hydrostatic method for measuring fat.

5. _____ Hydration and mineral content influence bioelectrical impedance.

6. _____ The Symmetrometer test was designed to measure physique changes.

7. _____ Most mesomorphs are great at endurance events.

8. _____ Subcutaneous fat is measured in inches.

Multiple Choice

9. _____ What percentage of fat content, as related to health, is considered to be very high?
   a. Males more than 31%, Females more than 35%
   b. Males more than 20%, Females more than 25%
   c. Males more than 10%, Females more than 14%
   d. Males more than 35%, Females more than 31%

10. _____ What percentage of body fat should an athletic person have?
   a. Males 3%-6%, Females 4%-8%
   b. Males 10%-14%, Females 14%-18%
   c. Males 20%-22%, Females 25%-27%
   d. Males 31%-22%, Females 35%-37%

11. _____ Which of the following pertain to essential body fat?
   a. Minimum amount of fat is needed for physiological function
   b. It is important for childbearing
   c. Regulates energies needed for human development
   d. Answers "a" and "b"

12. _____ A female's percentage of essential body fat is sex-specific because
   a. Childbearing
   b. Menstruation
   c. Functions relating to hormonal changes
   d. All of the above

13. _____ Which ways are appropriate methods to measure body fat?
   a. Body Mass Index and Skinfold
   b. Hydrostatic weighing and Bioelectrical Impedance
   c. Whole-body potassium method and Dual Energy X-ray absorption meter
   d. All the above

14. _____ What is the function of knowing body composition?
   a. To know your body type
   b. To know if you are obese
   c. To know if you have any disease and/or health issues with being overweight
   d. To compute exact fat-to-muscle mass composition

15. _____ Where in the body is essential fat stored?
   a. Bone marrow, heart and lungs
   b. Central nervous system and spleen
   c. Kidney, intestine, muscle, and liver
   d. All the above

16. _____ Which test is the best for physique measurement?
   a. Body Mass Index
   b. Symmetrometer
   c. Hydrostatic
   d. Bioelectrical Impedance

17. _____ The hardest part of weight training is
   a. Finding out what works for your body type
   b. Keeping a training log book
   c. Having a mesomorph body type
   d. All the above

18. _____ Which method of body fat measurement is based on the subcutaneous fat?
   a. Hydrostatic
   b. Skinfold
   c. Body Mass Index
   d. Bioelectrical Impedance

19. Place a letter in column B next to the appropriate descriptions in column A.

Column A	Column B
_____ 1. Measure body composition based on ratio of body weight and height.	a. Dual Energy X-ray Absorption
_____ 2. Uses the principle of displacement to determine body volume.	b. Whole-body potassium method
_____ 3. Body mass, lean muscle mass, connective tissue: organs and water are measured.	c. Bioelectrical Impedance
_____ 4. Based on a measure of subcutaneous fat.	d. Hydrostatic Weighing
_____ 5. Resistance to current is measured.	e. Skinfold
_____ 6. Emission of potassium-40 is measured.	f. Body Mass Index

20. Match the body characteristics in column B with correct body type in column A.

Column A

_____ 1. Mesomorphs

_____ 2. Endomorphs

_____ 3. Ectomorphs

Column B

a. Slender, slim arms and legs

b. Athletic with broad shoulders

c. Pudgy with thick arms and legs

NOTES

Please feel free to write on this page

Name _____

Date Started _____

	LB												LB													
	REPS												REPS													
_____	SET												SET													
	LB												LB													
	REPS												REPS													
_____	SET												SET													
	LB												LB													
	REPS												REPS													
_____	SET												SET													
	LB												LB													
	REPS												REPS													
_____	SET												SET													
	LB												LB													
	REPS												REPS													
_____	SET												SET													
	LB												LB													
	REPS												REPS													
_____	SET												SET													
	LB												LB													
	REPS												REPS													
_____	SET												SET													
	LB												LB													
	REPS												REPS													
_____	SET												SET													
	LB												LB													
	REPS												REPS													
_____	SET												SET													
	LB												LB													
	REPS												REPS													
_____	SET												SET													
	LB												LB													
	REPS												REPS													
_____	SET												SET													
	LB												LB													
	REPS												REPS													
_____	SET												SET													
	LB												LB													
	REPS												REPS													
_____	SET												SET													
	LB												LB													
	REPS												REPS													
_____	SET												SET													
	LB												LB													
	REPS												REPS													
_____	SET												SET													
	LB												LB													
	REPS												REPS													
_____	SET												SET													
	LB												LB													
	REPS												REPS													
_____	SET												SET													
	LB												LB													
	REPS												REPS													
_____	SET												SET													
	LB												LB													
	REPS												REPS													
_____	SET												SET													

Name _____

Date Started _____

	LB										LB										
	REPS										REPS										
	SET										SET										
_____	LB										LB										
	REPS										REPS										
	SET										SET										
_____	LB										LB										
	REPS										REPS										
	SET										SET										
_____	LB										LB										
	REPS										REPS										
	SET										SET										
_____	LB										LB										
	REPS										REPS										
	SET										SET										
_____	LB										LB										
	REPS										REPS										
	SET										SET										
_____	LB										LB										
	REPS										REPS										
	SET										SET										
_____	LB										LB										
	REPS										REPS										
	SET										SET										
_____	LB										LB										
	REPS										REPS										
	SET										SET										
_____	LB										LB										
	REPS										REPS										
	SET										SET										
_____	LB										LB										
	REPS										REPS										
	SET										SET										
_____	LB										LB										
	REPS										REPS										
	SET										SET										
_____	LB										LB										
	REPS										REPS										
	SET										SET										
_____	LB										LB										
	REPS										REPS										
	SET										SET										
_____	LB										LB										
	REPS										REPS										
	SET										SET										
_____	LB										LB										
	REPS										REPS										
	SET										SET										
_____	LB										LB										
	REPS										REPS										
	SET										SET										
_____	LB										LB										
	REPS										REPS										
	SET										SET										
_____	LB										LB										
	REPS										REPS										
	SET										SET										